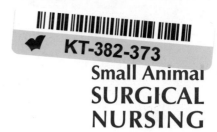

KT-382-373

Small Animal
SURGICAL
NURSING

Visit our website at **www.mosby.com**

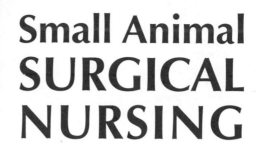

Small Animal
SURGICAL
NURSING

DIANE L. TRACY, B.A., Ed.M.

Practice Manager
Natick Animal Clinic
Natick, Massachusetts

THIRD EDITION

with 393 illustrations

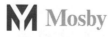

Mosby

A Harcourt Health Sciences Company

St. Louis   Philadelphia   London   Sydney   Toronto

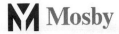

A Harcourt Health Sciences Company

Editor-in-Chief: John A. Schrefer
Executive Editor: Linda L. Duncan
Senior Developmental Editor: Teri Merchant
Project Manager: Patricia Tannian
Production Editor: Steve Hetager
Book Design Manager: Gail Morey Hudson
Cover Designer: Teresa Breckwoldt

Mosby, Inc.
A Harcourt Health Sciences Company
11830 Westline Industrial Drive
St. Louis, Missouri 63146

International Standard Book Number 1-55664-503-1

99 00 01 02 03 CL/FF 9 8 7 6 5 4 3 2 1

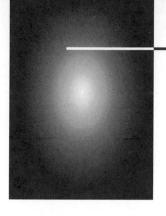

Contributors

ANDREA HOURIHAN, A.S., B.S.
Head Veterinary Technician,
Natick Animal Clinic,
Natick, Massachusetts

DANIEL LYNCH, B.S.
Veterinary Technician,
University of New Hampshire,
Durham, New Hampshire

DAVID McGRATH, M.S., D.V.M.
Owner, Natick Animal Clinic,
Natick, Massachusetts

MICHELLE M. SENNA, L.V.T.
New York State Licensed Veterinary Technician,
Affiliated with the Animal Medical Center and Animal
General Hospital,
New York, New York

To my
mother and dad

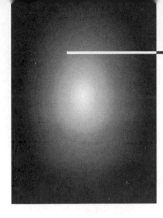

Preface

Since the inception of the first formal college-level training program for veterinary technicians in 1961, advances in veterinary science and technologies have ensured that educated and well-trained technicians will always be an integral part of the veterinary medical team. In 1975, the American Veterinary Medical Association assumed the responsibility for the accreditation of programs, thereby overseeing the quality of instruction and providing guidance and assistance to educators and practitioners. It has been my privilege, since the 1960s, to be part of this evolution as a technician, an educator, and a veterinary practice manager.

This book is intended to be a basic, practical text on small animal surgical nursing that can be used by students, educators, veterinarians, and technicians in practice. It can be blended with both formal and inservice training programs. It is not intended to be a comprehensive study of small animal surgery or of the complete research that has been done in this field.

The book is organized into five chapters:

- Chapter 1 contains information on the history and principles of asepsis. It includes an overview of the microbial world, the causes of disease, and the prevention and control of pathogenic organisms.
- Chapter 2 progresses to the practical applications of aseptic technique and concerns itself with the routine upkeep of the surgical areas, preparation of surgical areas, preparation of surgical packs and equipment, and preparation of the patient and the operating room personnel.
- Chapter 3 contains instruction on how to design, equip, identify, and maintain the instruments and materials commonly found in the small animal hospital surgery.
- Chapter 4 offers a survey of the basic principles of wound healing and describes selected common surgical procedures.
- Chapter 5 deals with common surgical emergencies and the technician's role in aiding the veterinarian with the management of the trauma victim.

Performance objectives are stated before each chapter, and review questions are given at the end of each chapter. Both of these pedagogical features are geared toward helping the reader grasp key content necessary for achieving passing grades on certification examinations.

The third edition has been thoroughly updated throughout, with the latest equipment and procedures included. The illustrations have also been extensively revised,

with nearly 100 new photographs. In addition, every effort has been made throughout all chapters to clearly define the veterinary technician's role in providing care.

ACKNOWLEDGMENTS

Past contributors have been pivotal in the evolution of this text. I would like to ac-
knowledge the work of Dr. Neal Andelman, Dr. Rhea Morgan, and Anne Bullied.
Special thanks go to Dr. Marjorie McMillan, who generously offered the facilities of
the Windhover Animal Clinic; to the Angell Memorial Animal Hospital for their pa-
tience and cooperation; to Dr. David McGrath, owner of the Natick Animal Clinic;
and to Carol Falk for her wonderful Labrador and Norfolk terrier models. I would
also like to thank Dr. Joanne Franks and Dr. Richard Jerram for their insightful
reviews.

My most special thanks go to my dear friend Donna Gallagher, who motivated
me, organized me, kept me focused, and chided me when I faltered.

Diane L. Tracy

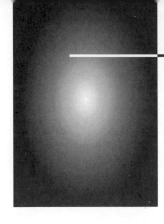

Contents

5 Surgical Emergencies, 323

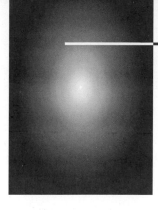

CHAPTER **1**

Principles of Asepsis

PERFORMANCE OBJECTIVES

After completion of this chapter the student will:

State the major events in the development of aseptic technique.

Discuss the meaning of aseptic technique.

State the means by which infectious particles are transmitted and the means of controlling transmission.

Describe the possible consequences of disregarding aseptic technique in the performance of surgical duties.

List the advantages and disadvantages of the various methods of controlling microbes in the surgical area.

Select the most advantageous method of microbe control for application in a given circumstance.

Describe the cumulative effect of consistent and repetitive application of control procedures in maintaining acceptably low levels of microbes.

The skill of the technician is enhanced by an understanding of *why* a procedure is done in addition to understanding *how* it is done. For this reason, a brief review of the historical development of aseptic technique as well as a short section introducing some of the basic concepts of medical microbiology are included in this chapter. The intention is to provide the technician, regardless of background or experience, with the basic knowledge necessary to develop a clear understanding of the rationale behind the procedures known collectively as aseptic technique.

A technician who clearly understands the reason why a procedure is performed, whether it is sterilizing surgical instruments or sanitizing waste receptacles, is more likely to perform these procedures willingly and thoroughly than someone who does not understand the potential dangers inherent in ignoring or insufficiently performing assigned duties. This is particularly true in medical and surgical applications in which consistently successful results depend on the control of the unseen microorganisms that surround us.

To aid the student in comprehending and studying the text, a brief discussion of essential words and phrases is given here.

Disease is any process that detrimentally interferes with the functioning of an organism.

Microbe and *microorganism* are commonly used to refer to living organisms too small to be seen with the unaided eye. *Pathogens* are microbes capable of causing disease.

Infection is the relationship between a parasite and its host that may cause disease if the parasite is a pathogen. *Infection* is commonly used to refer to the detrimental results of invasion by a pathogen. The disease is infectious (may be transferred by direct or indirect contact) as opposed to metabolic or inherited.

Microflora or normal flora refers to microbes that are normally found in healthy animals, such as *E. coli* of the intestinal tract. They may cause disease in debilitated animals or if transferred to other organs of the body. The microbe is then referred to as an *opportunist.*

Resistance is the sum of all factors contributing to the ability of an animal to overcome invasion by pathogens. When an animal is subjected to the physical trauma and mental stress of surgery, its resistance is lowered, and the animal must be protected against infection by aseptic technique. ·

In surgical terminology, *sepsis* refers to the presence of pathogens or their toxic products in the blood or tissues of the patients, and *asepsis* refers to the complete absence of living pathogenic microbes. The intention of aseptic technique is to prevent sepsis and the possible resulting disease. *Sterile* is used to describe the condition of any item that has undergone a cleansing procedure that results in the complete absence of microbes. *Nonsterile* is used to refer to an item that has not undergone a sterilization procedure and that may or may not be contaminated with microbes.

Surgical asepsis refers to the body of techniques that are designed to maintain an object or area in a condition as free of all microorganisms as possible. It is used whenever body tissues must be penetrated. *Medical asepsis* refers to the techniques used to reduce the number of microbes in general and the transmission of pathogens in particular. It is not expected to rid the immediate environment of all microbes.

In surgical applications, any item that has not been sterilized is considered *contaminated.* It may or may not be carrying microbes, but it cannot be proven to be sterile and is therefore considered to be contaminated. Any sterile item that comes in contact with a nonsterile item is considered contaminated; any sterile item left unattended or exposed to the open air for long periods is considered contaminated.

Three levels of intensity of care are recognized in the attempt to achieve asepsis. It is important to select the appropriate level of care in a given situation.

Sanitation is any cleansing measure intended to prevent disease and promote health, including the routine cleaning of such items as cages, floors, buckets, and sinks to remove soil, saliva, urine, and feces.

Disinfection is the application of an agent that possesses the property of destroying or inhibiting the growth of microorganisms. A given disinfectant will not necessarily kill all microbes but can be assumed to significantly reduce the level of contamination. The suffix *-cidal* refers to agents that kill microbes; the suffix *-static* refers to agents that inhibit the growth of microbes. For example, a disinfectant may be bacteriostatic or viricidal.

Sterilization is the use of a process proven to rid an object of all living microbes. The most intense level of care and therefore the most expensive, it is reserved for situations that pose the greatest risk of infection for the patient, the contact of tissues not normally exposed to air or inanimate objects that may carry pathogens. Informally, sterile items are "clean" and nonsterile items are "dirty."

Cold sterilization is the practice of immersing items in a disinfectant solution to reduce the level of contamination. Under ideal, controlled conditions, some chemical agents will sterilize; however, normal conditions of use are seldom ideal, and it is best not to rely on chemical disinfectants as sterilizing agents. Some items are cold sterilized because they will not withstand repeated exposure to high temperature sterilization. Items that have been cold sterilized should be handled as if they were sterile to prevent increased contamination.

Considering the ubiquity of microorganisms, it is fortunate that such a small percentage of microbes are capable of causing disease. Most are either beneficial or harmless, and only a minority of the thousands of species have disease-causing potential. It is against these pathogens that the numerous methods of sanitization, disinfection, and sterilization have been developed.

Surgical patients, who may be subjected to considerable stress because of the condition requiring surgery, must be able to withstand the trauma that occurs during surgery. This trauma can weaken a patient to the extent that the additional stress of an infection acquired during or after surgery could cause an unnecessary fatality.

Any facility in which procedures requiring aseptic technique are performed must develop a schedule of maintenance that will ensure a low level of microorganisms so that infection and subsequent disease will be avoided. The degree of contamination depends in part on the type of facility. Animal quarters housing only healthy animals that have been vaccinated against disease can maintain acceptably low levels of microorganisms by consistently using a combination of sanitizing and disinfecting methods. The surgical and medical areas of the same facility are exposed to increased numbers of pathogens, and the animals in these areas are at greater risk than healthy animals. The methods of microbe control must be intensified to include the sterilization of many items.

The methods used to control microbes and the scheduling of the application of such methods must be adapted to meet the needs of the animals that are being served and must be adhered to consistently. The instruments must be sterilized and gowns, gloves, and masks worn consistently, but if the floor is never scrubbed and the trash is improperly disposed of, the patient will continue to be subjected to an unnecessarily high risk of postsurgical infection. To ensure that the incidence of postsurgical infections remains as low as possible, it is essential that all personnel, regardless of how peripherally involved in the surgical procedure, perform duties in a way that minimizes the chances of infection.

In addition to the ethical aspects of preventing conditions that may bring harm to the animals entrusted to the care of the staff, the economic aspects must be considered. The cost of treating an infection must be absorbed by either the owner of the animal or the owner of the facility. Many of the aseptic procedures are neither time consuming nor costly when incorporated into a daily routine. Common sense housekeeping plays a large role in maintaining low levels of microbes. In addition to providing a safer, more pleasant environment for patients and staff, the routine performance of housekeeping duties ensures the longevity of all hospital equipment from floors to surgical instruments, thereby cutting down on replacement costs.

The surgeon's skill is necessary to perform the procedure correctly and to bring the greatest possible benefit to the animal; the skill of the technician is necessary to provide the surgeon with conditions that permit this to be accomplished.

■ HISTORICAL DEVELOPMENT OF ASEPTIC TECHNIQUE

Much of the mystique of the modern operating suite derives from the appearance of the personnel; capped, masked, gowned, and gloved, they handle equipment and instruments in what appears to be a ritual manner. In fact, almost every aspect of the appearance and movements of surgical personnel is a practical application of the scientific knowledge that forms the basis for aseptic technique, a relatively recent development in the field of medicine.

Until the nineteenth century, two factors that prevented the development of surgery were the lack of anesthetics and analgesics and the inability of medical personnel to prevent the high incidence of postsurgical infection. The inability of physicians to prevent the simplest surgical procedure from resulting in overwhelming infection derived from a lack of knowledge concerning the causes of infection (Table 1-1).

TABLE 1-1

Milestones in Medical Microbiology: Causes of Disease

Year	Contributor	Contribution
1546	Fracastoro	Suggested disease results not from "act of God" but from living organisms
1676	Leeuwenhoek	Provided means of direct observation of bacteria
1762	von Plenciz	Suggested specific disease is caused by specific organism
1838	Schleiden, Schwann	Discovered cell as basic unit of living organisms
1839	Schönlein	Related fungi to skin disease
1850	Davaine	Demonstrated transmission of anthrax from animal to animal
1864	Pasteur	Provided final refutation of theory of spontaneous generation
1868	Villemin	Demonstrated transmission of tuberculosis from animal to animal
1876	Koch	Isolated *Bacillus anthracis* and proved it caused anthrax
1882	Koch	Isolated cause of tuberculosis
1892	Iwanowski	Discovered viruses
1898	Beijerinck	Discovered viral nature of plant disease
1898	Löffler, Frosch	Discovered viral nature of animal (hoof-and-mouth) disease

Knowledge of the existence of disease-causing microbes depended on the development of magnifying lenses of sufficient strength to observe microorganisms. Credit for the development of these lenses is given to Anton van Leeuwenhoek. The progression from the demonstration of the existence of microbes to the proof of the role they play in disease was a long and difficult process, and it was not until the second half of the nineteenth century that a body of knowledge sufficient to convince the medical community was accumulated. A strong belief in the theory of spontaneous generation, which states that living organisms can generate from inanimate materials without the presence of parent organisms, prevented many scientists from appreciating the importance of the discovery that some of the microbes caused disease.

Several milestones in the nineteenth century discounted the theory of spontaneous generation and demonstrated the validity of the concepts of contagion and infection that we take for granted today. Ignaz Semmelweis, a Hungarian obstetrician, and Oliver Wendell Holmes, an American physician and poet, published their views on the contagiousness of puerperal (childbirth) fever. Semmelweis' beliefs were based on his observations that the incidence of infection in mothers of newborns was higher in those wards in which mothers were examined by physicians coming directly to the wards from the autopsy rooms. His views were independently supported by Holmes, and requiring scrupulous cleanliness in the wards and handwashing by personnel entering the wards, Semmelweis caused a significant drop in the mortality rates in these wards.

Louis Pasteur, a French chemist, disproved the theory of spontaneous generation, removing one of the major blocks to the development of the theory of aseptic technique. Pasteur's other contributions to the fields of science and medicine were immense. Among them were the development of a vaccine for anthrax, the first preventive treatment for rabies, and the process of pasteurization, which destroys the pathogens transmitted in milk. Much of his work was devoted to proving the link between microbes and the changes in organic material caused by the processes of putrefaction and fermentation.

The English surgeon Joseph Lister noted the similarities between the changes described by Pasteur and the changes he saw in wound infections and concluded that wound infections were caused by microorganisms. His use of dressings soaked with phenol (carbolic acid) and his insistence on operating procedures that he believed would destroy microbes caused a significant decrease in the incidence of postsurgical infections in his patients. His innovations spread from England until they were accepted by all practitioners of Western medicine. Lister is known as the father of surgical asepsis, and Semmelweis is known as the father of medical asepsis.

The contributions of Robert Koch, a German physician, helped to establish the development of techniques needed to work with bacteria (the preparation of slides, the dyes to stain the microbes, the technology to grow microorganisms in pure culture), allowing him to prove that a specific disease was caused by a specific microbe. This work resulted in Koch's postulates, which must be fulfilled to prove that a specific organism causes a specific disease. The postulates are still used today as a basis for the investigation of infectious disease.

Pasteur's work concentrated on finding practical solutions to some of the problems caused by microbes. Koch's work complemented Pasteur's by providing the laboratory techniques necessary to demonstrate the validity of the practical solutions. These men, in recognition of their contributions that remain in use today, have been called the fathers of bacteriology.

The work of all four "fathers" (Semmelweis, Lister, Pasteur, Koch), as well as countless others of their contemporaries, provides modern medicine with the body of knowledge necessary to develop aseptic technique to the level at which no one, layperson or professional, considers infection to be a preordained result of common surgical procedures (Table 1-2).

Even though the consequences of infection had been validly demonstrated, many members of the medical profession resisted the work of these men largely because of complacency and ignorance. The correlation between the application of aseptic measures and the lowered incidence of infection had to be demonstrated repeatedly before the practical application of aseptic theory became routine. The understanding

TABLE 1-2

Milestones in Medical Microbiology: Prevention of Disease

Year	Contributor	Contribution
1796	Jenner	Vaccinated against smallpox, using cowpox serum
1861	Semmelweis	Believed transmission of infectious disease could be controlled by hygienic measures and use of disinfectants
1870	Lister	Used carbolic acid as disinfectant in surgery
1881	Pasteur	Developed anthrax vaccine
1884	Metchnikoff	Demonstrated phagocytosis theory of immunity
1885	Pasteur	Treated rabies
1888	Roux, Yersin	Discovered bacterial toxin (diphtherial)
	Brieger	Discovered tetanus toxin
1889	Buchner	Discovered agents in blood and serum that are effective against bacteria
1890	Kitasato, von Behring	Discovered tetanus antitoxin (passive immunization)
1893	Sternberg	Established first school of modern hygiene in America
1894	Roux, Martin	Used horses in production of tetanus antitoxin
1898	Ehrlich	Demonstrated antigen/antibody (humoral) theory of immunity
1906	Ehrlich	Applied first chemotherapeutic agent
1910	Rous	Demonstrated link between a virus and a cancer
1913	von Behring	Used toxin-antitoxin to produce permanent active immunity
1928	Fleming	Discovered penicillin
1940	Florey, Chain	Demonstrated medicinal value of penicillin
1954	Salk	Conducted field trial of vaccine effective against viral disease (polio)

of the principles of aseptic theory is derived from a basic knowledge of medical microbiology. This was true for the physician of the nineteenth century, and it remains true today for anyone who is a member of the surgical team.

■ THE MICROBIAL WORLD

Today many biologists place microorganisms in a third kingdom (the protists) distinct from the plant and animal kingdoms. As a group, the protists demonstrate more biologic and biochemical independence than plants or animals (Table 1-3). They are primarily unicellular, capable of rapid growth, and because of their biochemical versatility, capable of rapid adaptation to changes in the environment. The protists include the groups known familiarly as the algae, the protozoa, the fungi, and the bacteria. Several small groups (mycoplasmas, chlamydiae, rickettsiae) appear to fit somewhere between bacteria and viruses in terms of organism complexity and are sometimes referred to as modified bacteria. Technically, viruses are not included because their structure does not conform to the definition of a cell and because they do not use their own components to reproduce (Tables 1-4 and 1-5). The algae, fungi, and protozoa (higher protists) are distinguished from the higher plants and animals by the fact that each cell has the potential to complete the entire life cycle of the organism. These higher protists are distinguished from the lower protists (bacteria and modified bacteria) because their cells have a distinct nucleus enclosed within a nuclear membrane. The lower protists do not have a distinct nucleus enclosed within a membrane, but all protists have both DNA and RNA like more complex organisms. A virus contains RNA or DNA but not both. Some authorities believe that viruses are not alive, whereas others believe they are because they are capable of replicating themselves. They are included here for convenience.

Text continued on p. 13

TABLE 1-3			
General Characteristics Differentiating Plants and Animals from Microbes			
Characteristic	Plants	Microorganisms	Animals
Outermost layer	Well-defined, rigid wall	Wall or membrane	Flexible membrane
Cell nucleus	Within nuclear membrane	May or may not be well defined	Within nuclear membrane
Stored food	Starch	Various, including starch and fat	Glycogen and fat
Energy source	Inorganic compounds (photosynthesis)	Inorganic and organic compounds	Organic compounds (food)
Motility	Nonmotile	May or may not be motile; some may be motile in one life stage and not in another	Motile

Modified from Hunter P: *General microbiology: the student's textbook,* St Louis, 1977, Mosby.

TABLE 1-4

Higher Protists

Group*	General characteristics	Classification based on	Nonmedical significance	Medical significance
Algae	"Simple" plants (photosynthetic). Unicellular and multicellular forms (colonies and filaments). Contain chlorophylls. Reproduction is asexual and sexual. Rigid cell wall. Size: 1 μm to 50 m.	Type of chlorophyll and other pigment; nature of reserve materials; method of reproduction.	Form part of planktonic soup, serving as basis of aquatic food chains. Source of polishing agents, filters, insulation, vitamins, and thickening and stiffening agents used in food and medicine.	A few species produce toxins that affect humans and animals.
Fungi	"Simple" non-chlorophyll-bearing plantlike organisms. Most are saprophytic, unicellular (yeasts) and multicellular (molds, mushrooms) forms. Reproduction is sexual and asexual. Size: cell diameter 1 to 20 μm.	Primarily on method of spore formation and type of vegetative cell.	Industrial production of alcohols, acids, antibiotics. Used in manufacture of cheese, bread, wine, and beer. Play role in decomposition of dead organic material. Plant pathogens responsible for crop losses.	The few pathogenic species cause superficial and systemic diseases of humans and animals. Source of antibiotics.

Yeasts

Mold

Protozoa

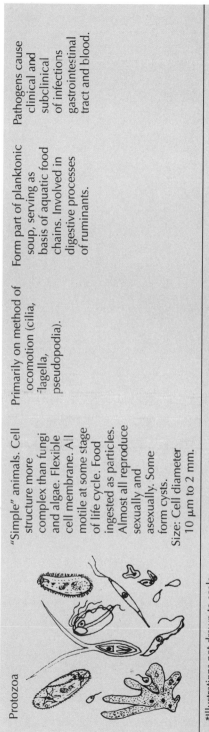

"Simple" animals. Cell structure more complex than fungi and algae. Flexible cell membrane. All motile at some stage of life cycle. Food ingested as particles. Almost all reproduce sexually and asexually. Some form cysts.
Size: Cell diameter 10 µm to 2 mm.

Primarily on method of locomotion (cilia, flagella, pseudopodia).

Form part of planktonic soup, serving as basis of aquatic food chains. Involved in digestive processes of ruminants.

Pathogens cause clinical and subclinical infections of gastrointestinal tract and blood.

*Illustrations not drawn to scale.

TABLE 1-5

Lower Protists

Group*	General characteristics	Classification within group	Laboratory media	Nonmedical significance	Medical significance
Bacteria	Rigid cell wall, motile and nonmotile forms. Reproduce by asexual binary fission. Include saprophytes, parasites, and pathogens. Some produce endospores. Susceptible to many antibiotics. Size: 5 to 100 μm.	Gram stain reaction, shape and arrangement of cells, growth requirements, biochemical and serologic properties.	Grown on artificial cell-free media.	Responsible for decomposition of dead organic matter, nitrogen fixation of plants, source of vitamins for animals. Improve soil fertility.	Include important pathogens of humans and animals. Source of antibiotics.
Mycoplasmas	Smallest free-living cells; intracellular parasites in host. No cell wall, very pleomorphic. Include saprophytes, parasites, and pathogens. Possess enzyme systems. Susceptible to antibiotics. Size: 125 to 250 nm (cell diameter), 10 to 250 μm (colony diameter).	Sterol requirement.	Can be grown on artificial cell-free media. As contaminant, often cause cytopathologic effects in tissue cultures of pathogens.	Little known.	Respiratory disease in humans, cattle, and poultry. Genital disease in humans.

Rickettsiae		Type of tissue infected in vertebrate host.	Tissue cell cultures, chick embryos, and lab animals.	Little known. Some apparently nonpathogenic forms have been identified.	Cause of disease syndromes in humans and animals affecting reticuloendo-thelial and blood cells.
WBC, RBC, Rickettsiae	Obligate intracellular parasites. Reproduce by binary fission, possess partial enzyme systems, and pleomorphic cell walls. Nonmotile. Gram-negative. Utilize arthropods as vectors and hosts. Most are retained by bacterial filters. Size: 0.2 to 0.5 μm in diameter.				

*Illustrations not drawn to scale.

TABLE 1-5

Lower Protists—Cont'd

Group*	General characteristics	Classification within group	Laboratory media	Nonmedical significance	Medical significance
Chlamydiae Nucleus Elementary bodies Inclusion bodies	Obligate intracellular parasites. Cell wall present. Gram-negative. Partial enzyme systems. Form inclusion bodies in host cells. Reproduce by formation of elementary bodies. Susceptible to some antibiotics. Size: 300 to 800 nm.	On basis of disease etiology.	Tissue cultures and chick embryos.	Little known.	Cause of disease syndromes of humans and animals involving many tissues and systems.
Viruses Brain cell (rabid dog) Nucleus Bacteriophage Plant Inclusion bodies (many virus particles) Animal	Obligate intracellular parasites. Contain either RNA or DNA, not both. No enzyme systems, no cell wall or membrane. Replicate at expense of host cell. Pass filters that retain bacteria. Some form characteristic inclusion bodies in host cell. Size: 20 to 300 nm.	Type of nucleic acid, sensitivity to physical and chemical agents, pathogenic characteristics. Type of tissue infected.	Tissue cultures, chick embryos, and inoculation of lab animals.	Little known.	Animal and plant pathogens. Many infections subclinical or latent. Implicated as cause of some cancer. Resistant to antibiotics.

*Illustrations not drawn to scale.

Infinite in variety and infinite in effect, the protists serve as the bottom rung on the food chain that eventually results in steak and peas for dinner. They permit more highly evolved plants to use nitrogen and to serve as food for meat-producing animals. Microbes cause the decay of dead organisms, permitting the recycling of components; they flavor our food, ferment our beer and wine, and provide us with medications. Because of the actions of microbes, termites digest wood, cows digest hay, and mammals are provided with the vitamin K necessary for the coagulation of blood. Without the activities of protists, our world would be unrecognizable, perhaps unimaginable. In recent years, humans have developed the technology to manipulate microbes for such tasks as the controlled digestion of oil spills, the synthesis of insulin, and the production of antibiotics.

Medical microbiology concentrates on the study of the relatively few species that are harmful to humans or animals (Fig. 1-1). A branch of science closely allied to medical microbiology is parasitology, which is primarily the study of multicellular parasites. Some scientists include protozoans in parasitology rather than in microbiology. Algae, the most plantlike of the protists, is the group that provides the least interest for medical microbiologists because few disease-causing organisms exist in this group.

Protozoa

Protozoa, the most animal-like of the protists, range in size from those just visible to the naked eye to those that are almost as small as the bacteria. They have the cell membrane typical of animals rather than the cell wall typical of plants, and all are motile in at least one stage of their life cycle. Protozoa form a cyst at some point of the life cycle that is relatively resistant to destruction. It is the cyst form of the

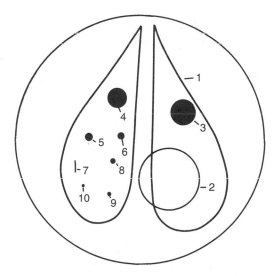

FIG. 1-1   Relative sizes of microbes. Largest circle represents erythrocyte. *1,* Protozoa *(Babesia); 2,* fungus (spore); *3,* bacteria (average); *4,* bacteria (small); *5,* rickettsia; *6,* chlamydia; *7,* virus (plant pathogen); *8* to *10,* viruses (animal pathogens).

pathogens that is usually transmitted from host to host and permits the survival of the protozoa when outside the host (Fig. 1-2). Examples of protozoan diseases are amebiasis, toxoplasmosis, and coccidiosis.

Fungi

The fungi can be described as non–chlorophyll-bearing plants and are commonly divided into the categories of molds and yeasts. Because they do not produce chlorophyll and cannot synthesize their own food, they must exist as parasites (dependent on a living host) or saprophytes (dependent on the remains of dead organisms). Examples of diseases caused by fungi are ringworm and histoplasmosis. The diagnosis of both protozoan and fungal diseases is usually based on demonstrating the causative agent in the appropriate specimen: feces, blood smears, tissue sections, or skin scrapings (Fig. 1-3).

Bacteria

Bacteria are generally unicellular with a rigid cell wall that defines one of three basic shapes: coccus (spherical), bacillus (rod), or spirillum (spiral) (Fig. 1-4). The composition of the cell wall is the basis for the reaction of the bacterium to the Gram stain, and bacteria are often referred to as gram positive or gram negative. The almost 2000 identified species of bacteria vary widely in conditions of temperature, pH balance, moisture, and sources of nutrition required for growth and reproduction. The majority of bacteria are free living, but many species are parasitic to plants and animals, and some of the parasites are pathogenic. The causative agents of tuberculosis, anthrax, and brucellosis are bacteria.

The endospore produced by some bacilli is the most resistant to destruction of all microbial forms, barring a few viruses, and bacterial spores are used as a standard to determine the effectiveness of microbial control methods.

The diagnosis of bacterial diseases is often based on clinical observation, and confirmation is provided by the laboratory isolation of the suspected microbe from an appropriate specimen.

Rickettsiae

The rickettsiae are a small group of microbes that are obligate intracellular parasites, being totally dependent on the cells of host tissues. At some point in the life cycle, rickettsiae use arthropods either as vectors or hosts. Rocky Mountain spotted fever, canine ehrlichiosis, and "heartwater" of cattle, sheep, and goats are caused by rickettsial agents, which characteristically attack the cells of the reticuloendothelial system. The genus *Bartonella* is composed of rickettsiae that are characterized by the ability to invade the red blood cells of the host. Feline infectious anemia is caused by a member of this group.

Chlamydiae

Microorganisms belonging to this group resemble rickettsiae in several ways. Their enzyme systems are not complete enough for an independent existence, and they are obligate intracellular parasites. Their life cycle in host cells is not completely understood, and under laboratory conditions they are handled in much the same way as viruses.

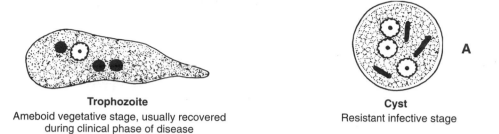

Trophozoite
Ameboid vegetative stage, usually recovered
during clinical phase of disease

Cyst
Resistant infective stage

A

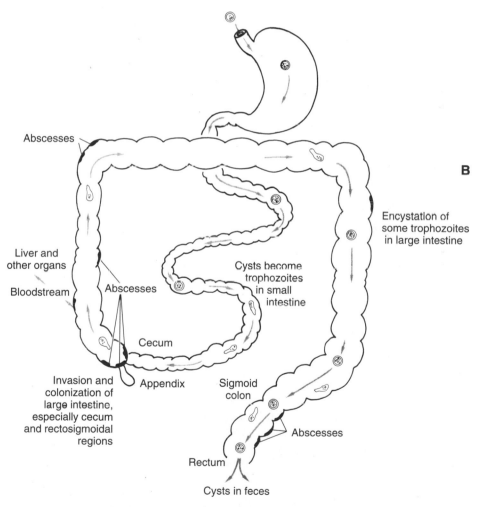

Abscesses

Liver and
other organs

Bloodstream

Abscesses

Cecum

Appendix

Invasion and
colonization of
large intestine,
especially cecum
and rectosigmoidal
regions

Encystation of
some trophozoites
in large intestine

Cysts become
trophozoites
in small
intestine

Sigmoid
colon

Abscesses

Rectum

Cysts in feces

B

FIG. 1-2   *Entamoeba histolytica,* protozoan pathogen. **A,** Vegetative and cyst stages of parasite. **B,** Passage of parasite through host. (From Hunter P: *General microbiology: the student's textbook,* St Louis, 1977, Mosby.)

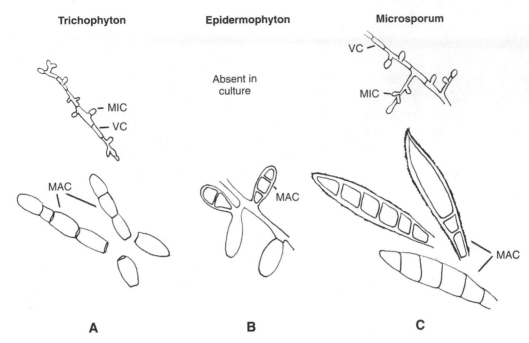

FIG. 1-3   Pathogenic fungi. Cultured under laboratory conditions, hyphae (vegetative cells) and microconidia (single-celled reproductive structures) or genera causing ringworm often look alike. Identification is often based on shape and arrangement of macroconidia (multicelled reproductive structures). Intertwined mass of hyphae and conidia makes up mycelium, visible to unaided eye as "mold." **A** and **C,** Pathogenic to many animals and humans. **B,** Pathogenic to humans. *VC,* Vegetative cell; *MIC,* microconidia; *MAC,* macroconidia.

The causative agents of cat-scratch fever in humans and feline pneumonitis are chlamydiae.

Mycoplasmas

The smallest free-living organisms discovered to date are mycoplasmas, which are so small that close to 10,000 might fit into one canine red blood cell. Mycoplasmas are sometimes referred to as pleuropneumonia-like organisms (PPLOs), and their role in disease is just beginning to be understood. They are found everywhere, frequently having a nuisance value as contaminants of viral cultures. They exist in saprophytic, parasitic, and pathogenic forms. Having no cell wall, they are relatively resistant to antibiotics. Mycoplasmas are among the causative agents of mastitis and pneumonia in domestic animals and have been implicated in arthritis.

Viruses

Living cells are characterized as containing both DNA and RNA and possessing at least some enzyme systems that carry on metabolic processes necessary for growth and reproduction. Viruses have either DNA or RNA, but not both, and have no en-

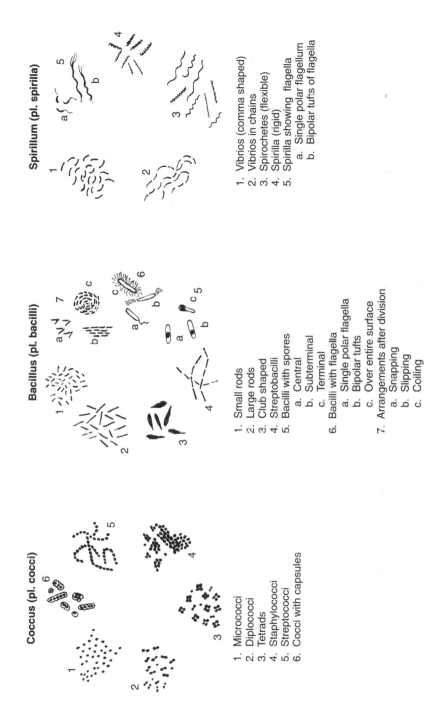

Coccus (pl. cocci)

1. Micrococci
2. Diplococci
3. Tetrads
4. Staphylococci
5. Streptococci
6. Cocci with capsules

Bacillus (pl. bacilli)

1. Small rods
2. Large rods
3. Club shaped
4. Streptobacilli
5. Bacilli with spores
   a. Central
   b. Subterminal
   c. Terminal
6. Bacilli with flagella
   a. Single polar flagella
   b. Bipolar tufts
   c. Over entire surface
7. Arrangements after division
   a. Snapping
   b. Slipping
   c. Coiling

Spirillum (pl. spirilla)

1. Vibrios (comma shaped)
2. Vibrios in chains
3. Spirochetes (flexible)
4. Spirilla (rigid)
5. Spirilla showing flagella
   a. Single polar flagellum
   b. Bipolar tufts of flagella

FIG. 1-4 Morphology of bacteria. Variation in cell shape, size, and arrangement and presence or absence of special structures can be used as aids in identifying bacteria. Other aids in identification include cultural characteristics and biochemical and serologic reactions.

zyme systems; therefore they do not conform to the commonly accepted definition for life forms. Composed of a nucleic acid coil surrounded by a protein coat, viruses are obligate intracellular parasites. In organization and complexity they occupy a place between the largest molecules and the smallest cells (Fig. 1-5).

Viruses use components of host cells to replicate. The viral nucleic acid enters a susceptible host cell and in effect directs the cell to manufacture hundreds of new virus particles instead of the normally manufactured cell components. These virus particles are then released to infect other cells.

In many instances, the cycle of viral infection causes no apparent harm to the host. Disease occurs when the host is harmed by the infection, but the mechanisms by which viruses harm the host are imperfectly understood. These mechanisms involve cell proliferation as well as cell destruction. Viral-induced hyperplasia has implicated viruses as a cause of cancer.

In contrast to other types of microbial diseases, viral infections often show no or minimal inflammatory response in the host.

Rabies, canine distemper, panleukopenia, and infectious canine hepatitis are caused by viruses.

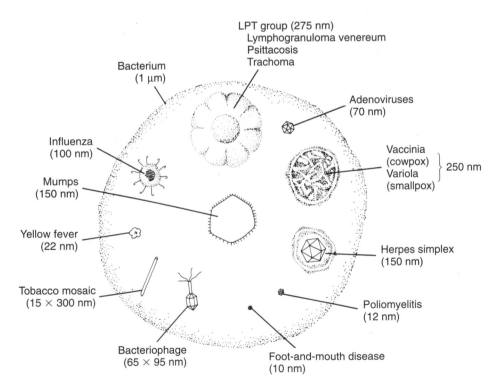

FIG. 1-5   Relative sizes of various common viruses compared to typical bacterial cell. (From Hunter P: *General microbiology: the student's textbook,* St Louis, 1977, Mosby.)

■ DISEASE
Causes of Diseases

Technicians should have a basic knowledge of common pathologic conditions and their causes. A previously existing disease may affect the ability of the animal to respond to the treatment of a subsequent condition. Regardless of the condition calling for surgery, no animal should be subjected to an infectious disease acquired in conjunction with surgery. The major efforts of aseptic technique are directed against the diseases in this category.

For convenience, diseases can be sorted into categories based on the type of cause.

Hereditary diseases are those transmitted genetically from parents to offspring. Hemophilia A of dogs is an example of a hereditary disease, and subluxation of the carpus has been closely linked with hemophilia A. For domestic animals, the major efforts in controlling these diseases are directed at identifying the gene carriers and discouraging the breeding of these animals.

Congenital diseases and prenatal malformations are disease states that occur during pregnancy and are present at birth. The exact cause of a specific disease of this type may be unknown, but factors that have been implicated include prenatal viral infection, exposure of the fetus to toxins ingested by the mother, vitamin deficiencies, and genetic factors. Prenatal malformations are relatively common. Animals that are severely affected by malformations, if they do not die shortly after birth, are usually euthanized. Polydactyly in cats and cleft palate are examples of congenital conditions attributed to genetic factors. The crooked calf syndrome, which includes cleft palate and scoliosis, was thought to be hereditary in nature, but the cause has now been identified as a toxin found in lupines eaten by pregnant cows. The importance of identifying the cause of a disease in this category is evident because the cause affects the method of controlling the disease. It should be understood that not all congenital diseases are hereditary.

Deficiency diseases are those resulting from the lack of a dietary substance or the inability to digest and use dietary substances. A large variety of dietary substances are required to maintain good health in the animal. Starvation is a deficiency disease, and some deficiency diseases result from the lack of a single substance, such as iron (anemia) or iodine (goiter). A deficiency disease caused by the lack of a dietary substance (or substances) can usually be handled by providing the missing or decreased substance. In some instances, although the diet is adequate, a dietary substance cannot be properly digested by the animal. In diabetes mellitus of dogs and cats, the animal is unable to use glucose derived from ingested carbohydrates because it lacks the necessary insulin to do so. The control of this disease is based on supplying the insulin necessary to use the carbohydrates in the diet.

Hereditary, congenital, and deficiency diseases rarely produce much reaction on the part of the animal's body defenses. Hypertrophy of tissues may occur in an attempt to compensate for the effects of the disease, such as goiter in an iodine deficiency.

Physical trauma diseases include injuries such as lacerations, fractures, crushing blows, burns, and gunshot wounds. Exposure to extremes of heat and cold can cause physical damage to body tissues. Because injuries such as these are often caused by objects contaminated by microbes or because microbes on the skin are carried to deep tissues when the injury occurs, infection may result. Injuries of this type are characterized by the production of an inflammatory response by the body. Many of the diseases in this category are accidental and are difficult to control. For those that are caused by the ignorance of the owners and handlers, education can play a large role in preventing repetition.

Poisons are substances that are toxic to living tissues. Ingestion, absorption, or inhalation of a toxic substance interferes with the metabolic functioning of the affected tissues. The degree of malfunction is determined by the nature of the toxin, the amount ingested, and the ability of the animal to eliminate or neutralize the poison before permanent damage occurs. The control of the occurrences of these disease states is based primarily on eliminating the source of the poison from the animal's environment or in preventing the animal from gaining access to the source. The affected animal is seldom able to offer significant resistance to poisons. Many ingested toxins are irritants, and vomiting and diarrhea rid the body of at least some portion of the dose.

The last category of disease-causing agents includes the infectious agents— metazoans (multicellular organisms) and microbes (unicellular organisms) that cause disease in higher animals. Because the diseases can be passed from animal to animal (by direct or indirect contact), these diseases are referred to as contagious or infectious. If a contagious or infectious disease can be transmitted from animal to human, it is referred to as a zoonotic disease (Table 1-6).

Some knowledge of these pathogenic states is important to the technician for two reasons. The existence of an infectious disease before surgery lessens the ability of the animal to withstand surgery. The prevention of nosocomial (hospital-acquired) infections is the desired result of aseptic technique.

A wide variety of metazoans and microbes are capable of causing disease by using varying mechanisms of disease production (Table 1-7). In general, it is of little benefit to the parasite if the disease that follows infection is so severe that all readily available hosts are killed. Many pathogens are able to achieve a balance with the host that allows both the host and the parasite to survive for long periods. The pathogenic metazoans (e.g., ticks, fleas, intestinal worms), the protozoans, and the fungi are noted for producing this type of disease. The ability of the individual host to resist succumbing to the pathogen plays a large role; very young, elderly, debilitated, or stressed animals are more likely to die from the effects of infestation or infection than mature, healthy animals who receive adequate care.

Protozoan diseases are often slow to progress, and death may occur only after a long period of infection. Almost all diseases caused by protozoans affect either the intestinal tract (coccidiosis) or the blood (babesiosis). Pathogens in this group may produce little or no inflammatory response in the host even if the injury to body tissues is severe.

Fungal diseases primarily involve superficial tissue, with a few exceptions. The majority of fungal pathogens are apparently unable to adapt to internal tissue environments. They are directly transmissible from one individual to another, maintaining a natural reservoir in susceptible species. Some fungal agents that cause systemic disease appear to originate from the soil, where they occur as saprophytes. Histo-

TABLE 1-6

Zoonoses: a Partial Listing of Diseases That Can Be Transmitted from Animal to Human

Disease	Dogs	Cats	Farm animals	Caged birds*	Poultry	Rodents†	Nonhuman primates	Reptiles‡
VIRAL								
Encephalitides			X	X	X	X	X	
Infectious hepatitis							X	
Rabies	X	X	X				X	
BACTERIAL								
Anthrax			X					
Brucellosis	X		X					
Chlamydial								
Cat-scratch disease§	X	X						
Psittacosis-ornithosis				X	X			
Leptospirosis	X		X	X		X		
Melioidosis			X			X	X	
Rickettsial—Q fever			X		X		X	
Salmonellosis	X	X	X	X	X	X	X	X
Tuberculosis	X	X	X		X		X	
Tularemia			X			X		
FUNGAL								
Ringworm	X	X	X	X	X	X	X	
PROTOZOAN								
Amebiasis	X						X	
Toxoplasmosis	X	X	X	X	X	X	X	
METAZOAN								
Roundworm infection	X	X	X			X		
Scabies	X	X						
Tapeworm infection	X	X	X			X		
Toxicariasis	X	X						

From Smith AL: *Principles of microbiology,* ed 9, St Louis, 1981, Mosby, p 134.
*Pigeons, parakeets, parrots, myna birds, canaries, and such.
†Mice, rabbits, rats, hamsters, and such.
‡Snakes, turtles, lizards, and such.
§Agent unknown, often discussed with chlamydial diseases.

TABLE 1-7

Representative Canine and Feline Microbial Diseases

Microbe type	Canine	Feline
Protozoan	Coccidiosis	Coccidiosis
	Entamoebiasis	Entamoebiasis
	Toxoplasmosis	Toxoplasmosis
	Babesiosis	
Fungal	Dermatomycosis	Dermatomycosis
	Cryptococcosis	Cryptococcosis
	Histoplasmosis	
	Blastomycosis	
Bacterial	Septicemia	Septicemia
	Enteritis	Enteritis
	Cystitis	Cystitis
	Pneumonia	Pneumonia
	Pyometra	Mastitis
	Mastitis	Conjunctivitis
	Conjunctivitis	Tetanus
	Nocardiosis	
	Tetanus	
	Brucellosis	
	Leptospirosis	
Rickettsial	Canine ehrlichiosis	Hemobartonellosis (feline infectious
	Hemobartonellosis	anemia [FIA])
	(splenectomized animal)	
	Rocky Mountain spotted fever	
Chlamydial	Polyarthritis (experimentally)	Pneumonitis
		Rhinotracheitis
		Conjunctivitis
Viral	Parvovirus infection	Feline panleukopenia (feline
	Infectious canine hepatitis (ICH)	distemper, FPL)
	Canine tracheobronchitis	Feline infectious peritonitis (FIP)
	(kennel cough)	Feline leukemia
	Canine distemper	Rabies
	Rabies	

plasmosis, a systemic mycosis, is often transmitted by birds, the agent being spread by droppings that contaminate the soil.

The bacteria are divided into the higher bacteria and the simple bacteria. The diseases that are caused by pathogens belonging to the higher bacteria resemble fungal diseases in that they are usually slow to progress, chronic in nature, and difficult to cure. Some of these pathogens, such as the bacilli that cause tuberculosis, produce toxins that will cause necrosis at the site of the infection.

The pathogenic simple bacteria are generally associated with acute diseases, often producing severe effects. The effect may be mechanical (the numbers of bacteria present are sufficient to interfere with tissue function), but it is more likely to be biochemical in nature. Bacteria may produce exotoxins *(Clostridium tetani)*, which are diffused out of the bacterial cell while it is alive, or they may produce endotoxins (*Salmonella* spp.), which are freed only if the cell integrity is disrupted.

In addition, bacteria produce a number of biochemical factors (termed accessory chemical substances) that contribute to the invasive capability of the bacteria by reducing the effectiveness of host defense mechanisms. Staphylococci and streptococci produce leukocidins and hemolysins. Leukocidins are toxic to white blood cells, and hemolysins dissolve red blood cells. These bacteria also produce kinases, which dissolve clots that are formed by the host in an attempt to restrict the spread of the pathogen. The capsules of the pneumococci enable these bacteria to evade the phagocytic action of the leukocytes.

The diseases of simple bacteria elicit a strong host response that causes the production of antibodies, which will provide protection against subsequent infection. The advantage of this is the ability to produce various vaccines. A specific bacterial pathogen may tend to localize in a particular tissue, exert its effect on a particular tissue, or diffuse throughout the body, affecting almost all tissues.

The development of vaccines and antibiotics has resulted in major advances in the control of bacterial diseases. Viral diseases present one of the remaining formidable problems in medicine. Few antibiotics are effective against viruses. Although they often elicit strong antibody response in the host, the rate of mutation in viruses is so rapid that new strains appear with alarming frequency. The mechanisms by which viruses cause disease are not well understood, but the diseases may be either destructive or proliferative in nature. Destructive viral diseases are often similar to simple bacterial disease in that infection is acute and severe. The effects of viruses causing proliferative diseases vary from hyperplasia to neoplasia; some viruses are implicated as a cause of cancer.

Sources of Pathogens

A disease-causing microbe may be exogenous (originating outside the body) or endogenous (normally found in the host). Endogenous infections occur when host resistance is lowered, microbial virulence is raised, or endogenous microbes are transferred to parts of the body in which they are not normally found.

With the exception of a few microbes that are soil saprophytes or are harbored by plants, the sources of exogenous pathogens are animals and humans used as hosts by the pathogens. A passive carrier is an animal that has been infected by a pathogen and discharges the pathogen for a long period without ever exhibiting clinical signs of the disease. Discharge of the pathogens may be continual or intermittent, which makes it difficult to detect the carrier. An active carrier discharges pathogens for a long period after it has recovered from clinical symptoms. A host may often transmit pathogens during the incubational or convalescent phase of a disease when clinical symptoms are not apparent, as well as during the active phase. For all these reasons, it is often not possible to pinpoint the source of infection in a given instance of a disease.

Endogenous microorganisms (microflora) may be commensals, opportunists, or pathogens. Resident microbes are commensals or opportunists, and transient microbes may well be pathogenic. Most of the microflora are obligate parasites, but not obligate pathogens, for the individual host. In healthy animals, several body regions have relatively high concentrations of microbes. These include the skin and mucous membranes, the conjunctivae, the upper respiratory tract, the mouth, the lower intestine, the external genitalia, and the anterior urethra. Each of these areas has its own microbial population that differs from other portions of the body.

Means of Transmission

An exogenous pathogen gains access to host tissues by entering through a portal of entry. The respiratory system, the alimentary system, the skin, the urogenital system, and the placenta are portals of entry. Direct contact between animals may allow microbes to transfer to a new host, but pathogens do not depend on direct contact and use various ways of gaining access to a new susceptible host. The most common means of transmission are shown in Fig. 1-6.

The goal of aseptic technique is to effectively break this chain of transmission, thereby preventing the pathogens from gaining access to a new host. The pathogens must be killed in body secretions and products, or they use the environment (fomites, vectors, air, food, water) to effect a transfer to a new host. The variety of ways in which microbes effect a transfer necessitate a variety of methods to control or eliminate the transfer of pathogens.

Invasion of the Host

The invasion of a host does not necessarily result in disease. Factors influencing the result include the portal of entry, the virulence and numbers of the pathogen, and the effect of host resistance on the pathogen.

Portal of entry. Many pathogens are unlikely to cause disease unless they gain access to a specific portal of entry. Some streptococci cause pneumonia if inhaled but are unlikely to cause any harm if ingested. A few microbes can enter by more than one portal or any portal. Microbes that are transmitted by insects depend in many cases on the creation of a skin lesion by the insect, which permits access to the blood.

Virulence of the pathogen. The capacity of the microorganism to invade a host and its capacity to produce substances toxic to the host contribute to the virulence of the pathogen (Fig. 1-7). The bacterium that causes tetanus has a low order of invasiveness, depending on such portals as puncture wounds and lacerations to invade the body and find conditions suitable for growth, but has a high order of toxicity because the toxin that it produces so severely affects the host. Opportunists are characterized by a high order of invasiveness, because it is relatively easy for them to establish themselves in at least one host tissue, but a low order of toxicity. High invasiveness and high toxicity would become self-defeating for the microbe because all potential hosts within a population would soon be eliminated, leaving the microbe with literally no place to go.

A sufficient number of pathogens must invade the host for disease to result. The local host response must be overcome for the pathogen to establish itself. The necessary number of pathogens depends on the virulence of the microbe and the resistance of the host.

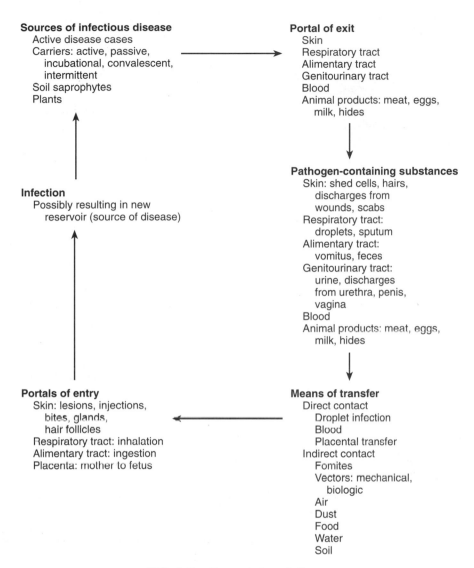

Sources of infectious disease
    Active disease cases
    Carriers: active, passive,
       incubational, convalescent,
       intermittent
    Soil saprophytes
    Plants

Portal of exit
    Skin
    Respiratory tract
    Alimentary tract
    Genitourinary tract
    Blood
    Animal products: meat, eggs,
       milk, hides

Infection
    Possibly resulting in new
       reservoir (source of disease)

Pathogen-containing substances
    Skin: shed cells, hairs,
       discharges from
       wounds, scabs
    Respiratory tract:
       droplets, sputum
    Alimentary tract:
       vomitus, feces
    Genitourinary tract:
       urine, discharges
       from urethra, penis,
       vagina
    Blood
    Animal products: meat, eggs,
       milk, hides

Portals of entry
    Skin: lesions, injections,
       bites, glands,
       hair follicles
    Respiratory tract: inhalation
    Alimentary tract: ingestion
    Placenta: mother to fetus

Means of transfer
    Direct contact
       Droplet infection
       Blood
       Placental transfer
    Indirect contact
       Fomites
       Vectors: mechanical,
         biologic
       Air
       Dust
       Food
       Water
       Soil

FIG. 1-6   Transmission of disease.

Infection. Assuming that the microbe has invaded the host and overcome host resistance, the resulting infection may vary. Local infections are confined to a restricted area of the body (abscesses), and generalized or systemic infections are those in which the pathogen has spread throughout the body by means of the bloodstream. The presence of bacteria in the blood is known as bacteremia. If bacteria grow and reproduce in the blood, the condition is called septicemia. Pyemia results when pus-

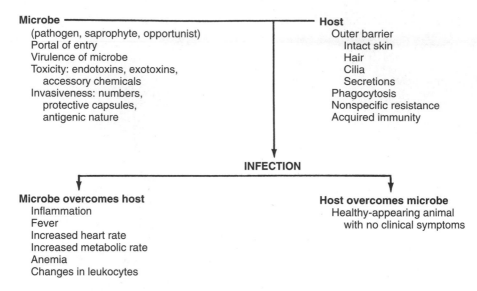

FIG. 1-7   Factors influencing infection.

forming bacteria use the bloodstream to spread to other areas of the body. If the disease causes toxic substances to enter the blood, the condition is called toxemia.

A subclinical infection is one in which no clinical signs appear. An infection may be present but is controlled by host defense mechanisms; if host resistance is lowered and the infection is manifest, it is said to have been a latent infection.

If one infection is present, lowering host resistance and thereby allowing the establishment of a second infection, the primary infection is said to be complicated by the secondary infection. The secondary infection may often be more serious than the primary infection. Terminal infections result in the death of the host animal.

Infections can cause both local and general changes in the host body. The local changes are associated with the inflammatory response that is discussed in the section on individual resistance. The general changes include fever and increased pulse and metabolic rates. Frequently, infections produce changes in the white blood cells— in the total number present, in the proportion of each type present, or in the appearance of individual cells. Many diseases are associated with characteristic patterns of change that aid in the diagnosis of the disease.

Host resistance. The ability of the host to successfully resist invasion by the pathogens depends on many specific and nonspecific factors. Nonspecific factors enable the host to control the general invasion by pathogens, and specific factors function against only particular pathogens (Fig. 1-8).

Species resistance. Many species of pathogens are limited to one or two species of host under normal conditions. For example, humans do not get canine distemper and dogs do not get whooping cough. The more closely two species are related, the

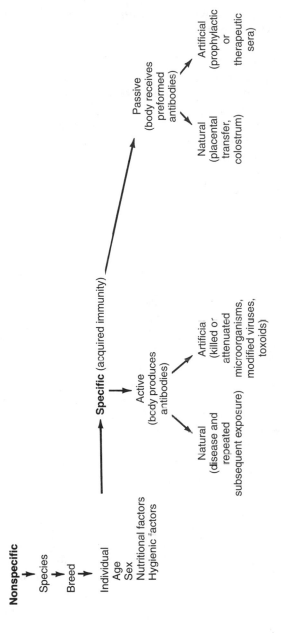

FIG. 1-8   Resistance to infection.

more likely they are to be susceptible to the same pathogen. There are nearly 200 diseases that are secondarily transmissible to humans from animals (zoonotic). It should be understood that species resistance is not axiomatic, and changes in diet and environment may affect the resistance of a species to a disease. If the natural host is nearly eliminated, the pathogen often will attempt to establish itself in a new host species. Anatomic and physiologic differences between species contribute to the maintenance of species resistance.

The nonsusceptibility of humans to many animal diseases often causes infectious animals to be handled with less care than infectious humans. Within limits this may be acceptable, but it is important to remain aware of which diseases can be transmitted to humans (for self-protection) as well as to remember that a human being can act as a mechanical vector in the transmission of disease from one animal to another (for patient protection).

Breed susceptibility may also vary. Dogs that do not maintain the outer ear in an upright position may be more susceptible to ear infections, because the covered ear canal provides a moist dark environment that is suitable for the growth of bacteria.

Individual resistance. The age, gender, nutritional state, and amount of stress vary from animal to animal within a species and can cause variations in the degree of susceptibility from one individual to another. Factors such as these affect the efficiency of the three major lines of defense available to the individual. The three lines of defense used by the individual to resist disease are anatomic barriers, phagocytosis and the inflammatory response, and humoral and cell-mediated immunity. The first two lines of defense are nonspecific in nature, and the third is specific.

The anatomic barrier. The first line of defense includes the mechanical barrier of the unbroken skin and mucous membranes and the antimicrobial substances produced by glands in these areas. Intact skin is difficult for most microbes to penetrate. Hair provides an additional barrier in the coat and in structures such as eyelashes. The mucous membrane of the upper respiratory system produces a slimy secretion that traps microbes and dust particles. Coughing and sneezing help to rid the body of these particles. Eyebrows, eyelids, and eyelashes provide mechanical protection to the eyes, and tears contain lysozyme, a bactericidal agent. In the gastrointestinal tract the acidity of the stomach kills many microbes, and those that reach the small intestine are subjected to the actions of enzymes, bile, and mucus in addition to phagocytosis. The vaginal tract is protected by a secretion that traps many microbes, and the acidity of the secretion repels many invaders. The acidity of normal urine, in addition to the flushing effect of urine as it leaves the body, affords protection to the urogenital tract.

Phagocytosis and the inflammatory response. If the barrier of skin and mucous membrane is broken, disease does not necessarily result. Phagocytosis and inflammation provide a second line of defense in preventing microbes from establishing themselves. Certain leukocytes, in particular the neutrophils, are capable of phagocytosis, ingesting and destroying microbes that penetrate the outer layers of the body, thus preventing pathogens from using the circulatory system as a transport to internal organs. If phagocytosis is successful and the ingested microbe is destroyed, disease is avoided or cured (Fig. 1-9). A serum component called opsonin enhances phagocytic action against some pathogens. Some anesthetics and drugs depress phagocytic activity, thus lowering resistance.

Inflammation is a local (surface) response to cellular injury (Fig. 1-10). It represents the body's defense against a harmful stimulus. Acute inflammation is characterized by the five cardinal signs of heat, redness, pain, swelling, and a disturbance of cellular function. For the most part, inflammation, like fever, is a protective device of considerable value to animals. It serves to bring phagocytes and antibodies to the site of the injury or infection. The successful result of inflammation is the healing of the injured tissue. On occasion, inflammation can be harmful, as in diseases such as systemic lupus erythematosus in which the inflammatory response harms rather than helps the host. Certain reactions between antigens and antibodies also result in inflammatory responses harmful to the animal.

Irritants that cause inflammation include physical agents, chemical agents, and microbial agents. Injuries that involve excessive heat (burns) and lacerations or blows

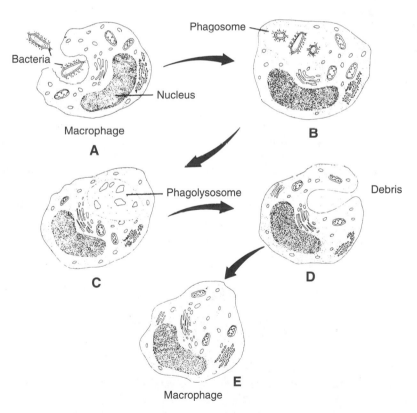

FIG. 1-9   Phagocytosis. **A,** Bacteria ingested by phagocytic cell. **B** and **C,** Bacteria digested inside cell. **D,** Digestive debris egested. **E,** Phagocytic cell returns to resting stage. Phagocytic cell may itself be destroyed. (From Smith AL: *Principles of microbiology,* St Louis, 1977, Mosby.)

Epithelium

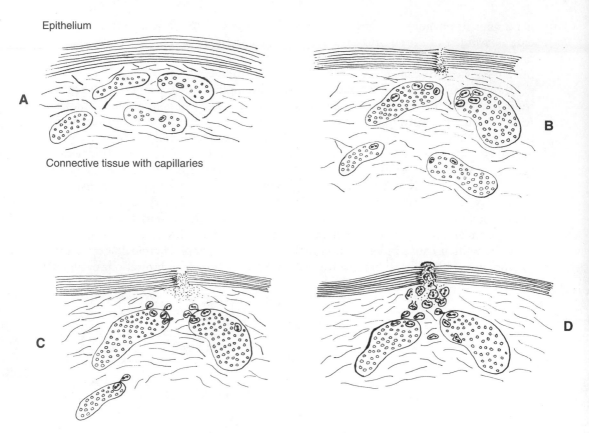

Connective tissue with capillaries

FIG. 1-10   Inflammation and infection. **A,** Normal tissue. **B,** Lesion occurs with contaminating bacteria; nearby capillaries dilate, and ameboid phagocytic cells in blood are attracted to site of injury. Capillary dilation causes redness. **C,** Phagocytic cells leave capillaries and migrate to site of injury; bacteria reproduce. Plasma exudate causes swelling. **D,** Phagocytic cells engulf bacteria and are themselves destroyed. Pus (destroyed cells and tissue debris) accumulates.

to the tissue initiate an inflammatory response, as do many chemical substances that are toxic or harmful to tissue.

Many pathogens act as irritants by producing substances that adversely affect the host tissue, eliciting an inflammatory response.

The classic (or cardinal) signs of inflammation include redness, heat, swelling, pain, and a disturbance of cellular function. Redness occurs because blood vessels in the vicinity of the irritant dilate, slowing the rate of blood flow and increasing the amount of blood in the area. Heat is also caused by the increased blood flow as it carries the higher internal temperature of the body to peripheral areas. The swelling is the result of increased amounts of blood and the accumulation of substances that pass from blood vessels to nearby tissues. The pain may be caused by increased pressure on sensory nerves or the irritating effects of toxins. Several chemical factors, such as histamine, serotonin, and the kinins, are found in the blood or released by injured cells; they play a role in the initiation of inflammation and the increased permeability of blood vessels. The increased permeability of the vessels allows phagocytes and antimicrobial substances in the blood to concentrate at the site. Serous fluid from the blood passes to the tissues, becoming the inflammatory exudate. Among the antimicrobial substances in blood are complement, which is bactericidal, and interferon, which is viricidal. The decreased rate of blood flow and the presence of coagulation factors in the exudate cause the formation of clots, which help to prevent the spreading of the process. Such a result is seen in abscesses and may prevent a local infection from becoming systemic. The movement of large numbers of phagocytes to the site of injury may result in the formation of pus, which is caused by the accumulation of phagocytes and tissue debris in the inflammatory exudate. An acute, intense inflammation is more likely to produce pus than a mild inflammation. Pathogens, not all of which are destroyed by phagocytosis or antimicrobial substances, accumulate in pus. Because of this, pus must always be treated as a highly infectious substance.

Humoral and cell-mediated immunity. Assuming that the microbe has penetrated the first two lines of defense, another means of defense is available in the animal: specific resistance or immunity. The body is provided with mechanisms that allow it to distinguish between "self" and "nonself." "Nonself" substances that invade the body provoke an immune response. The immune system of an individual consists of the elements that contribute to this discrimination of self from nonself. Phagocytosis is directed against components of dead tissue cells (self) as well as foreign invaders, such as bacteria (nonself). Many points regarding the immune system have not been clarified by science, and much work continues in the field of immunobiology. The term *nonspecific immunity* has been applied to the resistance to a specific disease for which there are no demonstrable antibodies. Individuals that have produced antibodies, or obtained antibodies already produced, are said to have *specific immunity* or *acquired immunity*. The production of antibodies (humoral immunity) does not occur unless an antigen (foreign substance) is present.

Active acquired immunity results when an antigen is introduced into the body and stimulates the production of antibodies. Because of the time lapse necessary for antibody formation, the protection is not immediate, but it is of long duration and may prevent reinfection for a lifetime (Fig. 1-11). Passive immunity results when the body obtains antibodies from an outside source. Because no antigens are present, the body does not produce antibodies itself and eventually the introduced antibodies are degraded and eliminated, causing immunity to disappear. Passive acquired immunity is immediately effective but of relatively short duration. Antibodies obtained by placental transfer and through colostrum protect the young animal for a period of months but subsequently disappear. To produce its own antibodies, the animal must be exposed to antigens, either during an attack of the disease or by vaccination. Infection will often produce immunity of longer duration than vaccination because the microbes used for vaccines must be modified so that they do not cause the disease they are intended to prevent.

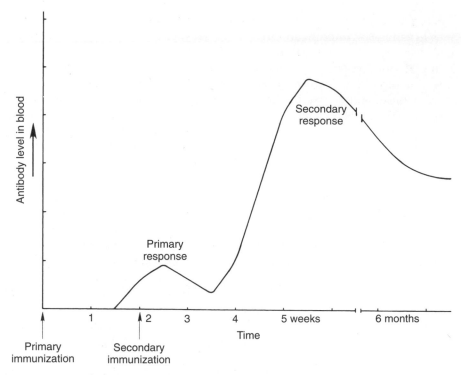

FIG. 1-11   A time lapse of several weeks is necessary for host to produce antibodies as result of exposure to antigen (either as result of infection or as result of immunization). (From Hunter P: *General microbiology: the student's textbook,* St Louis, 1977, Mosby.)

Certain types of leukocytes, particularly lymphocytes, play an important role in the production of immunity. The lymphocytes can be divided into the T cells (those that are processed by the thymus gland) and the B cells (those that are thymus independent).

B cells, which survive for only a few weeks, produce antibodies in the humoral system and provide protection against bacterial infection. T cells, which may survive for years, regulate cell-mediated immune responses. The mechanisms of a cell-mediated immune response are not as well understood as those of a humoral immune response; however, it is known to provide some protection against infections caused by fungi and acid-fast bacteria and against cancer.

Many hospitals require the owners of animals admitted for elective surgery to show a current vaccination certificate. This ensures the animal's safety, so that if exposed to an infectious disease during the hospital stay, it will be less likely to become infected.

Prevention of Infection

Safe and effective vaccines are not yet available for every possible infection of animals. Even if vaccines were available, it would be economically infeasible for the average pet owner to vaccinate a pet against every infection to which it might be exposed.

The advent of chemotherapeutic agents in the twentieth century (including sulfonamides and antibiotics) has enabled medical workers to significantly increase the amount of aid available to an individual when host resistance is overwhelmed by microbial virulence. The benefits of antibiotics to humans and animals in the struggle against disease cannot be overstressed. However, the fact that antibiotics are so effective has in some instances led to their overuse, and microbes have responded by selecting for resistant strains that are not easily or quickly destroyed. There are also many pathogens that are not particularly susceptible to antibiotic activity. Hospital personnel who have relied on the prophylactic administration of antibiotics to counteract an insufficient maintenance of sterility or inadequate aseptic technique procedures have discovered that they have contributed to the emergence of resistant strains of microbes. Although the problem may not be as acute in veterinary medicine, resistant strains have been isolated in animal facilities. The administration of antibiotics should not be relied on to protect animals from the consequences of inadequate control measures.

■ CONTROL OF MICROBES

It is against the microbial pathogens and opportunists that the efforts of aseptic technique are directed. The hospital environment may exhibit a high concentration of pathogens and house a large number of animals who have a decreased resistance to disease. Therefore it is imperative that the microbial population be decreased to the point at which nosocomial infection will rarely, if ever, occur. To control disease, efforts may be made in one or more of the following areas:

1. Eliminating or controlling the source of the disease
2. Increasing the ability of the host to resist disease
3. Preventing the transmission of the disease

Efforts to eliminate the source include isolation and the quarantine of animals with active disease. In some instances, domestic animals may be destroyed to control the spread of disease.

Efforts to raise host resistance include nonspecific measures such as applying basic hygiene practices to animal care and ensuring that animals receive an adequate diet. Specific measures include vaccination and the administration of chemotherapeutic agents.

The methods of control used to prevent the transmission of microbes vary in type and application. Simply providing adequate ventilation is a means of control in which microbes are dispersed in large volumes of air and are therefore less likely to contact a new host before dying in the atmosphere. The incidence of airborne disease increases when animals are held in an enclosed space with little or no ventilation. Some methods of control are intended to decrease the overall microbial population in a large area. This results in fewer microbes being eliminated from small areas that must be made sterile and in fewer microbes being available to contaminate small areas that have been sterilized. An overall decrease in microbial population is just as important for the maintenance of sterility as the practice of aseptic technique when handling sterile items.

Both physical and chemical methods of control are used in the prevention of pathogen transmission. Both types of control are nonspecific in that they are effective not only against microbes but also against any other living cells.

Factors Influencing Methods of Control

A number of factors influence the effectiveness of any given method of control. An awareness of these factors enables the technician to effectively apply the appropriate method of control in a given circumstance.

Nature and number of microorganisms. Spore-forming bacteria are very resistant to destruction; therefore sterilization procedures must be capable of destroying endospores as well as heat-resistant viruses. The vegetative cells of bacteria are less resistant to destruction, but some produce a protective capsule that provides a measure of protection against disinfectants. The existence of large numbers of microbes means that a sufficient amount of the control method may not reach all microbes. In addition, large populations are more likely to contain individual microbes that are resistant to the control method than small populations.

Nature, mode of action, and concentration of agent. Dry heat has an oxidative effect on microbes, whereas moist heat hydrolyzes or coagulates cell proteins, thus interfering with or destroying the ability of enzymes to function. At relatively low temperatures, oxidation occurs more slowly than coagulation, and dry heat is less effective than moist heat.

Chemical agents use various modes of action to destroy or inhibit microbes, including the coagulation of protein, the oxidation of vital cell components, and the toxicity of the agent to enzyme systems. A given disinfectant may exert its effect with more than one mode of action, and in some cases the mode of action is unclear. The mode of action of a chemical agent depends on the nature of the chemical. For example, sodium chloride is of no practical value as a disinfectant, but the gas chlorine is extremely effective against microbes. Strong acids and alkalies are often highly bactericidal but may be too corrosive for wide use. Heat that is too intense or a chemical agent too highly concentrated may be harmful to metals and organic and synthetic substances and no more harmful to microbes than a lower concentration of the same method. The toxicity and the corrosiveness of the agent must be considered.

A disinfectant should not be used in a concentration stronger than that recommended. Solutions labeled as disinfectants should not be used as antiseptics. Antiseptics are often diluted disinfectants, but they should not be used interchangeably.

Environment. A number of factors other than those directly concerned with the microbe and the agent affect any application of a control method. Among them are temperature, time, and extraneous organic material.

Temperature. When using heat as a control method, a sufficient temperature must be attained to ensure the desired results. Warm disinfectants are usually more effective than cold ones because the heat speeds up the rate at which the necessary chemical reactions occur.

Time. Control agents, whether physical or chemical, do not work instantaneously. Sufficient time must be allowed. Temperature, pH balance, the ability of the agent to contact the microbe, and the concentration of the agent must be considered to determine the requisite period of exposure. No advantage is gained by unnecessarily prolonging the period, because increased exposure can frequently adversely affect the items being disinfected or sterilized.

Extraneous organic matter. Excretions such as blood, feces, mucus, vomitus, saliva, and urine are referred to as extraneous organic matter. Often chemicals used as disinfectants combine as readily with the organic compounds in the extraneous matter as they do with the organic compounds in the microbial cell. If a large quantity of extraneous organic matter is present, it will combine with so much of the disinfectant that an insufficient amount of the disinfectant will remain to destroy or inhibit all the microbes present.

Moist heat and some chemicals will coagulate the protein in extraneous organic matter, causing it to form a capsule around microbes in the extraneous matter that protects them from the effect of the agent. Items to be disinfected or sterilized should first be sanitized to remove as much of this matter as possible.

Physical Methods of Control

Dry heat

Drying. Microorganisms need water to complete their cycle of growth and reproduction, as do all living cells. The removal of water from the immediate environment will inhibit the growth of bacteria, protozoa, and fungi. Because many of these microbes are capable of producing a spore or cyst stage that allows the cell to survive long periods without water, the effect of drying is microbistatic, not microbicidal. The inhibitory effect of drying should be put to use in maintenance of the surgical suite.

Soiled garments (gowns, smocks, lab coats) should be washed and dried as soon as possible after being removed. Towels and blankets should be replaced if they become moist during use. Mops and cleaning cloths should be washed and dried on a regular basis and never left standing in containers of dirty water. Disposable cotton and gauze items that have been contaminated should be disinfected or burned. If the volume of such items is such that it is only practical to carry out cleaning or disposal procedures once daily, items should be held in covered containers lined with plastic bags. This also applies to items that (although soiled with feces, blood, or pus) dry before they can be decontaminated.

Soiled garments should be changed as soon as possible. As the moisture evaporates, minute flecks of matter, such as feces, pus, or blood, will drop off the fabric and be dispersed by air currents, even such minor currents as those created by the movements of the staff and the patients. Although drying inhibits the growth and reproduction of pathogens, it may also increase the dispersal of particles containing viable microbes. As moisture is removed from respiratory droplets, flecks of blood, or drops of urine, the particles become lighter and are more easily transported. Dry dusting and mopping may add particles to the air rather than remove them. Vigorously shaking towels and pads adds more contaminants to the circulating air. Vacuuming and damp mopping are preferred to dry mopping and dusting, and movements should be carried out with no more vigor or briskness than is necessary.

Incineration. The complete destruction of material during incineration limits this method of sterilization to contaminated items that are of no value or that cannot be reused. The temperature within the incinerator must be high enough to ensure that the material is completely reduced to ash. Overloading the chamber and using inadequate temperatures for insufficient periods will result in partially burned lumps of material contained within the ashes. Microorganisms within these lumps may actually be protected from destruction by a layer of partially burned material that seals in moisture, provides darkness, and protects extraneous organic matter, which can be used as a source of nutrients; all these factors contribute to the growth of bacteria. If incineration is to be used, whether on or off the premises, personnel must be adequately instructed concerning the precautions to be taken when loading the incinerator, the size of the load, and the necessity of inspecting the ashes before final disposal.

Hot air ovens. Hot air ovens offer advantages and disadvantages (Fig. 1-12). The ovens are economic in terms of both purchase and running costs. Moderate heat does not dull the cutting edges of instruments, and there is no moisture present to corrode metal. Dry heat sterilizes some powdery substances that must remain dry throughout the sterilization process to avoid undesirable changes in consistency. Also, substances such as mineral oil, petrolatum, and waxes do not permit the penetration of moisture. Because the steam of the autoclave cannot penetrate these substances, they are best sterilized in small-quantity units by dry heat.

The disadvantages of dry heat sterilization include the extended time required and the fact that many items do not withstand repeated dry heat exposure. Paper and cloth are often scorched at the required temperatures, and most plastic and rubber

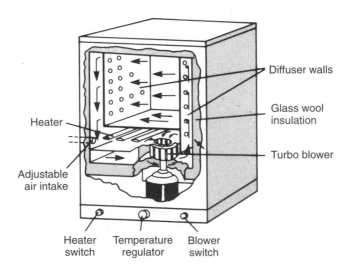

FIG. 1-12   Cutaway view of typical hot air oven. (From Hunter P: *General microbiology: the student's textbook,* St Louis, 1977, Mosby.)

goods are adversely affected (Fig. 1-13). Therefore dry heat is not recommended for items such as gloves, drapes, and towels (Table 1-8).

Guidelines for the use of hot air ovens for sterilization include the following:

- The temperature should be raised slowly to the required level and, after being maintained for the necessary time, should be allowed to drop slowly over a period of hours. This will minimize change in plastic containers and prevent the breakage of glassware.
- Metal items such as instruments should be clean and free of oily or greasy films. Sharp edges or tips such as needle points should be protected by gauze or cotton.
- Items must be placed in the oven in such a way that air can flow freely. The oven should not be overloaded, and items should not be packed in large, bulky units. The heat must penetrate to the innermost layers to ensure sterility.
- Glassware and metal items that do not have sharp edges should be held at a temperature of 170° C for 1 hour. Throughout the chapter, students are reminded of the following conversion factors:

$$°C = (°F - 32) \times 5/9$$
$$°F = °C \times 9/5) + 32$$

- Powders, oils, waxes, and petrolatum should be prepared in 1-ounce (29.57 ml) units and held at a temperature of 160° C for 2 hours.
- Sharp instruments should be held at a temperature of 150° C for 3 hours.

Today the smallest animal facilities, even those in relatively remote areas, have an autoclave, and hot air sterilization is not used as frequently as it once was. It can effectively be used as an emergency or substitute method of sterilization if an autoclave is not available.

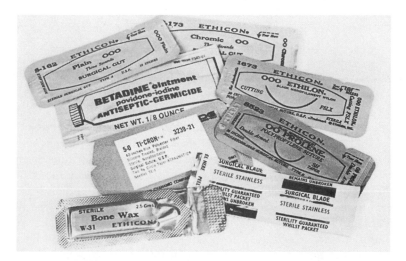

FIG. 1-13   Presterilized items packaged in aluminum. For average in-clinic use, aluminum is suitable wrapping for items sterilized by dry heat.

TABLE 1-8

Sterilization of Apparatus and Supplies

Article	Method	Time (min)
Aqueous solutions in glass	Autoclave	
2000 ml Erlenmeyer flask (Pyrex), thin glass		20
2000 ml Florence flask (Pyrex), thin glass		20
1800 ml Fenwal flask (Pyrex), thick glass		30
1000 ml Erlenmeyer flask (Pyrex), thin glass		15
1000 ml Florence flask (Pyrex), thin glass		15
1000 ml Fenwal flask (Pyrex), thick glass		20
500 ml flask, thin glass		12
250 ml flask, thin glass		10
125 ml flask, thin glass		8
2- to 4-oz bottles, thick glass		10
Test tubes, 150 × 18 mm		8
Rubber goods	Autoclave	
Catheters		20
Gloves		15
Sheeting		20
Tubing		20
	Autoclave	30
Scalpel blade holders and scissors	Autoclave	10
Tongue depressors	Autoclave	30
	Hot air	120
Trays	Autoclave	20
Utensils	Autoclave	15
Syringes (unassembled)	Hot air	90
	Autoclave	20
	Hot air	90
Glassware (test tubes, tubing, Petri dishes)	Hot air	120
Glycerin	Hot air	90
Needles (suture and hypodermic)	Hot air	60
Oils	Hot air	60
Petroleum jelly	Hot air	120

From Hunter, P: *General microbiology: the student's textbook,* St Louis, 1977, Mosby, p 188.

Additional methods of dry heat sterilization. Additional methods of using dry heat as a sterilizing agent have been developed to use the advantages and eliminate the disadvantages of ovens and autoclaves. These include heat transfer and heating items in oils, silicone fluids, low fusion solder, or containers of granular material such as sand, glass, or stainless steel beads. Each method appears to offer an advantage of either lower temperature or shorter exposure time. However, each method carries the disadvantage of being applicable to only a limited range of items or requiring that items be handled after sterilization, for example, to remove oil. Most of these methods do not seem to have overcome the problem of ensuring even heat distribution within the chamber. The practical application of these methods for the routine operation of a small animal hospital is limited.

Moist heat

Hot water. Water that has been heated to a temperature of 60° C or above is an effective sanitizing agent. The mechanical effect of agitation or scrubbing increases the sanitizing effect, as does the addition of detergents to the water. A combination of these factors applied over a sufficient period approaches disinfection.

Laundry machines and dishwashers are examples of the effective use of a combination of these factors that should be used wherever possible to decrease the potential for the transmission of infection. Items such as fiber mop heads, clothing worn while cleaning surgical areas, lab coats worn during preoperative and postoperative care, and blankets or towels used to pad surgical tables or cages can be effectively sanitized, almost disinfected, by the use of a washing machine. Trays or basins used to sort contaminated items, sponges (including mop heads), and brushes used to scrub instruments can be sanitized and partially disinfected by the use of an automatic dishwasher.

Clothes washers and dishwashers sanitize more effectively than manual washing. If automatic equipment is not available, these items should be manually washed frequently with hot water, detergent, and sufficient scrubbing to dislodge soil; thoroughly rinsed; and left to air dry, preferably exposed to sunlight.

Items such as these, which need not be sterile, should not be allowed to become reservoirs of microorganisms that may act as sources of contamination for items that must be sterile.

Boiling. The maximum temperature achieved by boiling water and the steam it produces is 100° C. Because some bacterial spores and viruses resist destruction at this temperature for extended periods, boiling cannot be considered truly effective as a sterilizing agent. However, boiling is an effective means of disinfection. Clean metal or glass items can be disinfected if completely submerged in boiling water for 20 to 30 minutes. They may in fact be sterilized, although it is not practical to determine whether this has occurred.

If the items to be boiled are soiled with matter such as blood, pus, or mucus, detergents should be added to the water. The use of boiling water alone will cause the protein in such fluids to coagulate, and bacteria in even minute clumps will be provided a protective coat against the effects of heat and moisture.

For practical application under modern conditions, boiling is of limited use. Under emergency conditions or where modern sterilization methods are not available, boiling can be used as a substitute method in the attempt to achieve asepsis.

Free-flowing steam. The use of free-flowing steam (live steam) as a method of sterilization has the disadvantage of boiling because the maximum temperature attained is 100° C, which is insufficient to kill all forms of microbial life. It has been used in the sterilization of fluids that would be harmed or rendered ineffective by prolonged exposure to higher temperatures or to chemicals. Fractional sterilization is a time-consuming procedure that involves exposing the fluid to steam for 30 minutes and incubating it for 24 hours. The process must be repeated. Spores not destroyed during the steam exposure will germinate during the incubation period and be destroyed during the next exposure to steam. This method is not effective in destroying all viruses. The use of membrane filters has largely replaced fractional sterilization as a method of preparing heat-sensitive sterile solutions.

Steam is sometimes used on a large scale to clean such items as stainless steel cages in a manner similar to the method used for steam cleaning engines. This application is limited to materials that will not be harmed by the heat and/or moisture.

Steam under pressure. Some viruses and the spores of a few saprophytic and parasitic bacteria can withstand temperatures of 100° C for a prolonged period, even hours. Because the highest temperature attainable by boiling water and free-flowing steam under atmospheric pressure is 100° C, these methods are not dependable for killing heat-resistant microbial forms. However, if the pressure is increased, the temperature can be raised and all microorganisms can be killed. Autoclaves incorporate this principle.

Atmospheric, or barometric, pressure is the pressure exerted by the atmosphere at a given point. Measured in terms of pounds per square inch (psi), the atmospheric pressure at sea level is 14.7 psi. Under this pressure, water boils and produces steam at a temperature of 100° C. At high altitudes, where atmospheric pressure is decreased, water produces steam at a lower temperature. If the pressure is increased, it is possible to increase the temperature of the steam. The increased temperature destroys spores and heat-resistant viruses and accomplishes sterility. This is achieved by allowing steam to flow into a steel chamber that is capable of withstanding increased pressure. As the steam enters the chamber, air is displaced or exhausted. When all air has left the chamber, exhaust vents are closed and steam continues to enter the chamber until the desired pressure is reached.

As the pressure increases, the temperature increases. The increased temperature will kill all forms of microbial life in a relatively short time. It is the increased temperature, not the increased pressure, that is the killing agent. The higher the temperature, the shorter the time necessary to achieve sterility.

At the normal atmospheric pressure of 14.7 psi at sea level and a temperature of 100° C, the time necessary to achieve sterility is so long that it becomes impractical. If the pressure is increased 15 psi above atmospheric pressure, the temperature is increased to 121.5° C. At this temperature, exposed heat-resistant spores are killed in 10 to 12 minutes. An increase in pressure allows an increase in temperature; an increase in temperature allows a decrease in time, thus making sterilization by moist heat practical.

To make efficient use of this principle, it is necessary that all air be exhausted from the chamber of the sterilizing unit. If the chamber contains a mixture of steam and air, the temperature will be lower than pure steam at the same pressure, because air is cooler, drier, and heavier than steam. The time necessary to achieve sterility would have to be lengthened, or the pressure would have to be increased to raise the temperature of the mixture. Because neither of these alterations is desirable, it is imperative that the equipment using steam under pressure as a sterilizing agent be maintained in excellent working condition.

The autoclave. The pressure cooker used in the preparation and preservation of food in the home illustrates the practical application of the sterilizing effect of steam under pressure. In hospitals and clinics the autoclave applies the same principle to sterilize items used during surgical and medical procedures that require aseptic technique. Autoclaves vary in size from countertop units (Fig. 1-14) to large, built-in units (Fig. 1-15) and can be purchased to satisfy the needs of the personnel in a given facility.

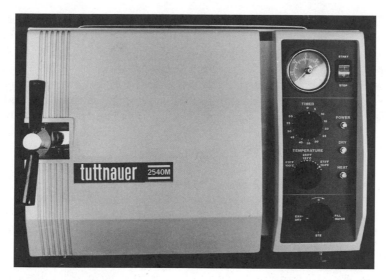

FIG. 1-14 Steam autoclave, countertop model. Chamber will hold one surgical gown pack or one surgical instrument pack each cycle.

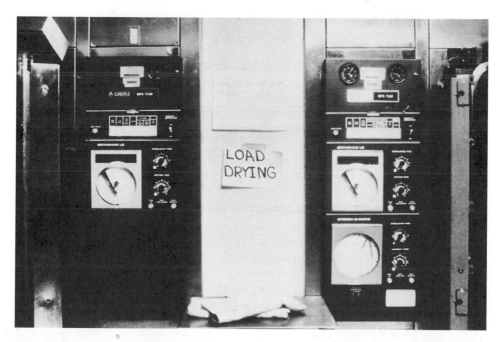

FIG. 1-15 Autoclave, built-in model. Large autoclaves that can hold wheeled racks with shelves capable of holding many packs are available for facilities that must process many packs daily. (Courtesy Ohio State University.)

The central sterilizing chamber of the autoclave is surrounded by a steam jacket. The items to be sterilized are placed in the sterilizing chamber and the safety-locked door is closed against a heat-resistant gasket. Autoclaves that are not connected to a central boiler supply of steam (as they may be in a large hospital or institution) use an electrically operated boiler that is incorporated in the autoclave as a source of steam.

During the cycle, the pressure in the steam jacket is raised 15 psi before any steam is admitted to the sterilizing chamber. This pressure in the jacket is maintained throughout the cycle so that the walls of the chamber remain heated and dry. When a pressure of at least 15 psi above atmospheric pressure has been attained in the jacket, steam is allowed to enter the central sterilizing chamber. At the time steam begins to enter the chamber, the chamber and items in the load are filled with air. A downward displacement gravity system causes air to be driven down and out of the chamber through vents, which allow the air to escape to the outside as the temperature increases.

Because steam is lighter than air, the air is displaced downward. If the air is not completely removed from the chamber, items in contact with air and not steam will not be exposed to the moisture necessary for achieving sterility at that temperature in the given period. Because the air is displaced downward, the sensing element of the thermometer that indicates the temperature reached during the cycle should be in the lower portion of the chamber. If any items do not receive the full benefit of exposure to steam, it will be items in the lower portion of the chamber, which are exposed to the cooler air.

As the last of the air leaves the chamber, steam will contact a temperature-controlled valve, which will close. Moisture-saturated steam entering the chamber condenses on the colder surfaces of items in the chamber. Moisture, which condenses on the portions of the chamber (the front and back walls) not encased by the steam jacket, drains to the bottom of the chamber and out to a waste line. Steam that condenses into water yields heat, which penetrates from the outer layers of the pack to the innermost layers, and the moisture caused by condensation increases the penetrability of the heat released by the steam. To ensure sterility, heat and moisture must be able to penetrate to the innermost layer of the pack in the allotted time. Guidelines for preparing the packs and loading the chamber must be followed rigidly.

The condensation of steam that permits the penetration of heat and moisture unfortunately also promotes the corrosion of metal and dulls the cutting edges of instruments. The use of a corrosion inhibitor such as sodium benzoate is recommended in preparing metal items for autoclaving. The cutting edges of instruments must be checked frequently. If the edges are no longer sharp, the instrument must be correctly sharpened or discarded.

If the autoclave is operating correctly and all air is displaced by steam, and if packs are correctly prepared and positioned in the chamber, a temperature of 121.5° C at a pressure of 15 psi (above atmospheric pressure) will kill all microbial life present on items in the autoclave in 10 to 12 minutes. The usual recommended time of 15 minutes at 121.5° C incorporates a safety factor to ensure sterility.

If the pressure is increased, the temperature will be increased and the time can be decreased.

The steam is allowed to remain in the chamber for the required period and is then slowly exhausted from the chamber. As the temperature drops, the pressure returns to normal. The door to the central sterilizing chamber should never be opened until the pressure gauge (if visible) records zero and the temperature gauge records less than 100° C (Fig. 1-16).

Modern automatic autoclaves incorporate a drying period at the end of the sterilization cycle by allowing heat-sterilized, filtered air to replace the exhausted steam. Because the effectiveness of textile and paper wraps is decreased if the material is moist, it is important not to remove packs from the chamber until they have dried.

If items to be sterilized will be used as soon as the cycle is completed, they may be processed unwrapped. They must be free from extraneous organic material and free from oily or greasy films; therefore they should be sanitized either by using an ultrasonic bath or by manually scrubbing with hot water and a detergent. The tray of the autoclave should be lined with a piece of autoclave paper or fabric to minimize

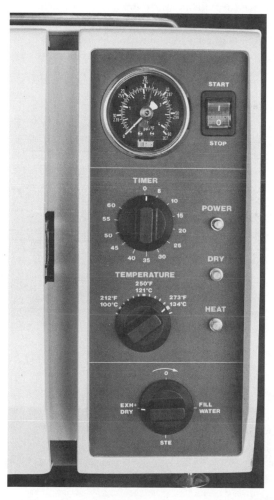

FIG. 1-16   Steam autoclave. The gauge on top indicates the temperature and the pressure inside the canula. The timer is manually set for cycle duration. The temperature gauge is adjusted to desired setting.

damage to delicate items, and items should be placed in the tray so that all possible surfaces are exposed. Open containers, such as basins for sterile solutions and cylinders for transfer forceps, should be positioned so that moisture from condensed steam cannot collect inside.

Items that will be stored for any period before use must be wrapped to prevent air contamination during storage. The proper wrapping procedures for various items are given in detail in Chapter 2.

The load should be packed loosely within the perforated metal trays or wire baskets that are placed in the chamber (Fig. 1-17). If the chamber is designed to hold more than one tray, packs in the lower tray should not touch the upper tray. Long, narrow packs of soft materials (drapes, gowns, gloves) should be placed on edge, not stacked on top of each other. The load should be distributed evenly on the tray. Even a small load of a few wrapped items, if piled tightly in the center of the tray, may not be sufficiently penetrated by the steam to ensure sterilization.

Step-by-step instructions for use of the autoclave are given in Chapter 2.

INDICATOR SYSTEMS. Modern autoclaves that have preset cycles include gauges to indicate the temperature and pressure within the chamber at any point of the cycle and timers. The temperature gauge is likely to be more accurate than the pres-

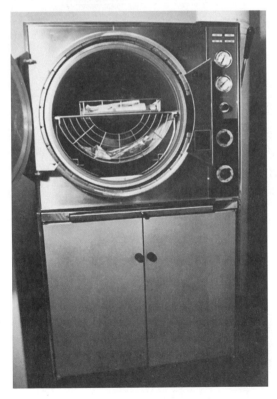

FIG. 1-17   Steam autoclave, free-standing. Chamber is large enough to process several packs in one cycle.

sure gauge because many pressure gauges indicate a pressure higher than the pressure that has actually occurred. Because sterilization is affected by the increase in temperature (increase in pressure serving only to achieve the increase in temperature), operation of the autoclave should be based on maintaining the required temperature for the required time, not on maintaining the required pressure for the required time.

Successful sterilization depends on three factors:

1. Proper operation of the autoclave
2. Proper preparation of the packs
3. Proper loading of the chamber

Assuming that the gauges are functioning correctly, they will reflect the degree to which the autoclave is functioning correctly. They will not indicate whether sterilization has occurred if packs are improperly prepared or positioned.

A number of indicator systems are used to monitor the effectiveness of individual autoclave cycles. These systems are based on the placement of a substance in the chamber with the load that will undergo chemical or biologic changes in response to some combination of time and temperature factors (Fig. 1-18).

Strips of paper that have been impregnated with chemicals will change color after a given temperature is maintained for a given period (such as 121.5° C for 15 minutes). A commercial system such as Steam-Clox incorporates a holder for the chemically impregnated paper that allows it to be inserted in the center of the pack

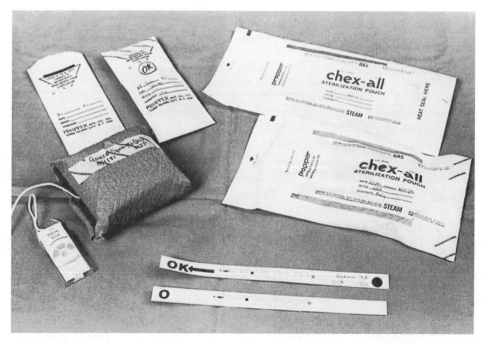

FIG. 1-18   Sterilization indicators. Compare pairs of envelopes, bags, and strips to note color changes that occur during steam sterilization.

before autoclaving and removed after autoclaving without contaminating contents of the pack. Correct interpretation of color changes allows the technician to determine the following:

- If steam has penetrated to the center of the pack, indicating the correct functioning of the autoclave and the correct wrapping procedures.
- If conditions have been attained that can be assumed to have sterilized nonporous materials, such as metal instruments, glassware, and rubber gloves.
- If conditions have been attained that can be assumed to have sterilized the innermost layers of soft packs, such as those containing drapes, gowns, or sponges.
- If conditions have been prolonged beyond the point necessary to ensure sterility. Because a prolonged exposure time confers no benefits and increases the rate at which materials deteriorate, it should be avoided.

In addition to systems based on color changes in a chemically impregnated paper, systems are available that use the heat-resistant bacterial endospores that autoclaving is designed to destroy. Strips of paper impregnated with the dried spores of *Bacillus stearothermophilus* are included in the load. After the cycle is completed, the strip is used to inoculate medium that encourages the growth of this bacteria, and the medium is incubated. If sterilization has been accomplished, the bacterial spores will have been killed and no growth will occur on the medium. If growth does occur, sterilization was not achieved and the operator must determine the reason by reviewing the wrapping and loading procedures and checking the operation of the autoclave. Spore systems are more accurate than chemical systems, but the delay in determining results because of the incubation time necessary for possible growth to occur is a disadvantage. A combination of both systems should be used; chemical indicators should be routinely included in at least a few packs in each load, and spore strips should be used at regularly timed intervals, depending on the volume of use.

Steam sterilization indicator autoclave tape (Fig. 1-19), which resembles masking tape, has been impregnated with a chemical that will change from colorless to gray-black when a temperature of 121.5° C has been reached. It should not be used to indicate sterility because it does not indicate that the temperature has been maintained for a sufficient period. It should be used only to indicate whether a pack has been processed through the autoclave cycle.

Vacuum displacement sterilizer. An improvement on steam pressure sterilizers that operate on a downward displacement gravity system, the vacuum displacement sterilizer incorporates a system that uses a vacuum, which rapidly evacuates air from the chamber at the beginning of the cycle. Steam (at 30 psi and at a temperature of 134° C) enters the chamber and penetrates to the innermost layer of packs so rapidly that sterilization occurs in 3 to 5 minutes. At the end of this short period, the creation of another vacuum quickly withdraws moisture deposited during sterilization and dries the load.

High-altitude sterilization

AUTOCLAVE. To maintain a temperature of 121.5° C, the pressure is increased 1 psi for each 2000 feet of altitude above sea level. At an altitude of 4000 feet, a pressure of 17 psi is necessary to maintain a temperature of 121.5° C.

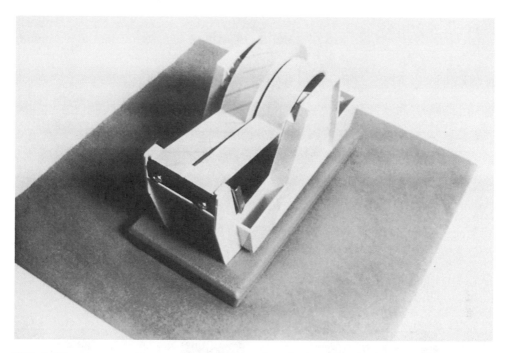

FIG. 1-19   Steam sterilization indicator tape. The roll of tape on left is impregnated with dye that will turn black when exposed to high temperature during sterilization. (Courtesy Ohio State University.)

BOILING. If boiling is used as a substitute or emergency method of sterilization, the boiling time should be increased 5 minutes for each 1000 feet of altitude. If the recommended boiling time is 30 minutes at sea level, at an altitude of 4000 feet the time should be extended to 50 minutes.

Ultrasonic vibration. Sound waves above the frequencies heard by the human ear are referred to as ultrasonic. The mechanical vibrations of sound waves in the ultrasonic range, if passed through a solution, produce innumerable minute bubbles that form and collapse thousands of times each second, producing a scrubbing effect on the surface of items immersed in the liquid. Particles that have been agitated from instruments are then suspended in the solution and are subjected to a negative pressure or suction effect. The result is that proteins are coagulated, cell walls are disrupted, and microorganisms are destroyed. The principle has been applied in laboratories as one of the first steps in isolating various cell components, such as specific antigens and enzymes.

It was once believed that this application of ultrasound would be useful as a means of sterilization. This has not proven to be true. However, ultrasonic baths can be effectively used to sanitize instruments in preparation for sterilization (Fig. 1-20). Machines are available that clean hundreds of instruments in about 10 minutes. The ex-

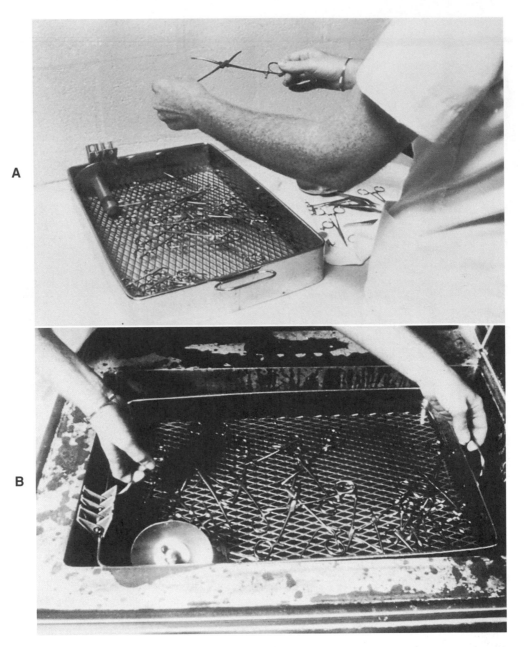

FIG. 1-20   Ultrasonic cleaner. **A,** Loading of instruments into tray. **B,** Placement of tray in tank. (Courtesy Ohio State University.)

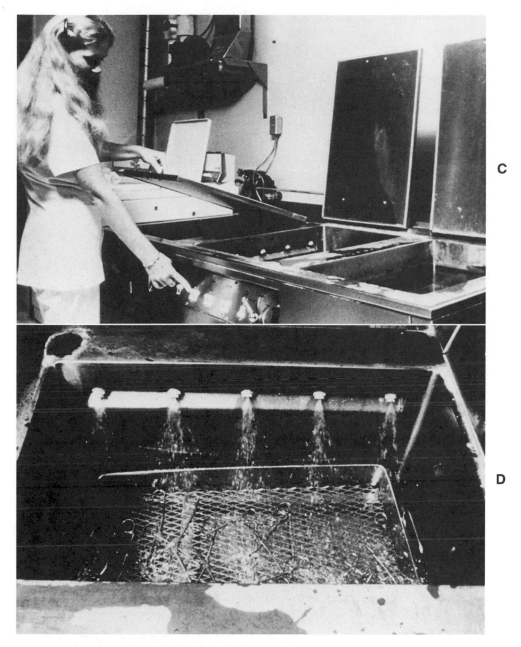

FIG. 1-20, cont'd   C, Operation of controls. **D,** Filling of tank.

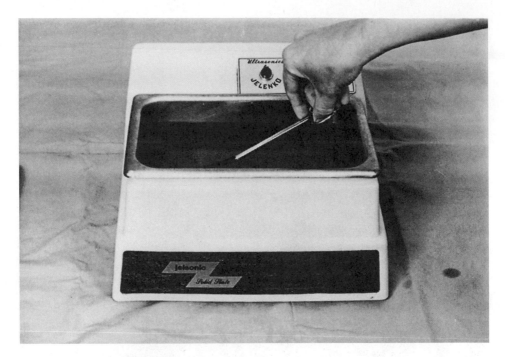

FIG. 1-21   Ultrasonic cleaner, countertop model.

pense of such units makes them uneconomical except for large institutions. Countertop units are available with tanks as small as 15 × 13 × 10 cm (Fig. 1-21). This of course limits the size of the items that can be sanitized.

If the volume of surgery requires instruments from several packs to be scrubbed on a daily basis, even a small unit may save enough time to justify the initial cost. Because the cycle is short, many cycles can be completed in a relatively short time and the period of the cycle itself can be used for other tasks.

Instruments with surfaces that are difficult to reach if manually scrubbed (hinges, box locks, clasps) are thoroughly cleaned by this method, and delicate instruments are subjected to less wear than is often the case in manual scrubbing.

Special solutions must be used in the tank, changed frequently, and rinsed off items that have been cleaned before they are sterilized. It is also important to follow the manufacturer's instructions concerning those items that can be safely processed in this manner.

Radiation

Ultraviolet light. Sunlight has long been recognized as having antimicrobial qualities. Part of the antimicrobial effect is caused by the drying action, but part is caused by the effect of the ultraviolet portion of the light spectrum. Light waves are measured by the length of the waves, the unit of measurement being the *angstrom* (Å). One angstrom is equal to 0.1 nanometer (nm). Within the visible light spectrum, the shortest waves are found at the violet end of the scale (4000 Å). Light waves that measure between 2000 and 4000 Å are said to be in the ultraviolet spectrum and are invisible to the human eye. Ultraviolet light waves in the range of 2500 to 2800 Å destroy many microorganisms, particularly bacteria. Ultraviolet light with a wavelength of 2800 Å is partially absorbed by components of microbial protein, and ultraviolet light with wavelengths between 2500 and 2600 Å is absorbed by nucleic acid. This absorption results in chemical modifications and mutations that may lead to cell death.

In addition to interfering directly with cell metabolism, ultraviolet light produces effects in air, water, and some organic compounds that are detrimental to microorganisms. In air, ultraviolet light causes the production of ozone; in water, the production of hydrogen peroxide; in some organic compounds, the production of organic peroxides. All of these products exert an antimicrobial effect.

One of the major disadvantages of ultraviolet light as a method of controlling microbes is its poor power of penetration; it is absorbed at the surface of most substances. Liquids and gases must be passed over the surface of the lamp that is used as a source of ultraviolet light in thin layers, and ultraviolet light cannot be effectively used to sterilize items of any complexity if all surfaces cannot be readily exposed to the rays. Ultraviolet light can be used to sterilize substances such as plasma that would be harmed by heat or chemicals.

Mercury vapor produces ultraviolet light with a wavelength of 2537 Å, and mercury vapor lamps are used widely in areas such as operating and treatment rooms, nurseries, and animal holding areas. The acts of coughing and sneezing, even breathing, discharge large numbers of respiratory droplets that may contain pathogenic microbes. These droplets dry when exposed to air and are easily dispersed on air currents in enclosed spaces. Mercury vapor lamps installed over entrances to halls connecting various areas of a clinic or hospital can decrease the number of microbes spread through the air. The ultraviolet light is not as effective against organisms on dust particles or on surfaces such as countertops.

Prolonged exposure to ultraviolet light can cause irritation or permanent damage to the cornea and is implicated as a factor in the formation of skin cancers. Eyes that are light in color are more susceptible to this type of damage, as are fair-skinned persons. Care must be taken in positioning lamps intended to disinfect air. If used in ward areas, lamps must be placed so that it is impossible for caged animals to look directly at the source of ultraviolet radiation.

Because the lamps continue to glow after their production of ultraviolet rays has been reduced below the effective level, the radiation should be measured after every 1000 hours of use.

Ionizing radiations. Other forms of radiation of shorter wavelength and greater energy than ultraviolet light can also cause the ionization of molecules in the path of the radiation. X-rays; neutrons; alpha, beta, and gamma rays; and cathode rays (of electrons) have all been investigated for potential use in routine sterilizing procedures. To date, all have been proven to have disadvantages in terms of safety, cost, and efficiency. Currently, these methods are reserved for experimental work performed under controlled laboratory conditions and in a small number of large facilities where the proper safety precautions can be taken.

Beta and cathode rays are used in industry for the sterilization of heat-sensitive, prepackaged surgical materials, such as rubber and plastic tubing, suture material, and gloves. Disposable needles and syringes are also sterilized with ionizing radiations. Gamma rays have been used in the production of safe, effective vaccines; cathode rays effectively sterilize selected antibiotics.

Filtration. Gases or liquids may be purified by passing them through a substance that retains undesirable components but allows the gas or liquid to pass unaltered. The applications of filtration in controlling microorganisms are widespread. For example, filtration is an important step in the purification of public water supplies.

Forced air ventilation systems employ filters to remove particles from the air before it is recirculated. Ventilation systems in areas where the possibility of infection is a concern can be equipped to filter particles of even submicroscopic size, thus reducing the possibility of the airborne transmission of disease. The air can be decontaminated by using high efficiency particulate air (HEPA) filters constructed of cellulose acetate pleated around aluminum foil. The incorporation of such filters in air-conditioning systems can provide almost 100% efficiency in removing particles as small as 0.3 μm in diameter. Regardless of the type of filter used to treat air, the continued efficiency of the system depends on reliable maintenance. Air filters clogged with dust and moisture will reverse the desired effects and emit a steady stream of dust particles and material from respiratory droplets into air being circulated through the hospital or clinic. The filters may even accumulate so much material that microorganisms will be able to use components of the accumulated scum as a source of food and will reproduce.

Fibrous materials such as gauze, muslin, and paper are used to filter air. Items such as instruments, needles, and syringes that have been sterilized must be maintained in a sterile condition until they are used. For this reason, these items are wrapped in fabric or paper that will filter bacteria when packs are exposed to air, hands, or counter surfaces after sterilization. The ability of these materials to act as filters is reduced if they are damaged by too high a degree of heat during the sterilization process. It is also important to ensure that the paper or fabric wrap remains dry. If the pores in the material become filled with moisture, they serve as an easy pathway for bacteria to permeate the outer wrap and reach the sterile contents.

Surgical masks are another example of the filtration of air designed to produce a two-fold effect. Microorganisms from the nose and throat of the wearer are prevented from contaminating sterile items or infecting the patient, and the wearer is protected from inhaling infectious microbes shed by the patient. This twofold purpose is achieved only if the mask is dry. Once the mask has become saturated with exhaled moisture, bacteria can travel easily along the pathways provided by moisture-filled pores in the material, negating the mask's effectiveness. During prolonged surgical procedures, moisture-laden masks should be exchanged for dry masks.

In addition to the employment of filtration to treat liquids on a large scale, such as the purification of public water supplies, filtration is used to purify liquids on a smaller scale. Pharmaceutical products such as intravenous medications, which would be rendered useless or even harmful if subjected to heat and/or chemicals, are purified by passage through a filter (Fig. 1-22).

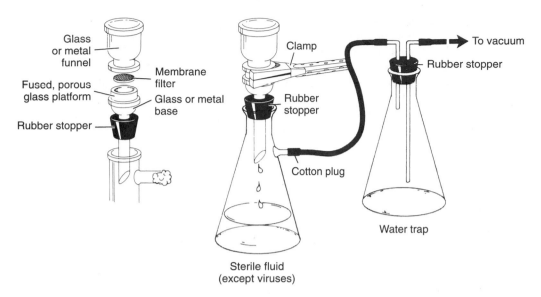

FIG. 1-22   Membrane filter, showing components *(left)* and typical setup for use *(right).* (From Hunter P: *General microbiology: the student's textbook,* St Louis, 1977, Mosby.)

Materials that have been used for filters include porcelain, diatomaceous earth, combinations of paper and asbestos, and sintered glass. In addition, membrane filters composed of cellulose esters can be manufactured with a pore size as small as 0.05 μm. These membrane filter systems (commercially known as Millipore systems) have advantages over the other materials. They are resistant to water, alcohol, ether, and hydrocarbons; can be autoclaved and stored indefinitely; and have a much faster flow rate. Cellulose membrane filters work by sieve action alone, whereas filters of other materials may exhibit absorptive qualities that will alter the concentration of certain components, such as organic compounds, or remove them from the fluid. Membrane filters are not absorptive and are therefore least likely to alter the composition of the fluid being filtered.

Technically, pharmaceuticals that have been purified by filtration are not sterile, because some of the molecules of organic compounds in these fluids may be as large as large viruses; a filter with pores small enough to filter these viruses would also filter out the necessary molecules. However, they have been made as microbe free as possible without altering the composition of the fluid, and they should always be handled using aseptic technique. The same organic compounds that make sterilization by heat or chemical methods impractical may provide bacteria with a source of food, and the fluid will then act as a culture medium for contaminating microbes.

Chemical Methods of Control

The ideal chemical agent. The ideal chemical agent for antiseptic and disinfectant use has yet to be discovered or invented. However, it is relatively easy to list the qualities of the ideal agent, and the newer agents on the market increasingly approximate the ideal.

The ideal agent will:

- Kill all pathogenic microorganisms, including resistant forms
- Work effectively in a short period over a wide temperature and pH range
- Exert residual action for extended periods
- Not corrode, dry, or stain inanimate materials, such as metal, glass, rubber, plastic, or fabrics
- Be stable in a dry form and dissolve readily in water to form a stable solution
- Be odorless and colorless
- Be nontoxic to and nonaccumulative in living cells other than pathogens
- Be easily and inexpensively manufactured and therefore widely available
- Not be affected by the presence of extraneous organic material
- Not be inactivated when used in conjunction with other agents that may be used for cleaning purposes

To achieve maximum effectiveness, it is necessary to recognize the advantages and disadvantages of the common types of agents and to know when a given agent should or should not be used. Instructions should be carefully followed, particularly regarding the proper dilution and the limitations of use. As well as being wasteful, the use of chemicals in too high a concentration will often harm the object being disinfected. In some cases, too high a concentration may under certain conditions result in the survival of microbes that would have been killed at a lower concentration. Attempting to save money by using an excessively diluted solution or to save time by shortening exposure periods may result in the emergence of microbial strains that are resistant to destruction.

Terminology. To discuss the categories of chemical agents used against microbes, it is helpful for the student to understand the meanings of some words frequently used when referring to these agents (Table 1-9).

Germicidal and *microbicidal* imply that the agent is effective against a wide variety of microbes. *Bactericidal* means that the agent can be expected to kill vegetative bacterial cells but not bacterial spores. *Sporicidal* commonly refers to bacterial endospores, which are the most resistant to destruction of microbial structures. *Viricidal* and *fungicidal* refer to the capability to destroy these types of microbes; viruses are difficult to destroy, and a given agent may be more or less effective against fungi than against bacteria. *Tuberculocidal* means that the agent is capable of destroying the vegetative bacterium that causes tuberculosis. This bacterium produces a waxlike coating that makes it difficult to destroy. Such terms as *bacteriostatic* and *fungistatic* indicate that the agent will inhibit the growth of the microbes but cannot be expected to destroy them.

Disinfectant refers to agents used on inanimate objects, *antiseptic* to agents used on living tissue. The same agent may be used as a disinfectant at one concentration and as an antiseptic at another concentration. If so, the solutions are not meant to be interchangeable. Antiseptics are often diluted disinfectants. The stronger solution may irritate or burn living tissue, but the weaker solution may not be effective on heavily contaminated objects. When used informally, the terms are often interchanged.

TABLE 1-9

Some Common Antimicrobial Chemical Agents

Agents	Major mode of action	Applications
Soaps	Disruption of cell membranes and increase in permeability	Cleansing, mechanical removal of microorganisms
Detergents	Disruption of cell membranes, by combining with lipids and proteins; leaking of N and P compounds out of cells	Cleansing, bactericidal action
Quarternary ammonium compounds	Cause changes in cell permeability, neutralized phospholipids	
Bisdiguanide compounds (chlorhexidine)	Alter cell-wall permeability, protein precipitation; rapid action broad spectrum	Routine skin preparation
Povidone-iodophor compounds	Damage cell wall, form reactive ions and protein complexes; rapid action	Routine skin preparation
Phenols		
Phenol, cresols, lysol, hexylresorcinol	Bactericidal; denaturation and precipitation of proteins	Disinfection of laboratory equipment, instruments, bench tops, garbage pails, toilets
Bis phenols (hexachlorophene)	Bacteriostatic	Deodorants in soaps, inhibition of gram-positive bacteria; require repeated use
Oxidizing agents		
Cl_2 and sodium hypochlorite (bleach)	Bactericidal, oxidation of $-SH$ and $-NH_2$ groups	Purification of water, kennel sanitation
Iodine	Bactericidal, oxidation of indole nucleus of enzymes or coenzymes	Skin disinfection, especially as tincture
H_2O_2 (hydrogen peroxide)	Bacteriostatic; mildly bactericidal	Antisepsis of cuts, minor wounds
Heavy metals		
$HgCl_2$ (zinc)	Highly bacteriostatic; precipitation of proteins	Antisepsis of cuts, minor wounds
$AgNO_3$, silver nitrate	Stops minor bleeding	

Modified from Hunter P: *General microbiology: the student's textbook*, St Louis, 1977, Mosby, p 191.

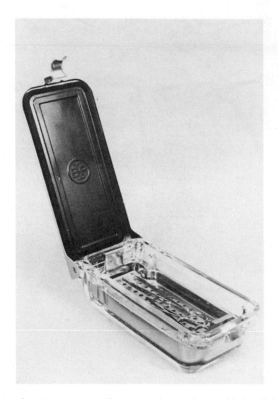

FIG. 1-23   Cold sterilization tray. Gasket on inner surface of lid will form seal when lid is closed, preventing air-carried microbes from contaminating contents and preventing evaporation of chemical disinfectant solution.

Cold sterilization refers to the practice of soaking objects in disinfectant solutions (Fig. 1-23). Few agents are so effective that with daily use their application will result in sterilization. It is better to avoid the use of these agents if possible. Some substances cannot be autoclaved and therefore must be cold sterilized in the average clinic. Such items should be handled as if they were sterile, but their sterility cannot be guaranteed.

Agents in solution form (Table 1-10)

Alcohols. If used properly, some members of this group of organic compounds exhibit strong bactericidal properties because of their ability to coagulate protein. Ethanol (ethyl alcohol or grain alcohol) and isopropanol (isopropyl alcohol or dimethylcarbinol) can be effectively used in a wide variety of applications. Methanol, because of its low molecular weight, is not a particularly effective germicide.

Absolute (anhydrous) alcohol has had all water removed, and dehydrated alcohol may contain up to 1% water. Denatured alcohol (referring to ethanol) has been rendered unfit for consumption in beverage or medicinal form by the addition of chemicals such as acetone or sulfuric acid and is intended for industrial not medical use.

TABLE 1-10					

Antimicrobial Activity of Commonly Used Cold "Sterilants"

	Destructive action against				
Agent	Bacteria	Tubercle bacilli	Spores	Fungi	Viruses
Alcohol-ethyl (70% to 90%)	+	+	0	+	±
Alcohol-isopropyl (70% to 90%)	+ +	+	0	+	±
Alcohol-iodine (2%)	+ +	+	±	+	+
Formalin (37%)	+	+	+	+	+
Glutaraldehyde (buffered, 2%) (Cidex)	+ +	+	+ +	+	+
Iodine (2% to 5% aqueous)	+ +	+	±	+	+
Iodophors (1%) (povidone-iodine complex)	+	+	±	±	+
Mercurials (Merthiolate)	±	0	0	+	±
Phenolic derivatives (0.5% to 3%)	+	+	0	+	±
Quats (benzalkonium chloride, 1:750 to 1:1000)	+ +	0	0	+	0

From Smith AL: *Principles of microbiology*, ed 9, St Louis, 1981, Mosby, p 239. After DiPalma JR, editor: *Drill's pharmacology in medicine*, New York, 1971, McGraw-Hill.
+ +, Very good; +, good; ±, fair (greater concentration or more time needed); 0, no activity.

Dilute alcohol is alcohol that has been mixed with a specified portion of water. Ethanol is generally used in a 70% solution, although it retains bactericidal properties in dilutions from 50% to 90%. Isopropanol is considered effective in concentrations up to 99%. Alcohol concentrations below 50% are considered to be bacteriostatic rather than bactericidal. Because alcohols are volatile, they evaporate faster than water from open containers, and solutions of alcohol rapidly lose effectiveness. An alcohol solution in an open container will quickly become bacteriostatic with no change in appearance. If the solution is contaminated, bacteria will not be killed, only inhibited, and will later be spread over the surfaces to which the alcohol is applied.

Isopropanol is considered to be somewhat more effective than ethyl alcohol and is more readily available because it is not subject to the government regulations that affect the sale and distribution of ethyl alcohol. Both alcohols are effective solvents for lipids and are frequently used topically as antiseptics (e.g., for the preparation of surgical sites). When used as a final rinse for the surgical scrub, they will temporarily reduce the number of microbes present on the skin surface.

Alcohol will remove the normal oils that form a protective shield on skin, and prolonged or repeated exposures should be followed by the application of a skin lotion or cream. The same property that allows alcohol to destroy bacteria by the coagulation of cell proteins renders it unsuitable for general use on severely traumatized tissues because further cell damage may result.

If properly used, alcohol solutions are effective against vegetative bacterial cells, including the bacteria that cause tuberculosis, but alcohol cannot be relied on to kill bacterial spores or viruses and therefore should not be used for cold sterilization. The addition of small amounts of iodine to alcohol solutions increases their effectiveness.

Aldehydes. Formaldehyde is available as formalin, a 37% solution of formaldehyde gas in water. For the purposes of calculating dilutions, this solution is treated as a 100% solution. Formalin acts by "fixing" or inactivating necessary cell proteins. Although it is sporicidal if properly used, it is injurious to skin and very irritating to mucous membranes, thus limiting its medical applications. Commercially available products of formalin compounded with alcohol and small amounts of alkalies are used as a cold sterilization agent for small, hard-surfaced items. Because both the alcohol and the formalin evaporate quickly, containers must be kept tightly covered and solutions changed frequently.

Histologic specimens obtained during surgery should be placed in a solution of 10% neutral buffered formalin, which will act as a preservative and prevent decomposition of the tissues during their transit to a laboratory. At least 10 ml of 10% formalin should be used for a specimen measuring $1 \times 1 \times 1$ cm.

The disadvantages of formalin preclude its use as an antiseptic and limit its usefulness as a disinfectant, but its mode of action (the inactivation of proteins) makes it useful in the sterilization of vaccines. Formalin can kill microbes without altering antigenic properties. After controlled exposure to formaldehyde, the pathogenic microbes are no longer capable of causing disease when injected as a vaccine but are still capable of stimulating antibody production.

Glutaraldehyde solutions are newer to the market than those made with formaldehyde. Used according to the manufacturers' instruction, they are bactericidal, tuberculocidal, and viricidal with as little as 10 minutes of exposure time. If exposure time is increased to several hours, the action is sporicidal. In dilute concentrations, glutaraldehyde is less toxic and less irritating to living tissue than formaldehyde, but repeated, prolonged exposure adversely affects items made of rubber and plastic. It is used to cold sterilize items that cannot be autoclaved, such as anesthetic equipment and accessories and lensed instruments.

Oxidizing agents. Oxidizing agents react with protein molecules of microbial cells, causing an oxygen exchange in which enzymes may be inactivated and cell processes disrupted. Agents in this group exhibit wide variations in terms of factors such as effectiveness, toxicity, and method of application.

Halogens. Iodine, chlorine, fluorine, and bromine are included in the halogen group of elements. They are strong oxidizing agents and are bactericidal, making them useful as antiseptic and disinfectant agents if used under controlled conditions. The use of iodine and chlorine is widespread, but the use of fluorine and bromine is more restricted.

INORGANIC IODINE SOLUTIONS. Because pure iodine is difficult to dissolve in water, iodine is dissolved in sodium or potassium iodide solutions for topical use as a 2% aqueous solution. It is also used as a tincture of iodine (iodine dissolved in alcohol). The iodine-iodide complex that is formed in solution releases free iodine, which acts as a disinfectant by inhibiting enzyme activity. It is capable of killing protozoans, fungi, vegetative bacterial cells, and some viruses, but it is not sporicidal at concentrations safe for routine use. Concentrations of iodine higher than 3.5% are not more effective than lesser concentrations and may burn living tissue. The use of strong solutions and old solutions (that may have become concentrated) should be discouraged. When tincture of iodine is used, care must be taken to prevent the evaporation of alcohol and the consequent increase in the concentration of iodine.

Because of the wide range of effectiveness and quick action, inorganic iodine solutions are used in the cleansing and surgical preparation of small areas of skin. These solutions are not as suitable for use on large areas of skin because of their staining properties and because of the care that must be taken to prevent skin irritation. They should not be applied to areas that will be tightly bandaged. Allergic skin reactions, although rare, may occur, and the technician should be aware of that possibility.

ORGANIC IODINE SOLUTIONS (IODOPHORS). Povidone-iodophor compounds are water-soluble complexes that allow slow, continuous release of the active ingredient, iodine. Povidone-iodine is a broad-spectrum bacteriocidal agent also effective against many fungi, viruses, and protozoans. Its action is rapid, but its effectiveness may be reduced by the presence of blood, fat, necrotic debris, and alcohol. Skin irritations are not uncommon.

BISDIGUANIDE COMPOUNDS (CHLORHEXIDINE [NOLVASAN]). Bisdiguanide compounds alter cell wall permeability, causing precipitation of intracellular material. They are broad-spectrum agents effective against many fungi and some strains of *Pseudomonas* spp. They have minimal activity against viruses and spores. Chlorhexidine has excellent residual activity and is effective in the presence of alcohol, organic matter, and soaps. Skin reactions are rare.

The ideal skin preparation agent is a broad-spectrum, bacteriocidal agent that rapidly kills skin pathogens. At this time, these standards are best met with chlorhexidine and povidone-iodophor products. The use of either of these agents is justified, although chlorhexidine's prolonged, residual activity when exposed to alcohol, organic matter, and soaps is an advantage.

CHLORINE. Chlorine compounds prepared in an aqueous solution release free chlorine, which combines with the water present to form hypochlorous acid, a strong oxidizing agent that is bactericidal.

Chlorine is in widespread use to disinfect public water supplies and to treat sewage. It is readily inactivated by extraneous organic material. As with iodine, care must be taken to ensure that the amount of chlorine used will be effective against pathogens that are likely to be present but will not be toxic to people or animals.

Sodium hypochlorite (laundry bleach) forms hypochlorous acid when mixed with water and is an effective disinfectant. Medical applications are not widespread because of its bleaching and corrosive properties. Calcium hypochlorite (chlorinated lime) results from the action of chlorine gas on calcium hydroxide. Highly diluted solutions are used as general disinfectants in animal housing facilities, slaughterhouses, and dairies because it so effectively disinfects feces. Care must be taken when using these products because they are irritating to living tissue and corrosive to inanimate objects.

BROMINE AND FLUORINE. Although bromine and fluorine are strong bactericidal agents, effective concentrations of these halogens are too toxic to living tissue for widespread use in the medical fields.

Other oxidizing agents. Hydrogen peroxide, used in a 3% solution, is weakly bactericidal compared to disinfectants containing one of the halogens, but it has the advantage of being far less toxic to living tissue. It is of little use as a general disinfectant but can be used as an antiseptic agent to clean wounds, particularly puncture wounds to the skin. When warmed, such as by contacting tissue, it degrades into water and oxygen with a strong foaming action that carries tissue debris, pus, and microbes away from the wound. In addition, the increase of oxygen in the wound environment inhibits the growth of anaerobic bacteria that may contaminate deep wounds and be capable of causing gangrene and tetanus.

Sodium perborate, potassium permanganate, and zinc peroxide are other oxidizing agents that have limited medical applications.

Surfactants and detergents. Agents that reduce surface tension are called surfactants. Molecules on the surface of liquids are held together by varying degrees of tension. Liquids with a high surface tension (oil, mercury) do not mix easily with other materials and tend to remain apart, separating from other substances. Liquids with low surface tension (water, alcohol) mix more easily with other materials and are more easily spread over other surfaces. They are "wetter." Surface-active agents (surfactants) lower the tension between molecules on both sides of a liquid interface, helping the liquids to mix easily. For example, a surfactant will increase the ability of oil and water to mix.

Technically, a detergent is any cleaning agent, including water, but the term is informally used to distinguish synthetic cleaning compounds from soaps.

Detergents (including soaps) are effective surface tension reducers, capable of emulsifying lipids. They are divided into three groups, depending on their ionization in water:

1. Anionic. The surfactant property is found in the negatively charged portion of the molecule, the anion. These are of limited disinfectant capability. Soap is an example.
2. Nonionic. These neutral detergents do not ionize in water and may be effective cleaning agents but are not antimicrobial and may even support microbial growth.
3. Cationic. The surfactant and disinfectant properties are contained in the positively charged portion of the molecule, the cation. These are the quaternary ammonium compounds sometimes referred to as "quats."

Soap. Soap, an anionic cleaning agent, is an effective cleaning agent with limited disinfectant capabilities. Its action is primarily mechanical, caused by the scrubbing motions that disperse oily and greasy films into tiny droplets, which can be lifted by the lather and rinsed away. The cleaning action depends on alkali, which suspends soot, dirt, microbes, tissue debris, and oil in water. It is inexpensive if not formulated with perfumes or antimicrobial agents and is available in many forms, but it combines with calcium and magnesium salts in hard water to form an insoluble scum. Because it is only mildly disinfectant, the use of soap in surgical suite applications should be followed by a suitable disinfectant, such as alcohol. Care must be taken that the disinfecting agent (Fig. 1-24) used after anionic soap is not a cationic quaternary ammonium compound because even minute traces of soap will neutralize the antimicrobial properties of the quaternary ammonium compound.

Cationic detergents. Cationic detergents are surface-active chemical agents that are effective against both gram-positive and gram-negative bacteria and are therefore

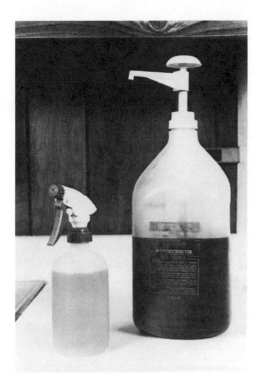

FIG. 1-24   Disinfectants can be purchased in concentrated forms and diluted as indicated for environmental use.

preferred over anionic detergents, which are mildly effective against gram-positive bacteria if disinfectant capability is considered. They are thought to act by dissolving lipids that are found in cell walls and membranes. Although effective bactericides, aqueous solutions of these compounds are not tuberculocidal, sporicidal, fungicidal, or viricidal, except possibly against lipid-rich viruses.

Quaternary ammonium compounds such as benzalkonium chloride (Zephiran) are nontoxic to tissue in recommended concentrations, odorless, colorless, nonstaining, readily soluble in water, and inexpensive. They are commonly used as antiseptics and disinfectants, but they must be used with care if they are to be effective. If the concentrate is purchased and diluted, hard water cannot be used because calcium and magnesium ions will inactivate the quaternary ammonium compound. This is true of iron-rich water, also.

It has been reported that in some instances benzalkonium chloride has increased rather than decreased bacterial growth, thus raising a question regarding the effectiveness of this agent. It should not be relied on for use as a cold sterilizing agent.

The quaternary ammonium compounds are inactivated by animal and plant proteins. If applicators (mops, swabs, gauze sponges) are immersed in the solution, the disinfectant will be absorbed and inactivated. It will be necessary to increase the concentration to 1:750 or 1:500 to compensate. If the solution is contaminated with soap, it may become neutralized and act as a reservoir for the growth and multiplication of bacteria. A quaternary ammonium compound should not be used as a surgical scrub rinse because even the traces of soap that remain after a long rinse in running water will inactivate the chemical compound.

Tinctures of benzalkonium chloride are more effective against fungi and viruses and less subject to contamination but are, of course, far more expensive and do not seem to be significantly more effective than alcohol alone.

Phenolic derivatives. Phenol (carbolic acid) was used by Lister as a surgical disinfectant and antiseptic. It is still used as a standard in determining the antibacterial capabilities of other agents but not as a disinfectant in surgical applications because it is irritating and corrosive to the skin. The phenolic derivatives (usually consisting of altered phenol molecules combined with a detergent) have for the most part replaced phenol itself. The derivatives are divided into two groups. The cresols are used primarily as general disinfectants on environmental surfaces, and the bis-phenols are generally intended for use as antiseptics.

Phenolics are bactericidal and not greatly affected by the presence of extraneous organic material. Thus they can be used to disinfect microbiologic cultures and proteinaceous material, such as feces, vomitus, pus, and phlegm. Phenolics are not sporicidal under ordinary conditions of use. They are often used in combination with detergents, which increases the tuberculocidal, viricidal, and fungicidal potential of the agent. They can be effectively combined with soap, unlike many other disinfectants.

Cresols such as saponated cresol solution, an alkaline solution of cresol in soap, are effective when used as a general disinfectant for walls, floors, furnishings, and equipment because of their residual action. When the film of water dries, the molecule remains active for a period of time, unlike the alcohols, which are extremely volatile.

The bis-phenols are so known because two phenol molecules are linked together when phenol is altered. They are nonirritating and noncorrosive when applied to skin but remain strongly bactericidal and residual in action because they are adsorbed to the skin surface. Unfortunately, they are also absorbed through the skin where they accumulate in tissues and may eventually exert toxic side effects. Studies have shown that hexachlorophene, the most common of the bis-phenols, accumulates in the brain tissue of rats. Soaps and detergents that incorporate hexachlorophene are now available by prescription only, and their use in hospital situations has been restricted. Because significant accumulation and possible toxic consequences occur only after repeated and prolonged exposure, these are not likely to be a problem for patients in veterinary hospitals, most of whom have fewer and shorter hospital stays than their human counterparts. However, if an agent containing hexachlorophene is used as a surgical scrub antiseptic, the possibility of long-term adverse effects should be noted, even if such a possibility is remote.

In addition to its disinfectant properties, hexachlorophene is an effective deodorant. Before the possible side effects are fully appreciated, it was incorporated into everything from toothpaste to dog food. At present, the use of this agent is more stringently regulated by the Food and Drug Administration (FDA).

Heavy metals. Living cells will readily incorporate the ions of heavy metals, causing an interference in enzyme activity that frequently leads to cell death. This toxicity applies to human and animal cells as well as to microbial cells, thus limiting the possible applications of heavy metal ions as disinfectants and antiseptics.

Silver nitrate is sold commercially in a pencil form intended to be used to cauterize small wounds. It is caustic, astringent, and antiseptic in action.

Zinc peroxide, zinc carbonate, and zinc hydroxide are combined in medicinal zinc peroxide, which is mildly antiseptic and astringent in action. It can be used in ointment or suspension form to combat infections caused by anaerobic microorganisms in gunshot or bite wounds.

Chemical sterilization using gases.
Sterilization (or disinfection) with gas has been used for decades, but it is a relatively recent development for these methods to be widely applied to the medical fields. Formaldehyde gas was at one time used to disinfect large, enclosed areas (rooms or cages) that were exposed to high levels of very virulent pathogens, but newer materials used in furnishings and equipment and newer disinfectants have made this practice largely obsolete.

In recent years the use of gaseous sterilization has been adapted to in-house medical applications for items that are damaged by exposure to steam autoclaving or available chemical solutions. Gas sterilization takes longer than steam and is more expensive. It is also more difficult to use because the techniques are not as standardized as those of steam autoclaving. Gas sterilizers range in size from those big enough to contain large items, such as mattresses, to small tabletop units that hold only a few instruments. The industrial use of this method is widespread, and many items that are purchased in a presterilized form and intended for disposal after one use have been gas sterilized.

Ethylene oxide. Ethylene oxide is *poisonous,* irritating to skin and mucous membranes, explosive, and flammable. It is also a very effective microbicide when properly used, capable of excellent penetration, and odorless, and it can be easily kept in a liquid form. It is thought to act by inactivating the DNA molecules in the microbial cells that have been penetrated, thus preventing cell reproduction.

The flammability of ethylene oxide can be reduced by mixing it with inert gases. Ethylene oxide–carbon dioxide mixtures are available in metal cylinders, and ethylene oxide–fluorinated hydrocarbon mixtures are available in disposable cans. The ethylene oxide–hydrocarbon mixtures can be used to sterilize items at room temperature and atmospheric pressure, and the ethylene oxide–carbon dioxide mixtures are used in units that are similar to steam autoclaves.

Several factors influence the ability of ethylene oxide to destroy microorganisms. These include temperature, pressure, concentration, humidity, and time of exposure.

As temperature increases, the ability of ethylene oxide to penetrate microbes and packaging materials increases. Because the method is used mostly for items that would be damaged by exposure to high temperatures, the temperature is usually no higher than 60° C so that plastics are not softened. Increasing the temperature allows the exposure time to be shortened.

The concentrations of ethylene oxide are measured in milligrams per liter of air. Instructions for use of the gas sterilizer will indicate what temperature and pressure must be attained to ensure a concentration of ethylene oxide sufficient to kill microbes. The correct temperature and pressure must be maintained throughout the entire exposure period for sterility to occur.

The amount of moisture present affects the ability of this gas to kill microbes: too little moisture may cause ethylene oxide to be unable to penetrate packaging materials and cell walls; too much moisture may cause ethylene oxide to hydrolyze to ethylene glycol, which is not as effective a microbicide.

The exposure time necessary depends on the temperature, pressure, concentration, available moisture, type of packaging material, and nature of the item being sterilized. One of the disadvantages of gas sterilizers is that they require longer exposure periods (up to several hours) than steam autoclaves. One of the advantages of ethylene oxide is that items can be sterilized at low temperatures if sufficient time is available (up to 24 hours for items treated at room temperature).

The following ranges of measurements are given as guidelines for practical use:

Temperature	120° to 140° F (50° to 60° C)
Concentration	500 to 1000 mg/L
Humidity	40% to 80%
Time	3 to 6 hours

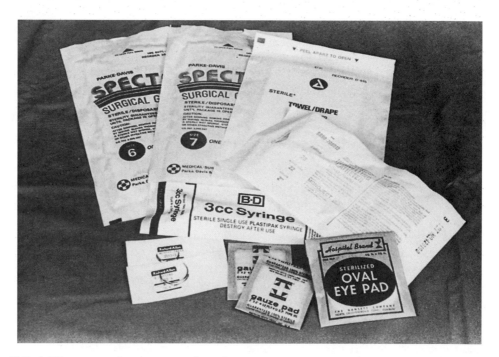

FIG. 1-25   Presterilized items packaged in paper. For average in-clinic use, paper is suitable for steam and gas sterilization.

The packaging materials recommended for use with steam autoclaves can be used with gas sterilizers (Fig. 1-25). In addition, a variety of plastic films (polyethylene, polypropylene, polyamide, nylon) can be used to wrap items so that they will remain sterile after treatment (Fig. 1-26). The manufacturer's instructions concerning exposure time and method of sealing should be carefully followed. If the instructions for a plastic film do not clearly recommend its use for gas sterilization, it should not be used for this purpose.

After sterilization, ethylene oxide dissipates slowly from the wrapping material. Because of its toxicity, items must be well aired before use. Usually it is assumed that a period of time equal to the exposure period will be sufficient to dissipate the gas, but some studies indicate that 24 hours may be necessary following 3 to 6 hours of exposure time.

Ethylene oxide is toxic whether it is in gas or liquid form. It should be used in well-ventilated areas and gloves should be worn. Even small accumulations in the atmosphere may prove harmful if inhaled, and the liquid form may cause severe burns. Any exposed portion of the body that comes in contact with ethylene oxide should be thoroughly rinsed with water. Medical attention should be sought following direct or indirect exposure.

Generally, the cost and the safety hazards connected to gas sterilization make it impractical in the small hospital.

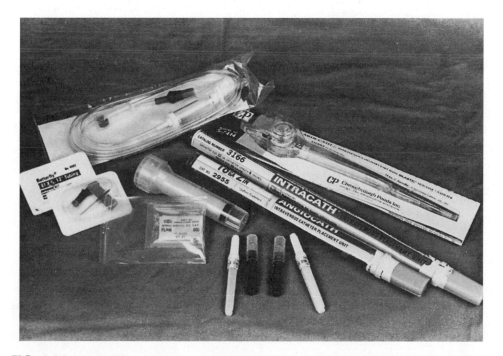

FIG. 1-26   Presterilized items packaged in plastic. For average in-clinic use, some plastic films are suitable for gas sterilization.

1. *Disease* is any process that detrimentally interferes with the functioning of an organism.
2. *Microbes* and *microorganisms* are living organisms too small to be seen with the unaided eye. *Pathogens* are disease-causing microbes.
3. *Infection* is the relationship between parasite and host; it commonly refers to detrimental results of a pathogen invasion.
4. *Microflora* or *normal flora* are microbes normally found in healthy animals. *Opportunists* are microflora that cause disease in debilitated animals or if microbes are transferred to other organs.
5. *Resistance* is the sum of all factors that enable an animal to overcome pathogenic invasion.
6. *Sepsis* is the presence of pathogens or their products; *asepsis* refers to their complete absence. *Sterile* is used to describe the condition of any item treated to become aseptic.
7. *Contaminated* refers to any item that is not sterile.
8. Three levels of intensity of care contribute to asepsis: sanitation, disinfection, and sterilization.
9. Semmelweis, Lister, Pasteur, and Koch are called the fathers of bacteriology.
10. *Protists* are the bottom rung on the food chain and include protozoa, fungi, bacteria, rickettsiae, chlamydiae, mycoplasmas, and viruses.
11. The most common categories of disease include hereditary diseases, congenital diseases and prenatal malformations, deficiency diseases, physical trauma diseases, contagious/infectious diseases, and poisonings.
12. A disease-causing microbe may be *exogenous* (originating from outside the body, such as animals or humans) or *endogenous* (normally found in the host, including commensals, opportunists, or pathogens).
13. Exogenous pathogens invade the host through a portal of entry (respiratory system, alimentary system, skin, urogenital system, and the placenta).
14. The goal of aseptic technique is to effectively break the chain of transmission, thereby preventing the pathogens from gaining access to a new host.
15. *Types* of infection include local infection, systemic infection, bacteremia, septicemia, pyemia, and toxemia. *Categories* of infection include subclinical, latent, primary, secondary, and terminal.
16. *Nonspecific factors* enable the host to control a broad range of invaders. *Specific factors* function against only particular pathogens.
17. The three lines of defense used by the individual to resist disease are anatomic barriers; phagocytosis and inflammatory response; and humoral and cell-mediated immunity. The first two lines of defense are nonspecific, and the third is specific.
18. The classic (or cardinal) signs of inflammation include redness, heat, swelling, pain, and disturbance of cellular function.
19. Histamine, serotinin, and the kinins aid in the initiation of inflammation and the increased permeability of blood vessels.

KEY POINTS

20. Immunity may be actively or passively acquired. *Active immunity* results when an antigen is introduced into the body and stimulates the production of antibodies. *Passive immunity* results when the body obtains antibodies from an outside source.
21. B cells are concerned with production of antibodies in the humoral system and provide protection against bacterial infection. T cells regulate cell-mediated immune responses.
22. Factors influencing methods of control include the following: nature and number of microorganisms; nature, mode of action, and concentration of agent in the environment; and extraneous organic matter.
23. Physical methods of control include dry heat, incineration, and hot air ovens.
24. Moist heat includes hot water, boiling water, free-flowing steam, and steam under pressure.
25. Successful steam sterilization depends on three factors: (1) proper operation of the autoclave, (2) proper preparation of the packs, and (3) proper loading of the chamber.
26. Although ultrasound is not useful as a means of sterilization, ultrasonic baths can be effectively used to clean instruments in preparation for sterilization.
27. Forced air ventilation systems use filters to remove particles from the air before it is recirculated.
28. The suffix *-cidal* refers to agents that kill microbes. The suffix *-static* refers to agents that inhibit microbe growth rather than destroy them.
29. *Disinfectant* refers to agents used on inanimate objects, *antiseptic* to agents used on living tissue.
30. *Cold sterilization* is the practice of soaking objects in disinfectant solutions.
31. Agents in solution form used in chemical control include alcohols, aldehydes, oxidizing agents, surfactants and detergents, phenolic derivatives, and heavy metals.
32. Gases used in chemical sterilization are principally ethylene oxide and formaldehyde, although other chemicals, such as beta-propriolactone, methyl bromide, and ethanol, are also used for gas or aerosol sterilization.

REVIEW QUESTIONS

Match the following terms on the left to the appropriate definitions on the right:

1. Disease
2. Microbe
3. Pathogen
4. Infection
5. Microflora
6. Opportunist
7. Resistance
8. Sepsis
9. Asepsis
10. Sterile
11. Contaminated
12. Medical asepsis
13. Surgical asepsis

a. Techniques to maintain a condition as free of microorganisms as possible, when body tissues are penetrated
b. The ability of an animal to overcome invasion by pathogens
c. Complete absence of living pathogenic microbes
d. Microbe capable of causing disease
e. Any process that detrimentally interferes with an organism's function
f. Condition of any item that has not undergone sterilization and that may or may not be contaminated with microbes
g. Living organism too small to be seen with the unaided eye
h. Technique to reduce microbe population in general and the transmission of pathogens in particular
i. Condition of any item that has undergone a cleansing procedure to rid it of all microbes
j. Presence of pathogens, or their toxic products, in patient blood or tissues
k. Relationship between parasite and host; commonly, the detrimental results of pathogen invasion
l. Microflora causing disease in debilitated animal
m. Microbe found in healthy animals

14. Identify and describe the three levels of intensity of care.

15. The suffix -cidal refers to _____ . The suffix *static* refers to

_____ .

16. Disinfectant refers to _____ , antiseptic to

_____ .

17. Cold sterilization is _____ .
18. Until the nineteenth century, what two factors prevented the development of surgery?

19. Identify the four "fathers of bacteriology."

20. What are the protists?

▼ REVIEW QUESTIONS—cont'd

21. Identify six of the more common categories of disease.

22. Name three factors that influence whether host invasion results in disease.

Match the following terms on the left to the appropriate definitions on the right:

23. Local infection
24. Systemic infection
25. Bacteremia
26. Septicemia
27. Pyemia
28. Toxemia
29. Subclinical infection
30. Latent infection
31. Primary infection
32. Secondary infection
33. Terminal infection
34. Nonspecific
35. Specific

a. Pus-forming bacteria spread to other areas of the body via the bloodstream
b. Results in death of the host animal
c. Infection with no clinical signs
d. Confined to a restricted area; abscess
e. Infection enabled by the presence of another
f. Infection that spreads throughout the body via the bloodstream
g. An existing infection manifest only when host resistance lowers
h. Presence of bacteria in the blood
i. Condition in which disease causes toxic substances to enter the blood
j. Bacteria that grow and reproduce in the blood
k. First infection, begun in the absence of others
l. Host resistance against only one or two pathogens
m. Host resistance against general invasion by pathogens

36. Identify the three lines of defense used by the individual to resist disease.

37. Identify three means of controlling disease.

38. What are the main factors that influence effectiveness of any given method of control?

39. List five physical methods of control, including specific methods for using some of these.

REVIEW QUESTIONS—cont'd

40. Describe the ideal chemical agent.

41. What is the difference between bactericidal and bacterostatic? between disinfectant and antiseptic?

42. Identify six categories of bactericidal agents available in solution form with examples of each type.

ANSWERS FOR CHAPTER 1

1. e   **2.** g   **3.** d   **4.** k   **5.** m   **6.** l   **7.** b   **8.** j   **9.** c   **10.** i   **11.** f
12. h   **13.** a

14. The three levels of intensity of care are: (1) sanitation (cleansing measure to prevent disease and promote health), (2) disinfection (applying an agent that can destroy or inhibit the growth of microorganisms), and (3) sterilization (ridding an object of all living microbes).

15. The suffix -*cidal* refers to agents that kill microbes. The suffix -*static* refers to agents that inhibit growth rather than destroy.

16. Disinfectant refers to agents used on inanimate objects, antiseptic to agents used on living tissue.

17. Cold sterilization is the practice of soaking objects in disinfectant solutions.

18. Until the nineteenth century, two factors prevented the development of surgery: the lack of painkillers and the inability of medical personnel to prevent postsurgical infection.

19. The fathers of bacteriology are Semmelweis, Lister, Pasteur, and Koch.

20. Protists are the bottom rung on the food chain and include protozoa, fungi, bacteria, rickettsiae, chlamydiae, mycoplasmas, and viruses.

21. Some of the more common categories of disease include (1) hereditary diseases, (2) congenital diseases and prenatal malformations, (3) deficiency diseases, (4) physical trauma diseases, (5) contagious/infectious diseases, and (6) poisonings.

22. Three factors that play a part in whether invasion of a host results in disease are: (1) portal of entry, (2) virulence and numbers of the pathogen, and (3) effect of host resistance on the pathogen.

23. d   **24.** f   **25.** h   **26.** j   **27.** a   **28.** i   **29.** c   **30.** g   **31.** k   **32.** e
33. b   **34.** m   **35.** l

36. The three lines of defense are: (1) anatomic barrier (unbroken skin and mucous membranes), (2) phagocytosis and inflammation (ingesting and destroying microbes that penetrate the outer layers of the body, preventing them from spreading to internal organs), and (3) humoral and cell-mediated immunity (identification and destruction of non-self-substances).

37. Disease control can be tackled in one or more of the following areas: (1) eliminating or controlling the source of disease, (2) increasing the host's ability to resist, and (3) preventing disease transmission.

38. Factors influencing the effectiveness of any method of control include (1) nature and number of microorganisms; (2) nature, mode of action, and concentration of the agent; and (3) environment (temperature, time, extraneous organic matter).

39. Five physical methods of control include (1) dry heat (drying, incineration, hot air ovens), (2) moist heat (hot water, boiling, free-flowing steam, steam under pressure, the autoclave, indicator systems, vacuum displacement sterilizer), (3) ultrasonic vibration, (4) radiation (ultraviolet light, ionizing radiations), and (5) filtration.
40. The ideal chemical agent will:
    • Kill all pathogenic microorganisms
    • Work quickly and effectively over a wide temperature and pH range
    • Exert residual action for extended periods
    • Not corrode, dry, or stain inanimate materials
    • Be stable in dry form and dissolve readily in water for a stable solution
    • Be odorless and colorless
    • Be nontoxic to and nonaccumulative in living cells other than pathogens
    • Not be affected by the presence of extraneous organic material
    • Not be inactivated when used with other agents
41. Bactericidal means that the agent can be expected to kill vegetative bacterial cells (but not spores); bacteriostatic means that it will inhibit the growth of bacteria but cannot be expected to destroy them. Disinfectant refers to agents used on inanimate objects, and antiseptic to agents used on living tissue.
42. Six categories of bactericidal agents available in solution form are (1) alcohols (ethanol, absolute alcohol, dilute alcohol, isopropanol), (2) aldehydes (formalin, glutaraldehyde), (3) oxidizing agents (any of the halogens, inorganic iodine solutions, the iodophors, chlorine, bromine, fluorine), (4) surfactants and detergents (anionic, nonionic, cationic), (5) phenolic derivatives, and (6) heavy metals.

SELECTED READINGS

Bojrab MJ et al: *Disease mechanisms in small animal surgery,* Baltimore, 1993, Williams & Wilkins.
Fossum TW: *Small animal surgery,* St Louis, 1997, Mosby.
Hunter P: *General microbiology: the student's textbook,* St Louis, 1977, Mosby.
Ikram M, Hill E: *Microbiology for veterinary technicians,* St Louis, 1998, Mosby.
Linton AH, editor: *Disinfection in veterinary and farm animal practice,* Boston, 1987, Blackwell Science.
Quinn PJ: *Clinical veterinary microbiology,* St Louis, 1994, Mosby.
Slauson D, Cooper B: *Mechanisms of disease: a textbook of comparative general pathology,* St Louis, 1990, Mosby.
Wistreich GA, Lechtman MD: *Microbiology and human disease,* ed 5, Beverly Hills, Calif, 1988, Glencoe.

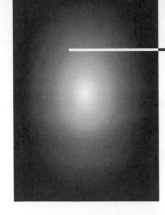

CHAPTER **2**

Practical Applications of Aseptic Technique

PERFORMANCE OBJECTIVES

After completion of this chapter the student will:

Apply a knowledge of aseptic procedures to the routine maintenance of the surgical area.

Describe the procedure for donning the sterile surgical gown and gloves.

List the steps involved in the routine surgical skin preparation of a patient.

Demonstrate the procedure for wrapping surgical packs.

Describe the sequence of steps in the performance of the surgical scrub.

Demonstrate the ability to place a patient in the basic surgical positions.

Identify the sterile boundaries for scrubbed and nonscrubbed personnel in the operating room.

Apply the rules of conduct for maintaining sterility before and during surgical procedures.

Identify the duties for each area of responsibility for surgical procedures.

■ ROUTINE MAINTENANCE OF SURGICAL AREA AND EQUIPMENT

Veterinary medical facilities are usually designed with separate areas or rooms for surgical procedures, the scrubbing of personnel, the preparation of the patient, the preparation of sterile packs, the performance of surgery, and the recovery of the patient. It is also possible to work in a facility in which all these functions must be performed in one or two rooms and where on occasion examinations and treatments are carried out in the same room.

Because of this diversity in facilities, it is impossible to give hard and fast checklists for the routine maintenance of the surgical area. For this reason, suggested protocols for the routine maintenance of various areas are given and can serve as a basis for the development of guidelines suited to the design, layout, and function of the individual facility. Regardless of the variations in construction and function that apply to an individual facility, it is vitally important to establish accepted procedures for routine maintenance to ensure that maintenance duties are completed. There

72

should be no doubt as to who is responsible for routine maintenance or when it should be performed.

Many facilities employ at least one technician whose primary responsibility is to function as an overall surgical assistant. Preparing the patient, assisting the veterinarian in surgical preparation, preparing sterile packs, scrubbing and assisting in surgery, and performing routine maintenance are some of the critical roles of that individual. Other facilities divide the duties among several people, and the same person may not perform the same duties on consecutive days. A list of equipment and supplies as well as guidelines for their maintenance should be readily available. A duty roster that indicates individual assignments and that can be initialed as assignments are completed is useful to ensure that adequate asepsis is constantly maintained.

Regardless of the amount of preparation the patient, the surgical team, and the instruments receive, asepsis will not be achieved unless the environment is equally prepared. The adequate maintenance of asepsis in the environment depends on the frequent repetition of cleaning procedures.

The following lists are based on the assumption that the facility has a separate surgical area, that one surgical session is scheduled daily Monday through Friday, and that sufficient staff are available to perform the procedures.

Cleaning Equipment and Supplies

Dry and wet vacuum. Dry vacuuming is preferred over sweeping the surgical area with a broom. Movement of debris across the surgical floor increases the amount of dust particles that become airborne. Ideally, the facility has a central vacuum system that exhausts directly outside the building, preventing further contamination of the surgery room environment. If a central vacuum system is not available, a canister vacuum with a high particulate exhaust filter should be used. When sanitizing the surgery floors, mopping is least desirable. Wet vacuuming is preferred. A disinfectant can be applied with an automatic spraying device or with a pump sprayer.

Mops. Although mops repeatedly have been shown to be a major source of infection, their widespread use continues. If mops must be used, a dry mop should never be used, and mop heads should be laundered and dried daily. Spare mop heads should be kept in supply so that a clean mop head can be used for repeated moppings or mopping in different areas. If a mop must be used more than once daily, it should be rinsed thoroughly after use and soaked for 30 minutes in a bucket of disinfectant. A mop that has been used should never be allowed to stand in a bucket of used cleansing solution.

A double-bucket technique should be used. Stands holding two buckets, each equipped with a wringer, are available. The mop is dipped in the floor disinfecting solution, wrung out, and moved from left to right across the body, never pushed back and forth at right angles to the body. After a few mop strokes, the mop is then placed back in the rinse solution and agitated, wrung out, and dipped again into the floor disinfecting solution. This procedure is repeated until all sections of the floor have been covered, starting with the area of the room that is farthest from the door. The floor should not be walked on until it is dry.

Disposable gloves. Disposable gloves should be worn to protect hands from prolonged exposure to disinfectants and to minimize additional contamination as furnishings are cleaned.

Disinfectant. A general-purpose disinfectant that is recommended for use on a variety of surfaces should be used. Quaternary ammonia compounds and iodophors are in widespread use. Instructions concerning dilution should be carefully followed. A stronger solution is not necessarily a more effective solution and may damage some surface finishes. A spray bottle of detergent/disinfectant solution can be used for the spot cleaning of dried blood or feces, and the spot can be wiped with a clean disposable towel. To attain the highest level of asepsis, one should follow the manufacturer's instructions regarding contact time of the disinfecting solution on the surface to be cleaned. Organic debris should be removed from the site before application of the disinfectant to maximize its disinfecting qualities.

Disposable cleaning cloths or sponges. Disposable cleaning cloths or sponges are helpful in maintaining asepsis because they can be completely removed and discarded after use, thus eliminating possible further contamination. If these are not disposable, they should be laundered and dried daily to minimize contamination.

Waste receptacle liner. All waste receptacles should be lined with disposable plastic liners. Liners should be changed frequently, and used liners should be tied shut and disposed of properly.

Operating Room

The operating room should be cleaned daily. Anyone entering the operating room should wear a cap, mask, shoe covers, and a clean smock or observation gown.

Before surgical session. One hour before surgery is scheduled to begin, wipe the flat surfaces of furnishings and lights where dust may have settled overnight. A cloth dampened with a disinfectant solution or spray bottle of disinfectant and clean cloth should be used.

Between surgical cases

1. Collect used instruments and place in a warm water and detergent solution to minimize the corrosive effects of blood. Many commercially available solutions contain enzymes or lubricating agents that maintain the integrity of surgical instruments.
2. Collect all waste materials and soiled linens and place in the proper container.
3. Check all surfaces of the Mayo stand and the surgical table for blood and other body fluids and spot clean with a disinfectant.
4. Move the surgical table to be sure there is nothing underneath it. Check the floor in the area of the table and the stand and spot clean.
5. Wipe the flat surfaces of the stand and the table with alcohol, which is quick drying. This procedure can be accomplished in approximately 5 minutes.

After surgical session
1. Collect all used instruments and soak in warm water and detergent solution.
2. Collect all waste material in plastic bags and place the bags near the door.
3. Collect soiled linen in bags and place the bags near the door.
4. If waste receptacles are kept in surgery, clean them with a disinfectant and dry them with a paper towel. Line them with plastic bags.
5. Check ceiling, walls, floors, cabinet doors, counter surfaces, and all furniture and spot clean as needed.
6. Follow the manufacturer's instructions regarding the maintenance of individual pieces of equipment, such as monitoring devices, anesthesia equipment, and surgical lights. If any problems with the equipment were noted during the surgical session, follow up with their maintenance.
7. Wipe all counter surfaces and cabinet doors with a disinfectant solution.
8. Wipe all exposed surfaces of the instrument stand and the surgery table with a disinfectant solution.
9. Check supplies; make a list of any items that need restocking.
10. Apply a disinfectant to a small area of the floor. Roll wheeled equipment such as the surgery table and anesthesia machines through the disinfectant.
11. Dry vacuum and damp mop or wet vacuum the floor after collecting and placing all cleaning supplies near the door.
12. Open the doors and remove the waste bags and cleaning supplies from the room. If light switches are inside the room, turn off the lights and wipe the switch plates with a disinfectant.
13. Wipe the push panels on the inside of the door with a disinfectant.
14. Mop the section of the floor immediately adjacent to the door and close the doors.
15. Remove cap, mask, and shoe covers and discard.
16. Properly dispose of waste bags and soiled linen.
17. Empty and disinfect mop buckets; launder and dry or discard the mop head.

After sterilization procedures are completed: restocking the operating room
1. Assemble packs to be returned to the operating room.
2. Check the list of disposable sterile items that are needed to restock the room and assemble.
3. Don cap, mask, and shoe covers and wash hands.
4. Take the items into the surgical area and store them in cabinets. Make sure to rotate sterile surgical supply such that previously sterile items are used before the supplies being added.

Preparation Room
Directions are given for cleaning both a scrub room that is used to prepare personnel for surgery and a preparation room that is used to prepare patients for surgery. If both functions are served by the same room or the same area, the lists can be consolidated.

Area used for the preparation of scrubbed personnel
Between scrubbing sessions
1. Properly dispose of wrappings from packs.
2. Properly dispose of debris in the scrub sink.
3. Spray the sink with disinfectant solution and rinse.

After surgical session
1. Remove waste. Wipe the waste receptacles with a disinfectant solution, dry them, and line them with plastic bags.
2. If an antiseptic immersion fluid is used during the scrub, dispose of the solution and clean the container as needed.
3. Check the walls, ceiling, and floor and spot clean if necessary.
4. Check the supplies and restock them if necessary.
5. Clean and refill the soap dispenser.
6. Wipe the counter surfaces, the cabinet doors, the wall area adjacent to the sink, the switch plates, and the door push panels with a disinfectant.
7. Disinfect and scrub the sink. Pour a disinfectant solution down the drain.
8. Dry vacuum the floor; then damp mop or wet vacuum with a disinfecting solution.
9. Empty and clean the mop bucket. Launder and dry or discard the mop head.
10. Return the supplies and equipment to the storage area.

Patient preparation area
Between patient preparations
1. Collect and dispose of waste material in covered containers.
2. If the bladder was expressed, properly dispose of the urine and disinfect the container.
3. Clean the clippers, according to the manufacturer's instructions.
4. Check the walls, counter surfaces, and cabinet doors and spot clean.
5. Spot clean the preparation table and wipe the surface with a disinfectant.
6. Check the floor. If hair clippings are present, vacuum. Spot clean if necessary.
7. Scrub the sink. Spray and rinse with a disinfectant.

After surgical session
1. Collect and dispose of waste material.
2. Wipe the waste receptacles, dry them, and line them with plastic bags.
3. Wipe the light fixtures and overhead supply lines with a disinfectant.
4. Clean the clippers according to the manufacturer's instructions.
5. If hair clippings are present in the area, vacuum. Unless a central vacuum system is used, move the vacuum to another area of the facility other than the surgical area and remove the bag from the vacuum. Replace the bag with a new one and clean the filter. Wipe the outside of the vacuum, including the hose and nozzle, with a disinfectant. The canister of a central vacuum system should be emptied when necessary.
6. Follow the manufacturer's instructions for the routine maintenance of other equipment used or stored in the preparation area.
7. Check the ceiling and walls and spot clean.

8. Using a disinfectant, wipe all counter surfaces, cabinet doors, the wall area adjacent to the sink, the switch plates, and the door panels.
9. Spot clean the preparation table. Wipe all exposed surfaces with a disinfectant.
10. Scrub the sink. Pour a disinfectant down the drain.
11. Check the supplies and restock.
12. Spot clean the floor. Dry and wet vacuum or damp mop the floor.
13. Empty the mop bucket and clean it with a disinfectant. Launder and dry or discard the mop head. Return the cleaning supplies to the storage area.

Pack Room

After sterilization of packs and supplies has been completed for the day, the following procedures are accomplished in the pack room.
1. Remove all waste, disinfect the receptacles, dry them, and reline with plastic bags.
2. Replace the materials used in pack preparation on shelves or in cabinets.
3. Collect the basins and trays used to clean and sort the instruments. Scrub them with a disinfectant, and leave them to air dry.
4. Clean the following equipment according to the manufacturer's instructions:
   a. Ultrasonic cleaning bath
   b. Sterilization units: autoclave
   c. Laundry equipment: washer and dryer
5. Wipe all exposed surfaces with a disinfectant.
6. Check the walls, cabinet doors, and other surfaces and spot clean.
7. Wipe the counter surfaces, the switch plates, the door panels, and the wall adjacent to the sink with a disinfectant.
8. Scrub the sink. Pour a disinfectant down the drain.
9. Check supplies and restock if necessary.
10. Spot clean the floor. Dry vacuum and wet vacuum or damp mop.
11. Empty the mop bucket and clean it with a disinfectant. Launder and dry or discard the mop head. Return the cleaning supplies to the storage area.

Recovery Room

Recovery room maintenance includes two areas: the routine maintenance of the room itself and the routine maintenance of the cages and animals. Animals in the recovery room should be disturbed as little as possible by the cleaning procedures. Only those procedures that directly concern the animals should be performed while the animals are in the room. Ideally, all surgery would be done in the morning, all animals would have a short, uneventful recovery, and all animals would have been transferred to wards at least 1 hour before the end of the shift, thereby allowing the day staff to clean the recovery room before leaving. This is rarely the case. When busy surgical schedules do not permit the day staff to clean the recovery area, an evening shift should be scheduled to clean the area before the next scheduled surgical session. In maintaining strict sanitation practices and preventing nosocomial infections, the surgical theater, surgical prep area, and recovery area should not go uncleaned until the following day.

Daily cleaning procedure

1. Remove waste, wipe receptacles with a disinfectant, dry them, and reline them with plastic bags.
2. Check the walls and ceiling and spot clean.
3. Spot clean the counter surfaces, the cabinet doors, the switch plates, the door panels, and the light fixtures. Spot clean all furnishings and equipment, such as intravenous poles, treatment tables, supply carts, and refrigerators if such items are kept in this area.
4. Wipe all exposed surfaces of the items listed in step 3, the wall adjacent to the sink, and the wall adjacent to the cages with disinfectant.
5. Check the supplies and restock if necessary.
6. Scrub the sink. Pour a disinfectant down the drain.
7. Spot clean the floor; dry vacuum and wet vacuum or damp mop.
8. Empty the mop bucket and disinfect it. Launder and dry or discard the mop head. Return all cleaning supplies to the storage area.

Patient care: concurrent and terminal disinfection. The terms *concurrent disinfection* and *terminal disinfection* are frequently used in the discussion of the care of animals with infectious diseases. Concurrent (or continuous) disinfection includes procedures that are carried out to maintain a low level of microbes while the animal is in the cage. Terminal disinfection refers to procedures that are carried out to eliminate residual microbes after the patient has left the facility. Although no infectious animals can be held in the recovery room, the same basic principles should be applied for two reasons.

First, animals that have undergone surgery are more susceptible to infection. Even if the animal is in good health, surgery causes stress, and any break in the intact skin, such as an incision, has a high potential for infection.

Second, animals in the recovery phase may produce copious amounts of extraneous organic material, such as saliva, mucus, serous fluid, feces, vomitus, urine, or possibly blood and pus. These body products contain moisture and often nutrients that can be used by microbes for their growth and reproduction. If they do not contain microbes when produced, they will soon become contaminated with microflora classified as opportunists.

Guidelines for concurrent disinfection. If an animal's cage is found to be soiled with organic material, the animal should be moved to a clean cage in the recovery area. If the animal is in critical condition and the surgeon has left orders that it is not to be moved unless specific instructions involving nursing procedures are given, the staff member responsible for the care of the animal should be notified. Any matter that has drained or has been projected from the cage should be picked up with paper towels and the contaminated area should be wiped with a disinfectant.

When a staff member is handling extraneous organic matter such as vomitus, feces, or pus, the following procedure should be used:

1. Wear an economical, disposable, nonsterile glove or insert the hand in a small plastic bag.
2. Hold a paper towel in the gloved hand and pick up the matter.

3. Pull the cuff of the glove downward over the hand, turning the glove inside out and forming a bag containing the waste matter and paper towel.
4. Use a paper towel and spray bottle of disinfectant to wipe the area. Allow the appropriate contact time of the disinfectant on the contaminated surface according to the manufacturer's instructions.
5. Dispose of the bag and the cleaning towel in a covered container.
6. Wash hands.

If the padding, paper, or fabric in the cages becomes soaked with urine, saliva, or blood, it should be changed. If this is not possible for medical reasons, several thicknesses of paper or a towel should be placed over the wet area. If the cage is not padded, several thicknesses of paper should be used to absorb moisture as it accumulates.

All staff members should meticulously and promptly dispose of waste, such as gauze sponges, cotton balls, used needles and syringes, scalpel blades, and used adhesive tape, as soon as it is no longer needed. Because of the potential for infection, all sharp objects and contaminated materials should be disposed of in a regulation biohazard container and removed by a company authorized to dispose of hazardous waste.

Guidelines for terminal disinfection. After the animal has been returned to the ward, the following procedure should be accomplished:

1. Remove all padding from the cage. If the padding is paper, dispose of it in a covered container. If it is fabric, remove any organic matter, and wash and dry properly.
2. Spray the cage interior surfaces with a disinfectant and allow the appropriate contact time according to the manufacturer's instructions.
3. Spray the cage door with a disinfectant. If dried organic matter is on the door, scrub with a brush and respray.
4. If a thermal recirculating water pad was used, spray with disinfectant spray, allow for contact time, and wipe dry.
5. If items such as intravenous poles or examination lights were used, spot clean them.
6. If a treatment table was used, wipe it with a disinfectant.
7. Scrub the cage and the door. If there are any crevices, use a brush or a pointed tool to clean them.
8. Spot clean the floor area adjacent to the cage.

Frequently, a number of animals will be transferred from the recovery area to the wards, allowing several cages to be cleaned at one time.

These guidelines are primarily used to maintain a consistently low level of microbes within the surgical area. Although it is not directly concerned with patient care, the meticulous care of the areas in which animals are quartered will minimize the chances of the patient acquiring a nosocomial infection.

Treatment Room

If only one operating room is feasible because of space and economics, it should be reserved for sterile procedures. In this case, nonsterile procedures are usually performed in a treatment room, which should be considered a part of the surgical area.

Procedures such as those involving dentistry or the draining of abscesses release large numbers of microbes, which may be pathogenic or opportunistic. This room will therefore be subjected to more contamination than other areas, and the same measures used to clean the other rooms in the surgical area should be used here. Overall, it is most beneficial to employ the same sanitation standards throughout the entire veterinary facility to maintain a low level of microbes.

Between procedures

1. Dispose of all waste. Disinfect the waste receptacles, dry them, and reline them with plastic bags.
2. If hair was clipped, vacuum the clippings.
3. Clean the clippers according to the manufacturer's instructions.
4. Spot clean the treatment table, the counter surfaces, and the sink area.
5. Instruments that were used should be rinsed in cool water followed by washing in warm water and detergent solution. It is important to rinse the instruments before soaking in detergent solution because the extraneous organic material will nullify the effect of the disinfectant. A soft-bristled toothbrush or filamentous pipe cleaner can be used to gently scrub the lock box or teeth of the surgical instruments to remove extraneous organic material. After scrubbing, rinse thoroughly and drain dry on paper towels or a drying rack.
6. Scrub the sink and pour a disinfectant down the drain.
7. Spot clean the floor.

Daily cleaning

1. Collect and dispose of waste material. Wipe the waste receptacles with a disinfectant, dry them, and reline them with plastic bags.
2. Vacuum clipped hair.
3. Clean the clippers according to the manufacturer's instructions.
4. Spot clean the walls.
5. Spot clean and wipe with a disinfectant all surfaces of the treatment table, the wall area adjacent to the sink, the cabinet doors, the counter surfaces, the switch plates, the light fixtures, the door panels, and any item of equipment used during the day.
6. Empty the cold sterilization trays. Clean the trays, refill with fresh solution, and replace covers.
7. Take any items to be autoclaved to the pack area for processing.
8. Scrub the sink. Pour a disinfectant down the drain.
9. Check the supplies and restock as necessary.
10. Spot clean the floor, and dry vacuum and wet vacuum or damp mop.
11. Empty the bucket and clean with a disinfectant. Launder and dry or discard the mop head. Return the cleaning supplies to the storage area.

Weekly Cleaning

In addition to the daily cleaning, all areas should be thoroughly cleaned on a weekly basis using the following guidelines.

Surgical room

1. Wipe the ceiling with a disinfectant solution, using a sponge mop reserved only for this purpose. If the ceiling is made of material that will not withstand water, dry vacuum it and use an aerosol disinfectant on the vacuumed area.
2. Damp mop the walls. Use a sponge mop reserved for this purpose.
3. Check the sterile packs and supplies. Remove outdated supplies to the pack preparation area for reprocessing. Supplies and instruments are generally considered outdated when the current date exceeds the expiration date stamped on the item or when the current date exceeds the autoclaved date by more than 6 weeks, assuming the supplies are stored in closed cabinets.
4. Change the filters in the ventilation systems. Since many ventilation systems use specialized filtration to remove microscopic airborne particles in the surgical area, it is important that filters be changed at regularly scheduled intervals.
5. Spray the floor with a disinfectant detergent solution and scrub with a bristled scrub brush on a handle or use a rotary scrubbing machine. Scrubbing will remove any buildup of organic debris that may accumulate in crevices of the floor. After scrubbing, the floor should be rinsed with a damp mop or sprayed with water and wet vacuumed.

Other rooms of the surgical area

1. Spot clean the ceilings.
2. Wash the walls with a disinfectant.
3. Check the supplies to note outdated items and items that need to be reordered.
4. Wipe the shelves of the open supply lockers with a disinfectant.
5. Clean the interior of the refrigerators. Defrost them if needed.
6. Scrub the floors as in step 5 above.

Special Care of Equipment

Throughout the surgical area are many items of equipment that should be maintained according to the manufacturer's instructions, not only to maintain a consistently low level of microbes, but also to keep the equipment in efficient working order and to extend the life of each item as long as possible. These items should also be checked frequently for things such as frayed cords, burned-out bulbs, and rubber gaskets that have deteriorated with age.

A file of maintenance manuals should be kept, and a checklist should be established listing the equipment, the required maintenance, and the intervals at which procedures should be performed. Spaces should be provided for personnel to initial on completion of each maintenance procedure.

A file should also be kept that includes the following information for each piece of equipment. File cards can be used for this purpose.

- Name of equipment
- Location in facility
- Model and serial numbers
- Name of manufacturer

- Name and telephone number of company from which it was purchased
- Name and telephone number of salesperson
- Name and telephone number of person to call for servicing
- Date of purchase
- Period of warranty
- Dates of routine maintenance

Taking a few minutes to record the information when a new piece of equipment is received will save time in the future if the equipment malfunctions or if parts must be ordered.

Items that should be listed for maintenance of this type include the following:

- Anesthesia equipment
- Monitoring devices
- Suction equipment
- Respirators
- Surgical lights
- Surgical tables
- Ultraviolet lights
- Ventilation system units
- Air conditioning/heating system units
- Dental scaling equipment
- Clippers
- Ultrasonic cleaners
- Thermal recirculating water pad
- Autoclaves
- Vacuum cleaners and central vacuum system
- Laundry equipment: washer and dryer
- Refrigerator

Aside from maintenance of equipment, special surgical tools such as drills and saws used in orthopedic surgery require meticulous care to ensure their proper function and sterility. Such equipment should be maintained regularly and tested before sterilization. To promote the working integrity of the equipment, it is important to follow the manufacturer's instructions for regular maintenance. Specialized surgical equipment requires more detailed cleaning and preparation than do most surgical instruments.

■ PREPARATION OF STERILE PACKS

When the need for asepsis was first understood and accepted by the medical profession, little was available in the way of methodology or materials to help the medical worker achieve asepsis. Soap, water, a few disinfectants, and a few ways of using heat were the only materials available, and subsequently organization, meticulous attention to detail, and a lot of "elbow grease" were indispensable. Today the technician is faced with a wide variety of methods and materials that can be used to sterilize the increasingly complex items required during surgery. As in so many other areas, advances in technology have resulted in a decreased need for long hours of physical labor, but the need for organization and attention to detail has remained the same. Proper initial organization will ensure that packs are available when they are needed, and consistent attention to detail will ensure that contents are sterile at the time of their use.

Because more methods and materials are available, more decisions must be made and a system of pack preparation and processing should be established. No system will consistently run smoothly if unattended, and therefore periodic reviews should be performed to establish whether objectives are being attained and whether improvements could be made.

Because of widely differing circumstances among small animal facilities, no single system can adequately serve all facilities. This increases the need for all staff members concerned to participate in adopting a system that is tailored to fit the needs of an individual clinic or hospital.

Factors to be considered when establishing a system include patient safety, cost volume, availability of materials and personnel, and personnel preference. No facility remains static for long periods. The volume of business increases or decreases, the staff changes, and new surgical techniques or pieces of equipment are introduced. With forethought, a system can be instituted that will maintain a balance among patient safety, the needs of the facility, and the capabilities of the staff. Planning should also establish guidelines to be used when making changes. It is often possible to rent large or complex pieces of equipment for a short period before deciding whether to buy them. With this option, it is possible to determine whether anticipated savings in time, energy, and money are real or imaginary without a large initial investment. Smaller, less expensive items can be purchased in small quantities for a trial period during which their suitability can be assessed before large lots are purchased. With the commercial availability of sterile disposable surgical supplies, small quantities can be purchased for trial use and later procured in larger quantities.

Regardless of the system used, the overall process should be as simple as possible. Too complex a system usually results in too many errors. The same system should be used by all involved personnel, not necessarily because one system is better than all others in every detail, but because the fewer variations and "surprises" that occur, the fewer errors there will be. If three technicians wrap packs three different ways, all the methods may result in sterile pack contents but may also result in an increase in accidental contamination of pack contents on opening.

Ideally, the preparation of sterile packs should be carried out in an area reserved for that purpose alone. For many small animal practices this is not feasible because of economic considerations and the limitations of available space, and pack preparation must take place in a multipurpose area. Because all packs should be prepared before the preparation for surgery, it is often convenient to combine the pack preparation area and the area used for preparation of operating room personnel, an activity that takes place immediately before surgery. The area should be compact and well organized with sufficient storage space for supplies and sterilized packs. Traffic to and from the area should be minimized, and routine cleaning procedures should be carefully followed so that the microbial load of the area is reduced as much as possible.

As a general rule, all contaminated reusable items from one surgical session should be repacked and processed before the start of the next scheduled session. If presurgical preparation has achieved the aim of as low a microbial load in the environment as possible, the occasional breaks in aseptic technique that occur because of human error during surgery are less likely to result in infection.

The technician preparing sterile packs assumes a twofold responsibility: (1) to follow recommended guidelines designed to ensure that the contents of each pack are sterile at the time of use and (2) to inspect each item before it is sterilized to ensure that the item will function as intended at the time of use. The surgeon and the assistant should be able to assume at the start of the surgical session that items in sterile packs are functional as well as sterile. No patient should have to be maintained under anesthesia for extended periods while missing or broken instruments are found, replaced, and sterilized so that the surgical procedure can be completed.

Procedure Manual

A procedure manual for the preparation of packs should be developed and updated as necessary. One technician may assume the responsibility for pack preparation and sterilization, or several staff members may divide the responsibility. In the first instance, employees with little or no experience may be required to prepare packs during any time the responsible technician is absent. In the second, it is important to ensure that all concerned personnel are adhering to the same guidelines, which are aimed at achieving consistently reliable results.

The following information should be included in the procedure manual and/or should be posted in the pack preparation area:

- Supplies that are necessary for pack preparation. Information should include the manufacturer's guidelines for use, the source of supply, and the minimum amount that should be stocked.
- Instructions for the use and the routine maintenance of equipment. Such information as the supplier, the date of purchase, the length of warranty, and the telephone number to call for service should be included.
- Printed material that can be used to identify instruments. Manufacturer's and supplier's catalogs are a good source of illustrations.
- Contents of packs. For each instrument pack, the name of the pack (e.g., emergency or abdominal), the names of the instruments to be included, the number of each instrument to be included, any additional items that should be included, and information on how the pack is to be wrapped (whether instruments should be placed on a stainless steel tray, single wrapped in an autoclave envelope, or double wrapped with muslin) should be listed.

If more than one surgeon performs surgery and their draping preferences differ, towel clamps can be sterilized separately and supplied only when they will be used. Instruments that are frequently used may be sterilized separately, and large instruments may be wrapped one to a pack because of the space limitations of the autoclave chamber. Extra instruments that must be available to replace any instruments contaminated during surgery may be sterilized singly or in pairs to avoid the necessity of contaminating a large pack of many instruments to replace one contaminated item.

For packs containing fabric or soft goods, information on how many of the items should be included in each pack (e.g., 1 gown and 1 towel, or 20 sponges), how to fold (or a source of information on how to fold), and how to wrap each pack (e.g., single wrap with paper, double wrap with muslin) should be provided.

Supplies Needed in Pack Preparation

The following supplies should be readily available for use in the pack preparation area:

- A detergent or enzymatic solution that is recommended for use on glassware and metal items.
- Brushes that are soft bristled, to be used in scrubbing the grooves on instrument tips.
- Pipe cleaners of various sizes for lumen instruments.
- Plastic containers (basins or trays) that are adequate to soak, wash, rinse, and sort instruments. For sterilization packs, stainless steel trays should be used.
- Wrap material. Several types of fabric and paper products are available for use as wrapping material. See the following section for more detailed information. In addition to paper products in precut sheets of various sizes and in bulk packaging (so that any desired size can be cut), paper, plastic pouches, and tubes are available to expedite packaging of small items.
- Instrument milk should be used by following the manufacturer's instructions to maintain the lubrication of instruments. Substitutes such as mineral oil should not be used because the substitute may provide a medium for bacterial growth.
- Autoclave indicator tape should be used for sealing linen- and paper-wrapped packs. Lines in the tape will change color when the pack is steam sterilized, indicating that the pack has been processed. This change in color does not necessarily mean that sterilization of the pack contents has been achieved.
- Sterilization indicator strips. Indicator strips should be placed inside the instrument pack when the pack is wrapped. During autoclaving, the indicator strip changes color verifying that the instruments have been steam sterilized. Autoclave tape should not be relied on exclusively to ensure that sterilization has been accomplished.

Sterile Pack Wrapping Materials

Wraps used for sterilizing instrument packs are commonly made of cotton or linen textiles and paper or plastic sleeves that are able to sustain the heat and moisture of steam sterilization. Newer methods of sterilization, some of which are economically feasible only when done on a commercial basis, and advances in paper technology have led to a marked increase in the variety of products that can be used as wraps. Plastics, metals, glass, textiles, and new papers are used to provide protection to the inner contents of packs through maximum integrity of the pack exterior. The selection of the wrap material used depends on the contents of the pack and the method of sterilization.

For the technician working in a small animal facility that relies on steam sterilization for in-house procedures, the choice is usually among a textile, paper, or plastic wrap. The ideal wrap should have the following qualities:

- Selective permeability. Steam or gas must be able to penetrate the wrapping for sterilization to occur and must be easily exhausted from the pack once the sterilization process is completed. Microbes and/or dust particles must not be able to penetrate from the outer surface of the wrap to the inner surface.

- Resistance. The material should be resistant to damage when handled. If rips, punctures, or worn areas do occur, the damage should be readily visible to avoid using contaminated instruments.
- Flexibility. The material should conform to the shape of the pack.
- Memory. After the pack has been opened, the wrapping material should return easily to the original flat position. This will alleviate accidental contamination of the pack contents.

In addition to these considerations, the availability and expense of the wrap and the type of sterilization used must be considered when a selection is made. Paper, plastic, and textile wraps are commercially available in various sizes to accommodate a wide range of surgical instruments. In general, these materials can be used for steam or gas sterilization but not for heat sterilization.

Textile wraps. Traditionally, cotton textiles have been used as wrapping materials and as drapes. Cotton muslin (a fabric with a thread count of 140 threads per square inch) and other cottons (with thread counts of up to 288 threads per square inch) can be used today as wraps if guidelines are followed. When woven textiles are used, more layers of wrap must be used than when paper wraps are used. This adds to the bulk of items that must be processed and stored and requires that a relatively large number of wraps be available for a relatively small number of packs. Textile wraps must be prepared in predetermined sizes; it is usually not convenient to have wraps made up in more than three or four sizes, although a large variety of textile wraps are commercially available. Paper wraps, however, can be cut to the most convenient size for each pack.

Textile wraps must be laundered, dried, and inspected for any damage before reuse as an instrument pack wrap. The advantage of using textile wraps is that they are more resistant to rips and punctures than paper and generally have a higher degree of flexibility and memory.

Packs wrapped in textile material should be wrapped with a double-wrap technique. Two double-layer wraps should be used if they are muslin. Two single-layer wraps may be used if the wraps are of high-count fabric. One double-layer muslin wrap and one single-layer, high-count fabric may be used, but all packs wrapped with textiles must be double wrapped.

When purchasing textile wraps, the following points should be kept in mind. Select cottons. Synthetics may contribute to static electricity in the operating room. Gray, medium tones of green, or medium tones of blue are often preferred because they result in less eyestrain over a period of time than does white.

Select fabric by the thread count, not by the weight or feel of the fabric. In some instances, manufacturers put a finish on the fabric that will make the material feel more substantial but that will wash out.

Mending textile wraps. Because of the high initial investment, technicians are often reluctant to throw out textile wraps that become worn or ripped and attempt to mend the wrap. This is not recommended because each stitch in the body of the wrap creates a passage for microbes. If heat-sealed patches are used, steam cannot penetrate the patches during sterilization as easily as it penetrates the body of the wrap.

Paper wraps. A number of different types of paper have been used as wrap materials. Of the types that are currently available, those papers that are referred to as crepe are preferred over the noncrepe papers. Crepe produces a crimp in the fibers during the manufacture of the paper that causes a greater degree of flexibility and stretchability during use. These papers are easier to work with than papers with flat fibers, are less subject to rips and punctures, and have a better memory than noncrepe papers. They are also more expensive than noncrepe papers. Manufacturers of autoclave paper do not recommend reuse, because continuous autoclaving can destroy the integrity of the paper fibers.

Although papers are produced in a variety of sizes and bulk packaging, a local distributor may carry only a limited line of paper wraps. The availability and cost must be considered in addition to the suitability of the paper. If more than one type or brand of paper is readily available, small lots of each can be purchased and compared before a decision is made.

When sealing paper-wrapped packages, some technicians will attempt to use ordinary masking tape instead of indicator tape, again for reasons of economy. This is not advisable because the adhesive on masking tape will not adhere adequately during steam sterilization.

The most economical way to purchase paper is by the roll or by accordion-pleated bulk packaging, but time will be necessary to cut the paper to the correct size. If some care is not taken in establishing the correct sizes for the various packs, time and paper will be wasted when the piece is initially cut the wrong size. Too small a wrap does not provide sufficient overlap when flaps are folded; too large a wrap increases the difficulty of wrapping the package and adds to the bulk without providing any benefits. To make the most economical use of paper and staff time, some initial planning is necessary.

1. Determine what items will be wrapped in autoclave paper. For small items that are wrapped singly or for long, narrow items, it may be feasible to use disposable autoclave envelopes or tubing for steam or gas sterilization and limit the use of paper to larger packs or single items that are of considerable size.
2. Determine the largest size piece of paper needed by cutting a piece and wrapping the largest pack that will be commonly processed. If the initial cut was too large, the piece can be trimmed; if too small, it can be used for a smaller pack.
3. Once the size of the largest wrap is determined, note the size of the wrap and the pack contents.
4. Use this piece to wrap the second largest pack, adjusting the size of the piece by trimming if necessary, and write down the final size of the wrap.
5. Repeat this process until the wrap size of the smallest pack has been determined.

When it is practical for one size to do double duty because the variation in paper size is minimal, the list of sizes should be shortened. If pack A requires a 25- $\times$ 25-inch sheet and pack B a 24- $\times$ 24-inch sheet, a 25- $\times$ 25-inch sheet can be used for both. In most instances, four or five sizes will satisfy all requirements without the excessive waste of paper or time. When the list has been consolidated, it should be posted in the preparation area and included in the procedure manual.

To shorten the time required for measuring paper, waterproof paint or nail polish can be used to mark size guidelines on the counter where packs are prepared (Fig. 2-1).

Whether autoclave paper is used in a double or single wrap depends primarily on how long and under what conditions the pack will be stored after sterilization. For a pack that has been single wrapped in two-way crepe paper, sterility can be assumed for 6 to 8 weeks if the pack is stored in closed cabinets. Storage in open shelving cuts the safe shelf life in half. In addition, the contents of single-wrapped packs are more likely to be accidentally contaminated while being opened than are the contents of double-wrapped packs. Both these factors must be considered when choosing between double- and single-wrap methods.

Pack Preparation

The following guidelines should be followed in the preparation of packs for sterilization:

- All items to be sterilized must be clean and in good repair.
- The wrap material used must be suitable for the sterilization process, clean, dry, and in good condition. For textile wraps, double wraps must be used. For paper wraps, a single wrap may suffice.
- The contents of frequently used packs should be standardized so that the same packs can be used for the same surgical procedures from session to session.

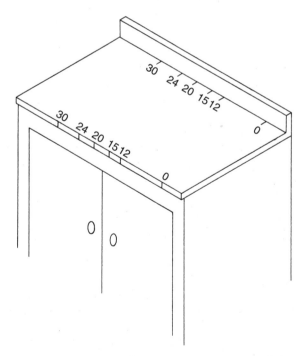

FIG. 2-1   To facilitate cutting autoclave paper to correct size, mark counter where paper is cut to indicate most commonly required sizes.

- Pack size must be suitable for the size of the autoclave chamber.
- Soft items, such as towels and drapes, should be folded using the accordion pleat technique (Fig. 2-2). Items that have been folded this way can be lifted by one corner and allowed to fall open. No elaborate unfolding or shaking is necessary, thus minimizing air currents that may circulate microbes.
- All packs should be wrapped by one method so that they can be unwrapped in the same way. A widely used method is shown in Fig. 2-3. The same method can be used for double or single wraps.
- A sterilization indicator strip should be placed on top of the instruments in the pack to verify sterility once autoclaving has been completed.
- The outer wrap should be sealed with autoclave tape to indicate that the pack has been autoclaved and to keep the pack from opening.
- The outer wrap must include a label that clearly identifies the pack contents and indicates the date on which the pack was sterilized. Some facilities indicate the expiration date of the sterile instrument pack on the label. The expiration date is determined to be a date that is 6 to 8 weeks from the date on which the pack was autoclaved.

Instrument packs. As soon as possible after surgery, instruments should be rinsed and soaked in warm water and detergent. Prolonged exposure to blood or saline will cause pitting on the surface of the metal.

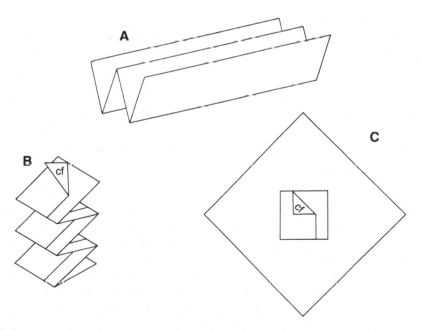

FIG. 2-2 Accordion pleat technique for folding soft goods before wrapping for sterilization. **A,** Fold lengthwise as shown. **B,** Then fold as shown. **C,** Position to wrap as shown. Corner fold *(cf)* will facilitate lifting drape when pack is opened and minimize chances of contamination.

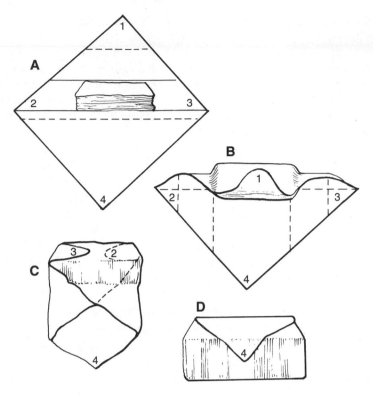

FIG. 2-3   General wrap. **A,** Position pack contents as shown. **B,** Fold flap 1 as shown. **C,** Then fold flaps 2 and 3 as shown. **D,** Flap 4 is folded as shown or folded under on dotted line. Pack is then ready to be sealed and labeled.

When instruments are handled throughout the preparation of packs, they should be placed gently in basins or on countertops, never dropped from heights or tossed into containers.

After the surgical session is complete, basins of instruments should be assembled. Large heavy instruments and fine delicate items should be handled separately so that they do not damage other instruments or are not damaged themselves. The instrument should be disassembled, if it is so designed. Instruments used in orthopedic surgery are commonly intricate in design and require special disassembling and cleaning.

Instruments should be soaked by using the following procedures:

1. Prepare a basin with warm water and detergent.
2. Open box locks and unlock ratchets as each instrument is gently placed in the basin.
3. Wash all surfaces of each instrument. A soft-bristled toothbrush serves this purpose well to clean grooves and teeth (Fig. 2-4). Make sure to open and close box locks when scrubbing surfaces with the soft-bristled brush to remove debris that may have become dried and lodged in the box lock.

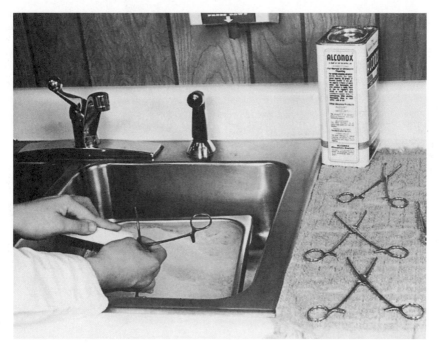

FIG. 2-4 Washing surgical instruments. Instruments should be handled with care, paying particular attention to grooves and crevices. Instruments should be soaked, washed, and dried in an open position.

4. Rinse each instrument thoroughly in clean water (if possible, use distilled or deionized water).
5. With locks and ratchets open, place instruments flat on an absorbent surface to drain.
6. If using instrument milk, follow instructions for dilution and exposure time. Do not use substitutes for instrument milk (Fig. 2-5).
7. Cover the draining instruments with another layer of lint-free absorbent material and blot dry.
8. When instruments are clean and dry, check each for its general condition and its ability to function properly. Box locks should open and close smoothly, ratchets should engage and disengage easily, and jaws and teeth should mesh as designed. Scissor blades should close properly, and cutting surfaces should be sharp. Instruments with broken, missing, or malfunctioning parts and instruments with pitted, discolored, or rusted surfaces should be set aside for repair or replacement. When purchasing new instruments, it is wise to buy high-quality instruments that will withstand repeated and excessive use.
9. If large numbers of instruments are being processed, separate them into specific types, such as all straight Crile forceps, or separate into specific groups, such as spay pack or biopsy pack.
10. If packs are not going to be assembled immediately, place instruments in a covered, dust-free storage area.

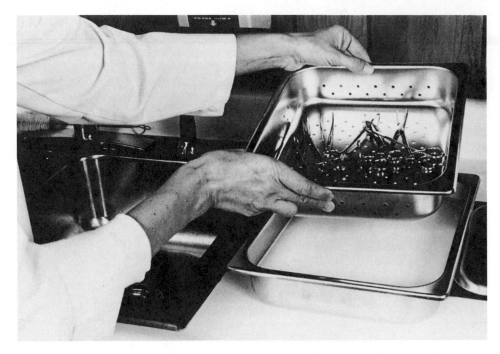

FIG. 2-5   Instrument milk. Use of perforated pans will facilitate application of instrument milk.

Multiinstrument packs
1. Check the procedure manual to determine the type and size of the wrapping material, the size of the stainless steel tray, and the types and numbers of instruments to be included in the pack.
2. Assemble the instruments in a tray. Keep all instruments of a kind together and place heavier instruments near the bottom and lighter instruments near the top. Hinged instruments should be placed in the open position.
3. Follow the procedure in Fig. 2-6 if a single-wrap method is desired. For a double-wrap method follow the procedure in Fig. 2-7. Sterilization indicator strips should be placed in the pack according to instructions (Fig. 2-8).

Single instrument packs. Use paper wrap, autoclave envelopes, or tubes according to instructions (Figs. 2-9 and 2-10), or place the instrument or a small group of instruments in the center of the wrapping material. Fold, wrap, place a sterilization indicator strip on top of the instruments, and seal using guidelines for multiinstrument packs. If instruments with cutting edges are to be autoclaved, protect the cutting edge to prevent penetration of the wrap material after sterilization. Insert the open tips of scissors into the folds of a gauze sponge and thread needles through a commercially available spring needle holder or autoclavable rubber tubing.

If instruments are wrapped loose (not in a stainless steel tray), always use a double wrap. Wrap tightly enough so that there is minimal room for instruments to shift when the pack is handled, but not so tightly that tips and points will puncture the wrap material.

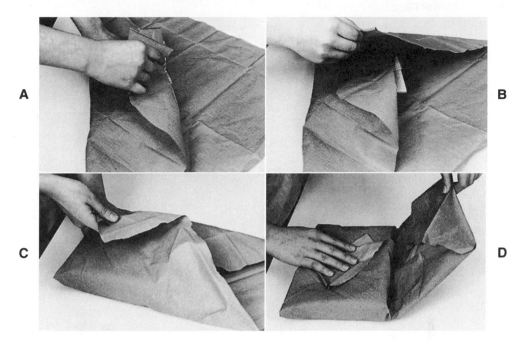

FIG. 2-6 Single wrap. Folds should always be performed in same sequence (**A,** proximal; **B,** left; **C,** right; **D,** distal) so that sterile packs can always be opened with same sequence, lessening chances of contamination.

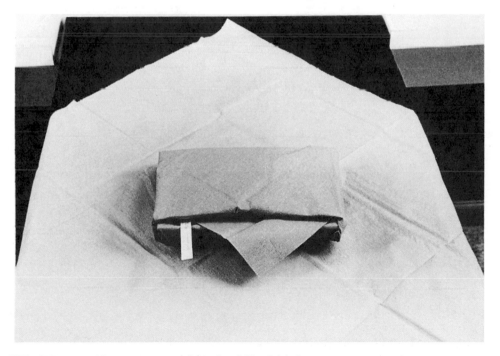

FIG. 2-7 Double wrap (inner). Flaps should be folded in same sequence shown in Fig. 2-6, but fourth flap is tucked as shown here instead of being taped. When pack is opened there is less chance of accidental contamination. Only sterile personnel open inner wrap. Outer wrap is done as shown in Fig. 2-3 and can only be opened by nonsterile personnel.

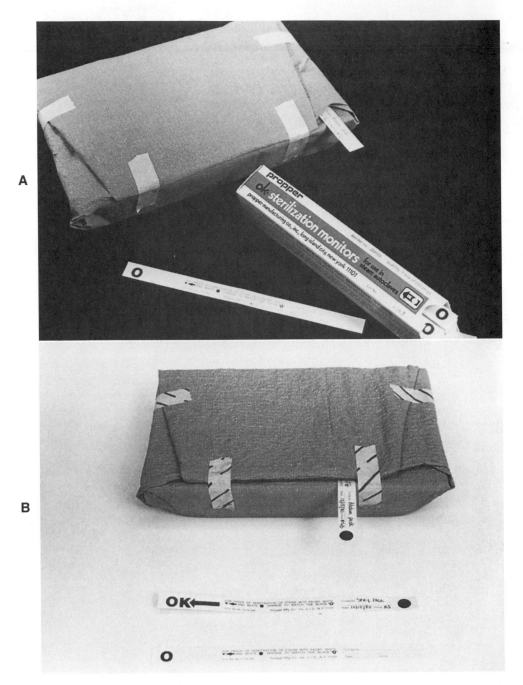

FIG. 2-8   A, Prepared pack. Pack has been correctly wrapped, sealed, and labeled and is ready for sterilization. **B,** Sterilized pack. After sterilization process is complete, color changes will have occurred on tape and indicator strips.

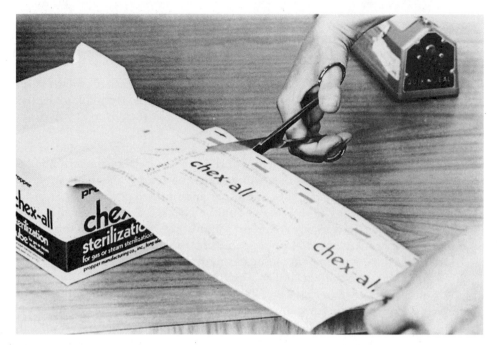

FIG. 2-9   Paper tubing and envelopes can be used to sterilize single instruments, syringes, and so on. Even if one side is transparent, the label should be correctly filled in, indicating pack contents and date of processing. Sterilization indicator areas are incorporated in paper.

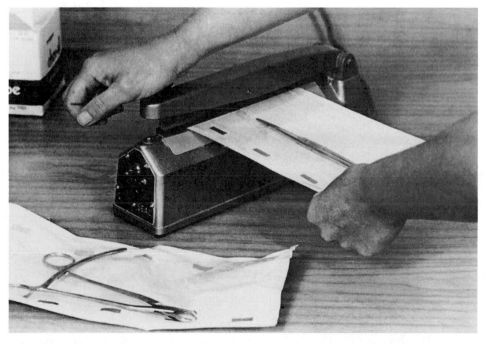

FIG. 2-10   Heat sealing is used to seal envelopes and tubes. Two applications, ½ inch apart, at each open end will increase chance of complete seal.

Soft goods packs. Fabric items (gowns, drapes, towels) that are going to be used again should be placed to soak as soon as possible after use. Cool water should be used to prevent stains from setting.

Before being wrapped for sterilization, all items should be washed and dried. The use of automatic washers and dryers is preferred. Although the use of bleach and the heat in the drying cycle will cut down on the microbial load, their overuse will weaken fabrics.

If manual methods must be used, a low-sudsing alkaline detergent should be used. The fabrics should be agitated sufficiently to remove stains, but hard scrubbing actions should be avoided because they will weaken the fabric. The items should be rinsed thoroughly in two changes of clean water and hung to dry.

When items are clean and dry they should be checked carefully for rips, holes, and unraveled seams, or worn areas that may permit the passage of microbes.

Fabric or paper items should be wrapped using the following guidelines:

1. All items to be wrapped should be clean, dry, and in good repair.
2. To fold fabric items, the accordion pleat method should be used. Gowns should be folded as shown in Fig. 2-11. The outside of the gown, which includes the sterile area when the gown is worn, is innermost. When the gown is lifted from the pack after opening, the inside of the gown, the nonsterile area, will be facing the person donning the gown, minimizing the chances of accidental contamination of sterile areas while donning the gown. To ensure that the finished pack is small enough to fit in the autoclave chamber it may be necessary to fold the gown again lengthwise. If so, after the gown is folded as shown in Fig. 2-11, *B*, it is folded again lengthwise from the left to the center and from the right to the center before it is accordion pleated as shown in Fig. 2-11, *C*. When the gown is completely folded, the technician should check to be sure the neck ties are lying loose on top of the gown. An indicator strip should be placed on top of the gown so that once it is unwrapped, the indicator strip is visible. The indicator strip will fall to the floor once the gown is picked up for donning.
3. Bulky items should be wrapped one to a pack to ensure steam penetration during sterilization. The final size of the pack must be small enough so that the pack does not touch the sides or the top of the autoclave chamber. If a countertop autoclave is used, it may not be possible to sterilize more than one bulky item at a time. A soft pack should not be larger than 30.6 × 30.5 × 52 cm (12 × 12 × 20 inch) regardless of the size of the chamber. Steam penetration of larger packs may not be sufficient to ensure sterilization.
4. Items that are used one at a time (fenestrated drapes) should be packaged singly to prevent waste regardless of size.
5. Items of moderate size (towels, drapes) can be wrapped two to a pack if both will be used when the pack is opened.
6. Gauze sponges should be packaged in standardized quantities (20 to a pack, or other multiples of five if varying quantities are needed) to facilitate counting procedures.
7. After the item is properly folded, it should be placed in the center of the wrap and the wrap should be folded as shown in Fig. 2-3. The outside of the pack

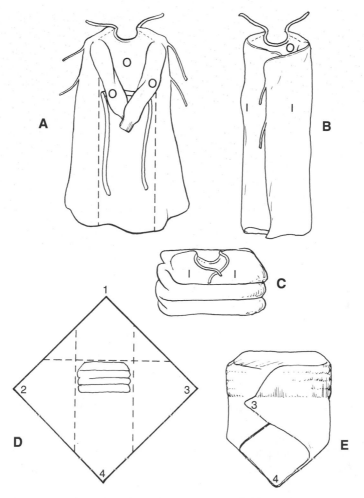

FIG. 2-11 Instructions for folding surgical gown. **A,** Lay gown on flat surface. Avoid large wrinkles because they may affect donning gown. **B,** Fold lengthwise. **C,** Accordion pleat. **D,** Position gown in center of wrap. **E,** Wrap by folding flaps in sequence. *O,* Outer (sterile) surface of gown when worn; *I,* inner (nonsterile) surface of gown when worn.

is secured with tape and labeled. The label should include the size and quantity of the contents (Gauze sponges 2 × 2—10) as well as the date of processing and expiration date.

Sterile rubber and plastic supplies. The increased availability of sterile, disposable catheters, drains, and other rubber and plastic accessories has greatly decreased the need to sterilize and reuse these items. Many surgical accessories are available presterilized in individual disposable packages. The advantage of using disposable items is that the preparation of these items is time consuming for the technician, and therefore it is more economically feasible and sterility is guaranteed. If a plastic or rubber item must be sterilized, the technician must check to see if the instrument can withstand steam autoclaving or must be cold sterilized. If steam sterilization is used, the item should be wrapped as a single instrument as previously described. Plastic and rubber instruments should always be autoclaved singly wrapped to prevent damage to any other instruments should the plastic or rubber melt during the process. If cold sterilization is used, the items should be thoroughly rinsed in sterile normal saline to remove the disinfectant before their use. Overall, it is not recommended to cold sterilize instruments for surgical use unless absolutely necessary.

Fluids. Sterile fluids used during surgery can be purchased presterilized in single-use containers, thus reducing the time necessary to prepare them for surgery.

Fluids such as distilled water or normal saline can be sterilized in the autoclave by using the following guidelines:

1. Use only heat-resistant glass or plastic containers.
2. Containers must be chemically clean. Soak them in a detergent solution recommended for glassware, scrub all surfaces with a brush, especially the inner surfaces, and rinse thoroughly in running clean water to remove any detergent residue. Rinse in two changes of distilled water and invert to drain dry.
3. Use only flasks or bottles that are small enough to fit easily into the autoclave chamber.
4. When filling flasks or bottles, keep the top level of the fluid below the base of the neck of the container.
5. If using cotton plugs, do not pack the cotton so tightly that it must be forced into the neck of the container. If using screw caps, place them lightly on the neck of the bottle and do not tighten until after the autoclave cycle is complete. If using closures that consist of a rubber cap and a metal collar, assemble the closure before placing it on the container.
6. If using cotton plugs, place a strip of autoclave tape so that it runs up one side of the neck, over the top and plug, and down the other side of the neck. If using other caps or closures, place a small strip of tape on the container near the label.
7. The label should include the kind of fluid and the amount as well as the date the container was processed.

Use of the Steam Autoclave

When items are sterilized with a steam autoclave, the following guidelines should be used:

1. Study the operating instructions before using any autoclave for the first time. Do not use until the sequence of steps is understood and the instructions for the operation of the controls is clear.
2. Use only distilled water. Check the water level before each load. Do not overfill or underfill the water tank or the autoclave chamber.
3. Check packs for proper wrapping, sealing, and labeling (including date and expiration date) before loading.

4. Do not overload. Adequate space between packs and shelves is needed to ensure the free circulation of steam. Do not allow packs to touch the chamber walls (Figs. 2-12 and 2-13).
5. If possible, place packs in a vertical, not horizontal position. Do not put more than one layer of packs on a shelf (Figs. 2-14 and 2-15).
6. When the chamber is loaded, properly close and seal the door.
7. Start the autoclave. The timer for the sterilization period should not be set until the correct temperature and pressure have been attained.
8. When sterilization is complete, do not open the door until the steam has been exhausted and the temperature has fallen. Open the door 2 to 3 cm while standing to the side of the unit. If steam escapes, it will rise upward and the

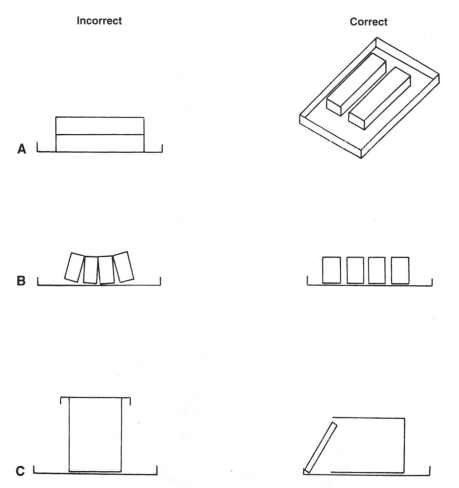

FIG. 2-12 Loading autoclave. **A** and **B,** Place packs in tray so steam can circulate freely. Do not pile packs on top of each other. Do not pile in center of tray. **C,** When sterilizing covered containers, place container on side and position lid so steam can enter interior of container.

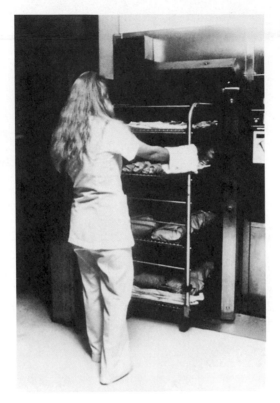

FIG. 2-13   Loading autoclave. Even when fully loaded, adequate space must remain between shelves of rack to ensure steam circulation and penetration.

operator will not be burned. As a safety precaution, the operator should wear safety goggles and thermal protective gloves when opening the autoclave to eliminate the risk of being scalded with steam.

9. Allow the packs to remain in the chamber until the drying portion of the cycle is complete. This will dry any residual moisture left in the pack and prevent wicking of the moisture to the outside of the wrap.

10. To ensure consistent results, follow operating instructions regarding the daily and/or weekly cleaning of the chamber and trays and the cleaning of the exhaust trap.

11. The time and temperature necessary to ensure sterilization will depend on the pressure setting of the autoclave and type of packs (Fig. 2-16). For most items commonly sterilized by autoclaving, 15 minutes at 121.5° C and 15 psi is adequate. If the pressure is increased to 18 psi, a time of 12 minutes will be adequate.

Storage of sterilized items. The conditions under which sterile packs are stored and the material in which packs are wrapped will affect the length of time pack contents can be assumed to remain sterile. As with other areas of preparation for surgery, if the system is kept as simple as possible, fewer errors will result.

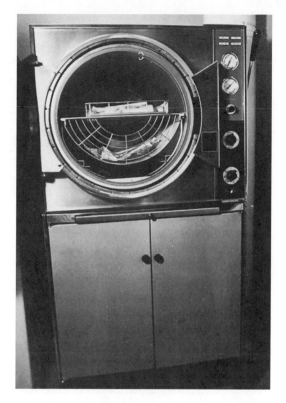

FIG. 2-14   Loading autoclave. Do not allow contact between packs on one shelf and packs on another shelf because this will impede free circulation of steam.

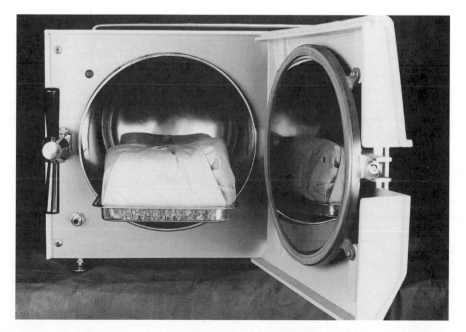

FIG. 2-15   Loading autoclave. If unit has small chamber, do not sterilize more than one bulky item at a time.

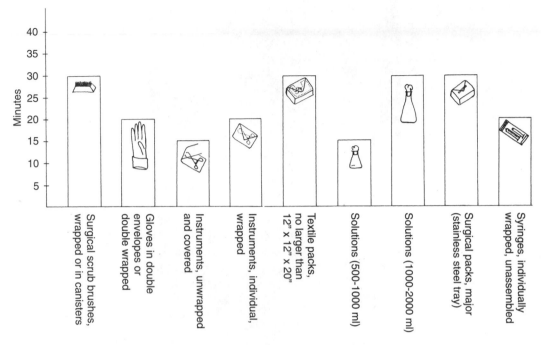

FIG. 2-16   Steam autoclave. Time necessary to ensure sterilization at pressure of 15 psi and temperature of 121° C (250° F).

A separate area should be reserved for the storage of sterile packs. Other items and contaminated articles should not be kept in close proximity to sterile packs. The storage area should be as dust free and as well ventilated as possible. Extremes of temperature, humidity, and altitude will shorten the safe storage time. In hot, humid climates, paper and cloth wrappings may remain constantly damp, contributing to the penetration of packs by microbes. Insect control measures must be meticulously followed in these areas because insects may be a major cause of pack contamination. In areas of high altitude or in arid regions, paper and adhesives dry and become brittle faster than at sea level. Heat seals and welds disintegrate more frequently.

Closed cabinets are preferred to open shelving for storage. In general, items stored on open shelves have a safe shelf life of only one-half the time of the same item kept in a closed cabinet.

When packs have been sterilized, they should be handled as little as possible. Necessary handling should be done with care. The most recently processed packs should be placed behind older packs on the shelves to ensure that the packs are used during the time they can be assumed to be sterile. This will reduce the time spent reprocessing packs that have become outdated before they have been used. As previously mentioned, it is beneficial to designate an expiration date on the pack label to assist with pack rotation.

A sterile pack is considered contaminated if any of the following conditions apply:

- It has become wet.
- The tape sealing the pack is broken or loosened.
- The date of processing is missing or illegible.
- Punctures or rips occur in the outer wrap.
- The pack has been dropped on the floor.

Assuming that packs are double wrapped in muslin (four layers) or single wrapped in two-way crepe paper and are stored in closed cabinets in a dust-free, insect-free, and well-ventilated area, they can be considered sterile for 6 weeks. Storage on open shelves will reduce the safe shelf life to 3 weeks.

Commercially sterilized packs should be stamped by the manufacturer with an expiration date because no pack can be assumed to remain sterile forever. It is commonly assumed that the methods of sterilization and quality control programs of manufacturers of sterile packs result in packs that will remain sterile for months or years when stored under the proper conditions. Commercially prepared paper packs will be affected by conditions of storage: temperature, humidity, altitude, the amount of handling, and the quality of ventilation. In the case of glass, metal, or plastic wraps, consideration must be given to the type of seal, such as rubber caps or heat-welded seams, and how long the integrity of the seal can be expected to be maintained. If commercially prepared packs are being kept for longer than 4 to 6 months before being used, it is an indication that too large an inventory is being maintained. For these reasons, a shelf life of 4 to 6 months is suggested for commercially prepared packs with no expiration date.

If goods must be purchased in large quantities and stored for long periods (for economic reasons or because an item is only available in relatively large quantities but is infrequently used) a portion of the packs can be wrapped in 3-ml polyethylene film and heat or tape sealed to extend the safe storage time up to 1 year or until the expiration date set forth by the manufacturer, whichever date arrives first.

If large quantities of packs of items in frequent use (basic surgical packs, gauze sponges) are found to be outdated before use, too large an inventory is being maintained, and storage space and processing time are being wasted. To increase efficiency, the inventory of these items should be reduced.

Items not frequently used (specialized surgical instruments and supplies) should be wrapped in double wrap (four layers of muslin or two layers of two-way crepe paper). The technician should be sure the drying cycle of the sterilization procedure is thorough and complete. The pack should be handled as little as possible, wrapped in 3-ml polyethylene film, and sealed. If stored in a dust-free cabinet, the pack can be assumed to be sterile for up to 1 year.

Certain specialized surgical items, such as orthopedic instruments and accessories, should not be stored for the length of time stated for other instruments. Many veterinary orthopedic surgeons will only use instruments that have been autoclaved within 48 hours before a scheduled surgery. Depending on the surgeon's protocol for orthopedic surgery, the technician should arrange for autoclaving of instruments under those guidelines. Since orthopedic surgery is invasive and breaks in sterility severely compromise the patient's health, the risk of unsterile instruments must be decreased by autoclaving in a timely manner.

If the item is for a procedure that is not considered to be an extreme emergency (the intent to do surgery is known at least 1 hour before surgery is done), the item can be singly wrapped and sterilized. When sterilization is complete, the instrument can be brought directly to the surgery, unwrapped, and transferred by the surgeon to the sterile field (Fig. 2-17).

Emergency Sterilization

Ideally, sterilization procedures will be so well organized and efficiently carried out that the need for emergency sterilization will not occur. The availability of sterile disposable instruments greatly decreases the need for emergency sterilization.

When the threat to life is immediate, no time is available for sterilization procedures. Under these conditions, the procedure is done without regard to the sterility of instruments and supplies and the effects of contamination are mitigated postoperatively by careful nursing procedures and the administration of antibiotics. This may occur (although rarely) in the most efficient hospital or clinic. However, if there is an increasing frequency of situations that are not truly emergencies and for which the proper packs are not available, then the processing system should be reviewed. It may be necessary to increase the inventory of some items, to purchase more presterilized items, or to assemble packs that are reserved for emergency use only.

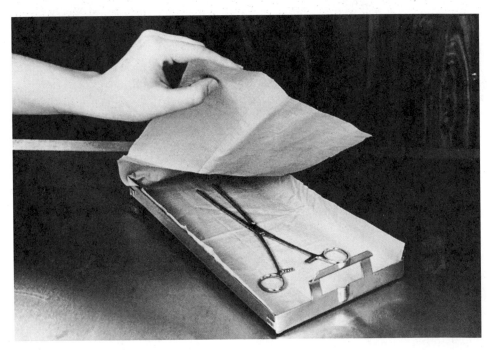

FIG. 2-17   To sterilize without wrapping, line tray and position instrument as shown. Cover instrument using aseptic technique.

In remote areas or during times of a natural disaster, facilities for sterilization may be absent or interrupted. If an emergency occurs under these conditions and time and circumstances permit, the following guidelines should be kept in mind:

- A sanitized item is preferable to a grossly contaminated one. Sealed packs of nonsterile gauze sponges should be opened rather than using the contents of open packs.
- Instruments should be washed and rinsed in clean water, if available, and boiled for 20 to 30 minutes or soaked in 70% alcohol for 1 hour if possible.

■ PREPARATION OF SURGICAL PATIENT

Before preparing the patient for surgery, it is the surgical technician's responsibility to ascertain several things concerning the animal. Only after the technician has completed the checklist does the actual preparation of the patient begin.

- *Verify* the patient's identity and the surgical procedure to be performed.
- *Confirm* that all fasting and other presurgical instructions have been carried out correctly.
- *Obtain* the results of all presurgical clinical, laboratory, and radiologic examinations.
- *Examine* the patient's history and permanent health record for any preexisting conditions that may affect the surgery and verify that the vaccine record is current.
- *Report* any existing conditions or behaviors that may interfere with the surgery or adversely affect the patient's surgical risk factor.
- *Confirm* the existence of a surgical release form or contract and a telephone number where the owner can be reached during the surgical procedure should any unexpected findings be encountered.

The animal is brought to the preparation room and receives a presurgical physical examination and evaluation by the veterinarian or technician. On completion of the examination, the technician will be ordered to administer preanesthetic drugs, such as tranquilizers and/or atropine. The veterinarian will administer the general anesthetic 10 to 15 minutes later. Once the animal has been anesthetized with a general anesthetic, the animal may or may not be intubated with an endotracheal tube (Fig. 2-18). For short, minor surgical procedures, an endotracheal tube may not be used. For long and invasive surgical procedures, the animal is intubated and anesthesia is continued with the use of an inhalant gas anesthetic. The technician may be instructed to insert an intravenous catheter into the patient for fluid and drug administration. The animal is then secured to the preparation table in a position that clearly exposes the surgical site and is conducive to the surgeon's needs. Intravenous fluid administration is begun, and monitoring devices are attached before preparation of the skin. Cardiac, respiratory, and body temperature monitors are commonly used to monitor the patient during surgical procedures (Fig. 2-18).

The skin of the surgical site is prepared by using the following steps:

1. Verify the sex of the animal if the procedure is an ovariohysterectomy or castration.
2. Express the bladder. If possible all animals should be allowed to eliminate before surgery. The bladder must be empty to increase space in the abdominal

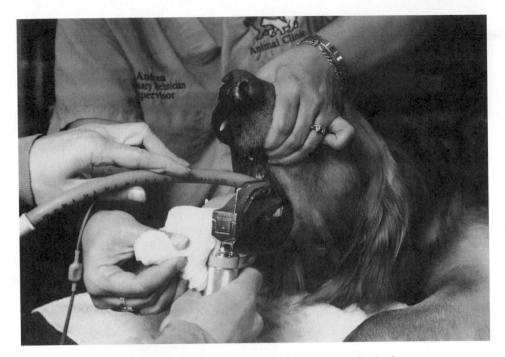

FIG. 2-18   Animal intubated with an endotracheal tube.

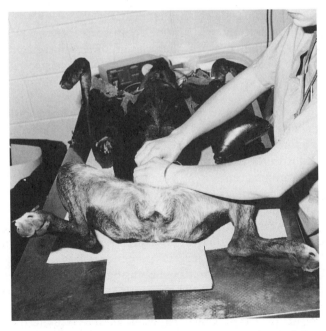

FIG. 2-19   Expressing the bladder of an anesthetized dog.

cavity, to avoid the possibility of the surgeon's incision accidentally puncturing the bladder, and to prevent soiling the table since the anesthetized patient will have little sphincter control (Fig. 2-19).

3. Clip all hair from the prescribed areas with a surgical preparation blade (#40). Fig. 2-20 shows hair removal patterns for abdominal, thoracic, cervical, limb, and tail procedures. As a general rule, always clip more rather than less hair. If an incision must be enlarged, it is dangerous and time consuming to have to "break scrub" to reprepare the surgical site. Fig. 2-21 shows the correct way to hold a small animal clipper. For maximum efficiency, the blade should be directed against the grain of the hair. Because the grain of hair changes direction in several places on the cat and dog abdomen, technicians must become adept at handling the clipper so that the skin is not unnecessarily abraded. Once the area is clipped, hair should be swept or vacuumed away immediately so that tufts and strands do not adhere to the scrubbed site (Fig. 2-22).

4. Wet the area with water (Fig. 2-23) and scrub away dirt and other debris with a surgical scrub preparation, such as povidone-iodine or chlorhexidine.

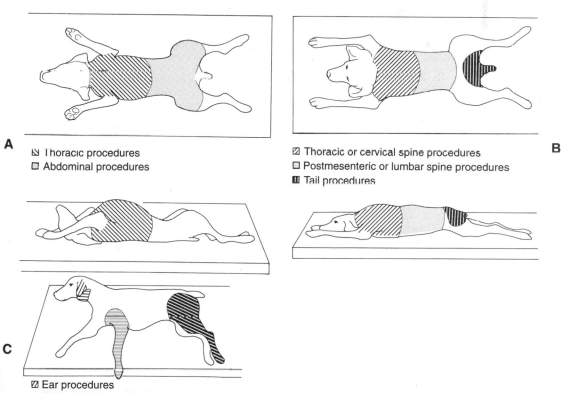

A

    Thoracic procedures
    Abdominal procedures

    Thoracic or cervical spine procedures
    Postmesenteric or lumbar spine procedures
    Tail procedures

B

C

    Ear procedures
    Pectoral limb procedures
    Pelvic limb procedures

FIG. 2-20   Hair removal patterns for selected surgical procedures. **A,** Dorsal recumbency. **B,** Sternal recumbency. **C,** Lateral recumbency.

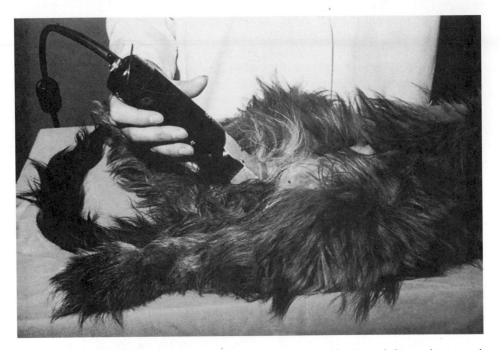

FIG. 2-21   Small animal clipper is held in a modified pencil grip and directed against the grain.

Chlorhexidine scrub is commonly used as a surgical scrub because it is less irritating to skin yet provides rapid bactericidal action. Scrubbing should be done with large pieces of sterile gauze sponges. Cotton will stick to hair stubbles and is not recommended. Do not use brushes or scratch the skin with fingernails because this will irritate and abrade the skin. Depending on the surgical scrub soap used, application and contact time may vary. If chlorhexidine is used, sufficient soap must be used to cover the surgical site and remain in contact for at least 2 minutes. During this period, a lather should be created with the soap on the surgical area. The soap is then rinsed with water, and the site is swabbed with alcohol-soaked sterile gauze pads or sprayed with alcohol and wiped with sterile gauze pads. If povidone-iodine scrub is used, approximately 1 ml should be used to cover 20 to 30 square inches. Excess scrub soap on the surgical site is not necessarily more potent at killing microbes nor is it economically wise. Contact between the povidone-iodine and skin should last approximately 5 minutes. During this period, a rich lather should be created with the soap on the surgical area. Proper disinfection of the skin results from contact time and effectiveness of the surgical scrub soap, and friction produced by scrubbing action. Following the 5-minute scrubbing period with the povidone-iodine, the area is rinsed with water and sprayed or swabbed with alcohol and gauze. This sequence of scrubbing with surgical soap, rinsing with

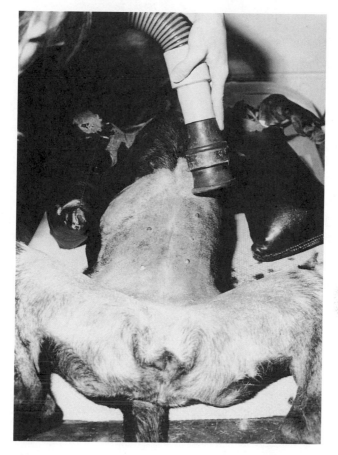

FIG. 2-22   Clipped hair should be removed before skin scrub is started.

water, and spraying or swabbing with alcohol and gauze should be repeated at least three times on the surgical site (Fig. 2-24).

5. To prepare a limb for surgery, the limb should be shaved 360 degrees by the methods previously described. How much of the limb is shaved can be determined by the surgeon according to the area of the surgical site, or the entire leg can be shaved as illustrated in Fig. 2-20, C. The pattern for skin preparation is described as follows. The surgical site is viewed as a rectangle. The first stroke made with the gauze is done vertically down the incision line. Subsequent strokes are made either to the right or left of the incision line, alternating outward toward the borders of the shaved area. Again, no stroke is retraced with the same wipe, and the technician must take care not to allow the gauze to drag over already prepped areas. An alternative method is to begin with the first stroke in the center of the surgical site. From the center, a circular motion is made that widens as the circular swab covers more of the surgical site.

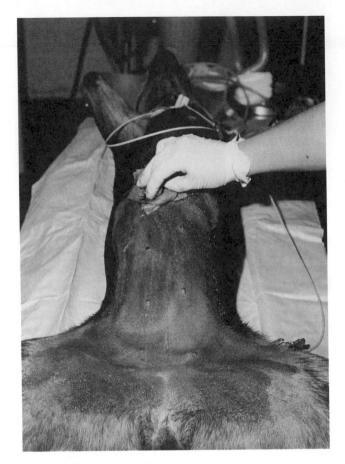

FIG. 2-23   Application of surgical scrub preparation.

Eventually, the circular swab will lead to the surgical site boundary, where the swab is removed and discarded. Subsequent swabs retrace the same pattern as the first and continually move outward so that the pattern is not retraced with the same swab.

6. Transfer the animal to the surgical theater. Take care not to contaminate the prepped surgical site. Once the animal has been secured to the operating table, paint the surgical site with a germicidal agent, such as 1% iodine and 70% ethyl alcohol with sterile gauze and sterile gloves or sterile sponge forceps. A germicidal agent applied as a spray is less effective than the same agent applied with friction. The final paint is not removed. It is allowed to dry 3 or 4 minutes to reach maximum antiseptic effect.

Overall, it is crucial that the chosen scrub pattern be performed at least three times for the time previously described. When performing either of the scrub pat-

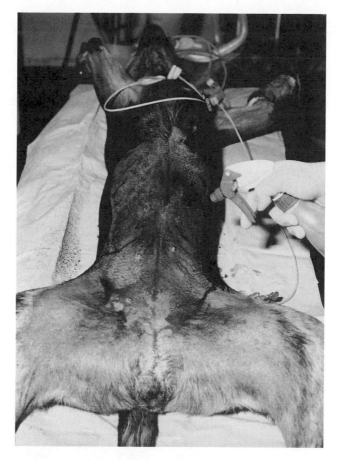

FIG. 2-24   Final paint is sprayed on surgical site.

terns, one must not retrace a stroke with the same wipe. Attention to detail must be followed to maintain surgical aseptic technique.

Positioning the Patient

The choice of position is usually made by the surgeon, but a nonsterile technician must always actually position the patient.

The type of position in which the patient will be placed is determined by the surgical procedure, the surgical approach, the type of anesthetic to be administered, and the size and condition of the patient.

Surgical patients are positioned only after the anesthetic has been stabilized. Care must be taken to maintain the airway and to support the head and neck. When the anesthetized animal is moved, it must be done slowly and cautiously.

An effective surgical position must provide maximum safety for the patient and convenience for the surgeon throughout the procedure. To be effective, the surgical position must allow for the following conditions:

- The maintenance of adequate respiratory function. The technician must remove any constrictions around the throat or chest and is responsible for maintaining a patent airway throughout the procedure.
- The maintenance of circulation. The technician must watch that blood flow is not constricted and that proper padding is provided under areas of the body that will receive excess pressure. Restraining straps should be checked periodically during the procedure and loosened if necessary.
- The maintenance of body temperature. The technician must monitor the patient's body temperature and adjust the thermal recirculating water pad under the animal such that a consistent body temperature is maintained.
- Exposure and visibility of the operative field. It is essential that the patient's position afford the surgeon maximum view of and accessibility to the surgical site.
- Access for the administration and monitoring of anesthetics. The team member monitoring the patient's condition and depth of anesthesia throughout the procedure must have access to the patient to observe airway function, measure membrane color and pupil size, and check monitoring devices.
- Noninterference with monitoring devices and intravenous lines. If the veins of the extremities have been punctured to administer anesthetics or fluids, it may not be possible to tie down the limb without interfering with the free flow of the agent. This is especially true in cats and small dogs (Fig. 2-25).

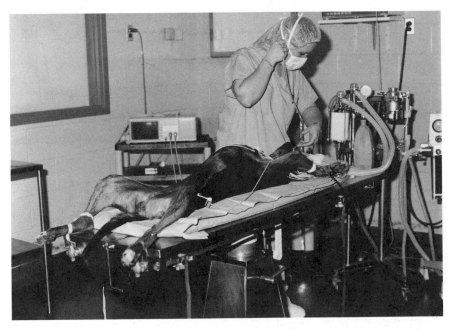

FIG. 2-25   Monitoring the anesthetized patient before surgery.

Positions for surgery. The surgery table is padded with a small mattress or conductive rubber pad covered with some type of disposable or easily laundered material. Also in use are warm water bags or a thermal recirculating water pad where the temperature of the animal can be controlled. The purpose of padding the table is to prevent undue pressure on the trunk and limbs and to minimize body heat loss.

Dorsal position. The supine or dorsal position, also called dorsal recumbency, is the usual position for entering the abdomen. At times, the surgeon may also access the chest cavity by means of a medial sternotomy. This position is achieved when the animal is placed on its back, and the pectoral limbs are extended anteriorly and secured to the table cleats. Some surgeons prefer to extend the front limbs caudally, securing them next to the body. The pelvic limbs are extended as much as possible and secured to the table. It is essential that the patient's body be properly aligned on the table. This is often a problem with thin animals or breeds with prominent vertebral columns. To assist with correct alignment, a U-shaped or V-shaped metal or plastic body positioner may be placed under the animal before securing it to the table. Sandbags, body rolls, wedge-shaped blocks, and V-shaped surgery tables are also used to aid in maintaining the patient's position.

Modified dorsal position. The modified dorsal position is sometimes used in abdominal surgery because it allows gravity to assist in keeping the intestines in the anterior portion of the cavity. The patient is positioned as in the dorsal position, and the top of the surgery table is tilted so that the head is lower than the tail. The surgeon will indicate the required degree of tilt, but if the tilt is to be more than 5 degrees, the patient may have to be restrained from sliding too far downward. While using this position, it is crucial that the technician monitor the patient's respiratory function and oxygen saturation, since this position may interfere with respiratory function because of the weight of the abdominal viscera pushing on the diaphragm.

Modified reverse dorsal position. The modified reverse dorsal position is used in neck surgery or upper abdominal surgery in large dogs. This position improves operative exposure by maintaining the intestines in the lower part of the cavity. A slight elevation of the head also improves hemostasis. When this position is used for neck surgery, a rolled pad or towel is placed under the shoulder, and the muzzle is taped or strapped to the table to hyperextend the neck. The patient is positioned as in the dorsal position, and the table is tilted so that the head is slightly higher than the tail. If more tilt is required, the patient must be restrained from sliding too far downward.

Sternal position. Animals scheduled for surgery on the dorsal aspect of the body are placed in sternal or prone position. Anesthesia is induced with the patient in a sternal position. Once fully anesthetized, the patient's body is further aligned using a positioner, body rolls, or sandbags. The pectoral limbs are abducted at the hip, flexed at the knees, and secured to the table. The head is positioned flat on the table and facing forward. Sometimes a small cushion is placed under the patient's head to level it with the trunk of the body, preventing the neck from arching downward. This position is also used in procedures involving the throat and mouth. In these cases, it may be necessary for the technician to pull the head up and prop open the mouth using loosened strips of sterile gauze behind the canine teeth of the upper and lower jaws.

Lateral position. The lateral position is sometimes used for procedures involving the thorax, hips, and extremities. Surgery on the chest cavity will necessitate directing and securing forelimbs away from the chest. The patient is placed lying on either side, depending on which side needs surgical access. The limbs are then tied to the table cleats. If surgery on the extremities is being performed, particularly if it is to be performed on a medial aspect of the limb, customized positioning may be needed.

Draping the Patient

The purpose of draping the patient is to create a sterile area around the surgical site. Depending on the structure of the surgical team, either the veterinarian or a scrubbed technician will drape the patient.

There are two types of draping procedures customarily used in small animal practice. One is a fenestrated sterile drape placed over the entire operating site and secured with towel clips (Fig. 2-26). The second type is the four-corner drape in which four drapes are applied one by one in a clockwise or counterclockwise manner and secured to the patient with towel clips.

Surgical drapes may be made of disposable paper similar to the paper wrap used for autoclaving instrument packs. Adhesive plastic drapes can also be purchased presterilized but cannot be steam sterilized. Plastic drapes are commonly used in human surgical settings because they conform to the contour of the patient, preventing gaps for possible contamination of the surgical site. Paper and plastic drapes can be ordered prefenestrated or plain, in which the surgeon cuts an opening to suit the size and location of the incision. Cloth drapes are also used and are prefenestrated, which presents a disadvantage if the opening is an unsuitable size.

Disposable materials reduce the possibility of contamination and are cheaper to use because linen drapes must be laundered and sterilized. Many surgeons prefer linen drapes because they are more absorbent, are easier to handle, and conform to the patient's body better than paper drapes.

Proper limb draping is essential in orthopedic surgery in which the likelihood of contamination must be kept as minimal as possible. A large sterile drape is placed over the entire patient with a fenestration to expose the limb requiring surgery. The foot of the animal is covered and wrapped with sterile rolled gauze or elastic wrap in a sterile manner. The covering of the foot should overlap onto the surgically prepped area so that unsterile areas are fully covered with sterile dressing. The surgically prepared limb is held or suspended upward by clipping a hemostat or towel clamp to a piece of tape or gauze that has been secured to the covered foot. A drape is then placed under the suspended leg and secured. A sterile stockinette is then inserted over the foot and limb. The leg is now lowered onto the sterile drape below, and three additional drapes are applied around the limb. The surgeon will cut the stockinette at the proposed incision site. As previously mentioned, plastic adhesive drapes are beneficial for use in orthopedic surgery, because they conform to the contour of limbs and extremities.

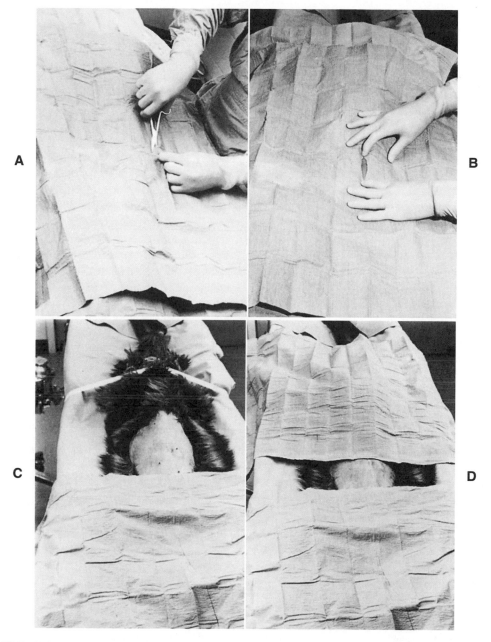

FIG. 2-26 **A** and **B,** Single drape method. Sterile drape is placed over patient, and fenestration is made over incision site. **C** to **H,** Four-corner drape method. Sterile drapes are placed on patient and secured with towel clips. It should be noted that drapes cover patient and hang over sides of operating table ensuring a sterile operative site.   *Continued*

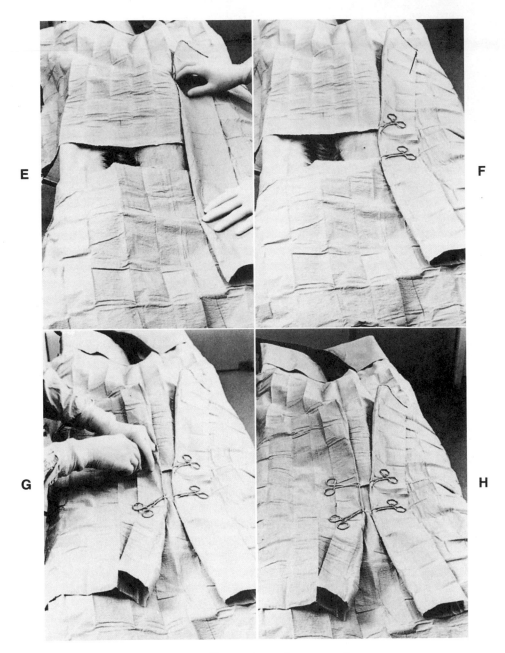

FIG. 2-26, cont'd   For legend see preceding page.

■ PREPARATION OF OPERATING ROOM PERSONNEL
All Personnel

Each person concerned with the surgical procedure, regardless of how peripheral the role played, should be expected to adhere to the following guidelines:

- Observe routine hygienic measures, such as bathing or showering daily and washing hair frequently.
- Keep nails clipped short and filed smooth. Do not wear polish.
- Do not wear cologne or perfume.
- Wear clean clothing for each session.
- Wear clean shoes for each session in the surgical area. If possible, reserve a pair of shoes for this use only.
- Remove all jewelry (rings, bracelets, chains, watches, earrings) before each session in the surgical area.
- Wash hands using the general handwashing procedure before each session, between each case, at the end of each session, and after handling waste material. If it becomes necessary to leave the surgical area during a session, wash the hands before leaving and on returning.
- Maintain hands and other exposed skin surfaces in good condition by the frequent use of lotion to counteract the drying effect of repeated exposure to heat, hot water, chemicals, and surgical gloves.
- Dispose of waste material as it is produced in covered containers. Do not allow waste to accumulate on counters, in open basins or pails, or in sinks.
- Organize the work to be accomplished in each session to minimize traffic to and from different areas of the surgical suite.
- Keep doors closed.
- Wear a cap, mask, shoe covers, and clean gown or scrubs whenever entering the surgical room, even if surgery is not in progress.

Visitors

Visitors should be expected to conform to the following guidelines:

- Refrain from entering the surgical area unless a definite need exists. The use of intercom systems will reduce the number of necessary visits.
- Wear a gown, clean scrubs, or a disposable lab coat over street clothing.
- Wear a cap, mask, and shoe covers when entering the surgical room, even if surgery is not in progress.
- Whenever possible, refrain from touching furnishings, equipment, and supplies.
- Wash hands according to the general handwashing procedure on entering and again before leaving the surgical area.

General Handwashing Procedure

To be effective, the general handwashing procedure should last between 1 and 2 minutes.

1. Turn on the water; adjust it to a comfortable temperature.
2. Hold the hands under a stream of water in a downward position, allowing water to drain from the wrists to the fingertips.

3. Clean the nails with a file or an orange stick. Many disposable surgical scrub brushes are packaged with a nail cleaning stick. This step may be omitted after the first handwashing of the day's first session, unless a need is apparent.

4. Apply a cleansing agent to the hands and spread it from the wrist to the fingertips.

5. Rub the hands together vigorously. Interlace the fingers and move them back and forth. Do not omit the backs of the hands.

6. Rinse, allowing the water to drain from the fingertips.

7. Repeat steps 4, 5, and 6.

8. Turn off the water. If the faucet controls cannot be operated by the elbow, the knee, or the foot, use a paper towel to turn off the water. Do not allow the hands to touch the faucets. Discard the towel.

9. Dry the hands thoroughly with paper towels. Discard the towels.

10. Apply a lotion and work in thoroughly.

Sequence of Events During the Preparation of Sterile Personnel

The following is the sequence of events to be followed during the preparation of surgical personnel who are participating in the surgical procedure:

- Remove jewelry.
- Change clothing. Personnel should change to a clean and dry, but not sterile, scrub suit.
- Don cap, mask, and shoe covers.
- Perform the surgical scrub.
- Don a sterile gown.
- Don sterile gloves.

Any person who will have direct contact with the sterile field or sterile supplies during the surgery is required to scrub and don sterile gloves and gown, along with mask, cap, and shoe covers. In two-handed surgery, only the surgeon will scrub; in four-handed surgery, the surgeon and assistant will scrub. The surgeon and the assistant are then referred to as scrubbed or sterile personnel.

Personnel who must be in the operating room during surgery but who are not required to have direct contact with the sterile field or sterile equipment and supplies are referred to as nonscrubbed or nonsterile personnel. They should wear caps, masks, shoe covers, and clean observation gowns and wash hands thoroughly before entering the surgical area.

Headgear. Caps and masks are not usually sterilized. Disposable ones are preferred. If caps and masks are reusable, they should be washed and dried after each use, folded loosely, and stored in covered containers, drawers, or cabinets.

Caps. Caps are available in a variety of styles. The simplest style resembles an ordinary shower cap with elastic around the edge to ensure a snug fit (Fig. 2-27). Other caps are cut to fit more tightly to the head and with ties in back for adjustment. When choosing a cap style, the amount of hair to be covered and the hair style must be considered. All hair should be contained within the cap, especially from the ears forward.

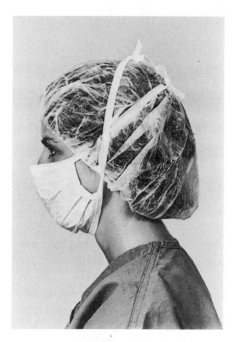

FIG. 2-27   Headgear for surgical session.

Personnel with sideburns and/or beards should wear a surgical bonnet that covers the cheeks, chin, and neck.

Masks. The typical mask is a rectangular piece of material with bound edges and a pleat that allows adjustment over the nose. There are two sets of ties, one at the upper corners and one at the lower corners. A pliable strip of metal in the center of the upper edge can be bent to fit over the nose. The mask must cover the nostrils and the mouth and should not have gaps between the seams of the mask and the face. The mask should fit so that all the seams meet with the face, especially in the cheek area (Fig. 2-27).

Handling masks

1. Hold the mask in position over the face and bend the metal strip to fit over the nose.
2. Tie the upper ties. Position the mask so that the ties pass from the cheekbones over the ears to the back of the head.
3. Gently pull downward from the middle of the lower edge to open the pleat, and fit the mask over the nose and mouth.
4. Tie the lower ties. Pass the ties below the ears to the back of the neck and tie, or pass the ties upward in front of or diagonally over the ears and tie on the top of the head. When using this position, be sure to conform the mask so that no gaps are formed between the mask and cheek area. The mask should be as comfortable as possible so that it is not a distraction during the surgical procedure.

5. After donning the mask, avoid coughing and sneezing and refrain from excessive talking.

Masks are not effective if in use for more than 30 minutes or if they become damp. It may not be possible to change the mask each time either of these conditions occurs, but if possible it should be changed. Masks should always be changed between surgical cases.

The mask is removed by untying the chin ties first and then the upper ties to prevent the mask from dropping on the gown or clothing. Only the ties should be handled. The mask should be discarded in a covered container.

Eyeglasses. Eyeglasses should be cleaned before each session. Personnel who must wear glasses often have difficulty with the fogging of lenses because exhaled moisture condenses on the glass. Products are available to prevent fogging of eyeglass lenses. Fogging can be minimized by following the steps listed.

- After cleaning and drying the lenses, apply a commercially available product to the lenses and wipe. The product will not interfere with vision.
- Bend the metal strip of the mask to conform as closely as possible to the contours of the face.
- If the lower rim of the glasses touches the upper edge of the mask, adjust the glasses so that they fit over the mask. Adhesive tape can also be placed on the upper margin of the mask to adhere to the area below the eyes and thus prevent exhaled breath from reaching the lenses.
- Special antifogging surgical masks can be purchased for individuals who wear eyeglasses.

The surgical scrub (Fig. 2-28). There are many variations that describe the exact conditions that constitute the ideal surgical scrub procedure for personnel. Studies can be cited to support almost any viewpoint regarding the necessary duration of the scrub, from those advocating a 20-minute scrub to a few that advocate omitting the scrub altogether. Most agencies find a comfortable compromise between the two extremes.

The surgical scrub is performed to ensure as high a level of cleanliness of the hands and forearms as possible. Both resident and transient microbes are found in large numbers on the hands, and the hands are the portion of the surgeon's body in most intimate contact with the surgical field and sterile equipment. It is not possible to rely entirely on gloves because gloves can accidentally tear or puncture during surgery and as many as 50% of all surgical gloves are found to contain holes by the time surgery is complete.

Directions for a routine scrub may be given in terms of strokes per surface area of skin or in terms of time to be spent scrubbing a given skin surface. Infinite variations have been used regarding the number of strokes, the time spent on a given surface, and the number of times lathering and rinsing are repeated.

Each surgical facility should formulate a policy regarding the conditions that constitute an acceptable scrub procedure, and guidelines should be posted and followed.

Before beginning the surgical scrub, the surgical personnel should check that all supplies are readily accessible. After the scrub is started, nonsterile items cannot be

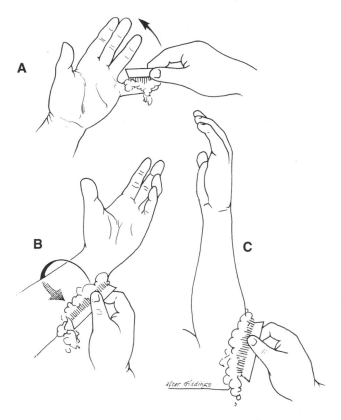

FIG. 2-28   Surgical scrub sequence. **A,** Starting with little finger and working across to thumb, scrub each surface of each digit. **B,** Scrub forearm, again scrubbing entire circumference. **C,** Scrub elbow area to 2 inches above elbow, including all surfaces.

touched. If this occurs, the scrub procedure must be repeated. Because the scrub, hand-drying procedure, and the donning of the gown and gloves are performed in sequence without interruption, all items necessary for this sequence should be available at the start of the scrub. These items include the following:

- A sink with elbow, knee, or foot controls. If these controls are not available, nonscrubbed personnel must turn the water off for the scrubbed person.
- A cleansing agent in a dispenser that has a foot control. Soap or iodophor solutions (Betadine) or chlorhexidine scrub is recommended. Chlorhexidine scrub solutions provide bactericidal action yet are less harsh and drying to the skin. This is beneficial to those individuals who must scrub frequently.
- A disposable nail file or orange stick.
- A sterile scrub brush. Individually wrapped and autoclaved reusable scrub brushes should be provided for surgical scrub. Disposable, individually wrapped scrub brushes bathed in an iodophor scrub solution can also be used.

Disposable scrub brushes tend to be economically beneficial because they reduce the number of surgical supplies that need to be reautoclaved.

- Sterile towels.
- Sterile gown.
- Sterile gloves.

The sterile brush pack should be opened before the scrub is begun. If nonscrubbed personnel are not available to open sterile towel and gown packs and the outer wrapping of glove packs as they are needed, these packs must be opened before the scrub is begun and placed so that they will not be splashed during the scrub.

Ideally, after donning the cap, mask, and shoe covers and performing the surgical scrub, the surgical team member enters the surgical room. Nonsterile personnel will have removed the outer wraps of gown and glove packs. The surgical team members will open the inner wrap and don the gown and gloves. If less than ideal conditions exist, this may not be practical. If it is not, the gown and glove packs are opened close to the scrub sink. Scrubbed personnel don the gown and gloves and move immediately to the surgical room or the area of the room where surgery is performed.

Directions are given here for a long scrub of approximately 7 minutes' duration. Variations are given for scrubs that require approximately 10 and 15 minutes to complete, should this be required. Another variation allows the scrub to be completed in 3 minutes. It is suggested that the 7-minute scrub be used at the beginning of the surgical session and the short scrub be used between cases. See Fig. 2-29 for the sequence of steps.

Seven-minute scrub

1. Turn on the water and adjust it to a comfortable temperature. The stream should be gentle to minimize splashing.
2. Wet the arms and hands.
3. Dispense a cleansing agent into the palms of the hands and spread over the hands and arms (to 2 inches above the elbows), working up a lather to remove surface dirt.
4. Holding the fingers under the stream, use a nail file or orange stick to clean under the nails. Discard the file by dropping it in the sink.
5. Rinse the hands and arms, holding the forearms higher than the elbows and allowing the water to drain off the elbows into the sink.
6. Obtain a sterile brush and moisten it under the stream.
7. Dispense the cleansing agent directly onto the brush.
8. Scrub the surfaces of one hand and forearm, using a straight stroke on fingers and nails and a circular motion on other surfaces. Clean the nails for 15 to 20 strokes. Position the brush so that the bristles clean under the nails. Clean the fingers using 20 strokes for each surface of each finger, including interdigital spaces. Clean the palm and the back of the hand for 20 strokes each, doing the palm first and working around to the back of the hand. Clean the arm using 15 strokes for each surface of each area of the arm. The first area extends from the wrist to 4 or 5 inches below the elbow. The second area extends from 4 or 5 inches below the elbow to 2 inches above the elbow. Scrub all surfaces of the first area before scrubbing the second area. Main-

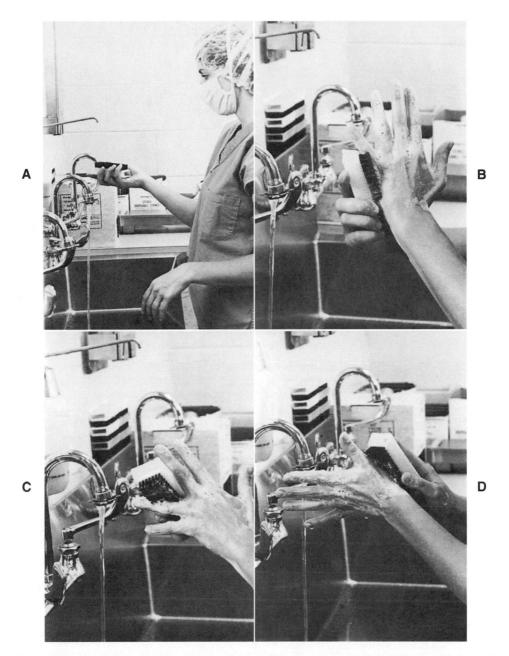

FIG. 2-29   Surgical scrub. **A,** Turn on water and adjust temperature. **B,** After wetting and working up lather, start scrub on little finger. **C,** Scrub each surface of each digit in turn. **D,** Be sure base of thumb is included.   *Continued*

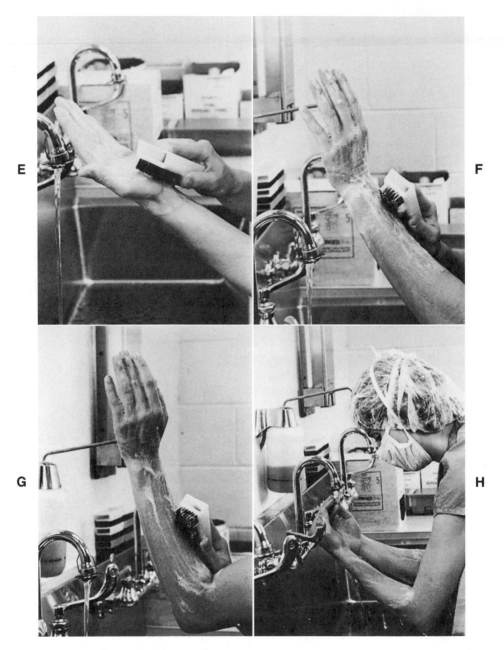

FIG. 2-29, cont'd   **E,** Scrub back of hand and palm. **F,** Scrub forearm. **G,** Continue scrub toward elbow. **H,** Hold hands upright under running water to rinse.

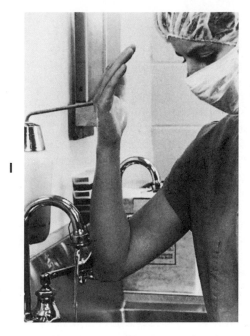

FIG. 2-29, cont'd   **I,** Turn off water using elbow. Once hands are rinsed, do not touch any nonsterile item.

tain a foamy lather while scrubbing, adding cleansing agent and water if necessary to prevent the skin surfaces from drying.

9. If using two brushes, discard the brush by dropping it in the sink and obtain a second brush with the scrubbed hand. If using one brush, rinse it and add a cleansing agent before transferring the brush to the scrubbed hand.

10. Scrub the remaining hand and forearm, repeating the sequence given in step 8 above.

11. Drop the brush into the sink.

12. Holding the hands above the elbows, with the arms over the sink, rinse the hands thoroughly under a stream of water. Do not allow the hands to touch each other.

13. Turn off the water using the elbow, knee, or foot control. If these controls are not available, an assistant should turn off the water.

14. Hold the arms above the sink and the hands above the elbows, to allow water to drain off the elbows and into the sink. Avoid allowing the water to contact clothing.

15. Holding the hands above the elbows with the arms in front of the body and the palms toward the chest, proceed to the gowning area to dry the hands and don the gown and gloves.

Ten-minute scrub
- Perform steps 1 through 10 of the 7-minute scrub. If using one brush, after scrubbing both arms, retain the brush in one hand. If using two brushes, discard the first brush after scrubbing both arms.
- Rinse both arms.
- Add a cleansing agent to the brush.
- Repeat the scrubbing procedure on each hand and forearm as follows. Clean the nails for 10 strokes. Clean the surfaces of the fingers, the palms, the backs of the hands, and the arm areas for 10 strokes on each surface.
- Perform steps 11 through 15 of the 7-minute scrub.

Fifteen-minute scrub
- Perform steps 1 through 10 of the 7-minute scrub.
- Rinse and retain the brush or discard it and obtain a new brush.
- Add a cleansing agent to the brush.
- Repeat the scrubbing procedure on each hand and forearm as given in step 8 of the 7-minute scrub.
- Perform steps 11 through 15 of the 7-minute scrub.

Three-minute scrub. Perform all steps of the 7-minute scrub. In steps 8 and 10, clean the nails for 10 strokes and the fingers, the palms, the backs of the hands, and the arm areas for 5 strokes.

Antiseptic rinse. Some hospitals may add a step to the scrub procedure by requiring the application of an antiseptic agent to the scrubbed surfaces after the excess water has drained and before the hands are dried. The antiseptic can be sprayed on and massaged into the skin, or hands and arms can be dipped in a solution.

The following antiseptics can be used: 70% ethyl alcohol, 50% isopropyl alcohol, or 1:1000 aqueous benzalkonium (Roccal). However, if soap is the cleansing agent used during the scrub, the soap will nullify the effects of the benzalkonium.

Emergency substitute for surgical scrub. In situations in which it is impossible to follow an accepted scrub procedure and surgery must be performed, the following procedure may be substituted only because it is better than no preparation at all.

Perform the general handwashing procedure, if possible prolonging the period during which the lather is rubbed over the skin surfaces. Follow by immersing the hands in an alcohol solution for 1 minute.

Drying hands after the surgical scrub. Sterile towels may be provided in the following ways: two sterile towels in a pack, one sterile towel in a pack, or one sterile towel included in the gown pack.

If one towel is included in the gown pack, the towel should be packed on top of the gown so that it can be removed without disturbing the gown. Sterile towels should be folded in the same way as sterile gowns (accordion pleated) so that it is easy to unfold the towel by picking up only one corner. Packs containing towels, if not opened by nonscrubbed personnel, must be opened before the scrub is begun. When drying hands, the scrubbed person should stand away from the surface holding the open pack. The towel should not be allowed to touch the surfaces of furnishings or to come in contact with clothing. Bending forward slightly will minimize the chances of contaminating the unused portion of the towel as the hands are dried.

Using one towel to dry the hands. When one towel is used to dry the hands, the towel should be mentally divided into four quarters, each strip running across the width of the towel and being one quarter of the length of the towel (Fig. 2-30).

1. Stand away from the surface holding the open towel pack. Lean forward and use the fingers of the right hand to pick up the uppermost corner of the towel.
2. Lift the towel (by the corner only) above the surface of the open pack. Do not shake the towel to open; allow the towel to fall open by gravity.
3. Allow the towel to fall over the fingers and the palm of the right hand.
4. Use the first quarter of the towel to dry the fingers, the palm, and the back of the left hand. Dry each finger separately; be sure that the areas between the fingers are dried.
5. Use the second quarter of the towel to dry the left forearm and the elbow. The left hand and the arm are now dry; the towel is draped over the undried right hand.
6. Use the dried left hand to pick up the towel by the fourth quarter (the end of the towel that is hanging free) and allow the towel to fall over the fingers and the palm of the left hand.
7. Dry the right hand, using the fourth quarter of the towel to dry the fingers and the palm and the third quarter of the towel to dry the forearm and the elbow.
8. Discard the towel and don the gown.

Using two towels to dry hands (Fig. 2-31)
1. Use one towel for each hand.
2. Pick up the first towel with the right hand, allowing the towel to fall over the fingers and the palm of the right hand. Use the entire length of the towel to dry the left hand and arm. Use approximately one third of the towel for the

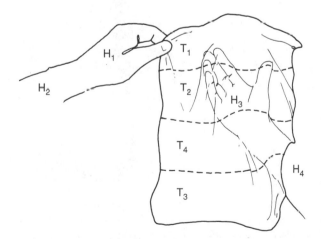

FIG. 2-30 To dry hands using one towel, left hand picks up towel from sterile field and drapes towel over right hand. Use T_1 to dry left hand, T_2 to dry left forearm and elbow. Dried left hand picks up towel at corner of T_3 and dries right hand using T_3, then forearm and elbow using T_4.

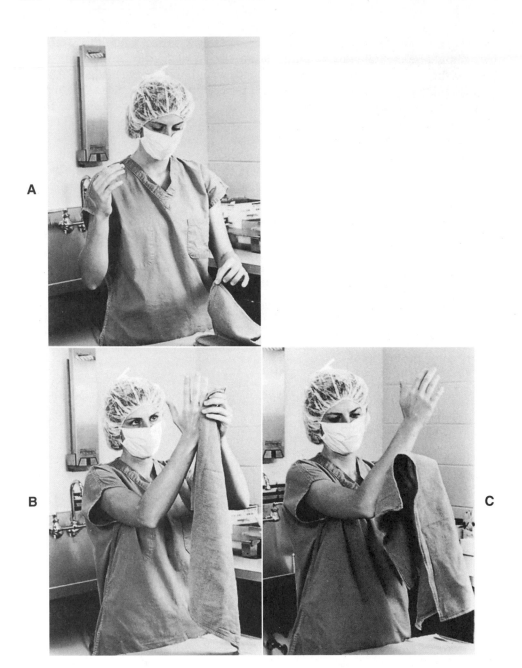

FIG. 2-31   To dry hands using two towels. **A,** Pick up sterile towel by corner. **B,** First third is used to dry hand. Second third is used to dry forearm. **C,** Last third is used to dry elbow area. Discard towel. Use dried hand to pick up second sterile towel and repeat on other hand.

fingers, palm, and back of the hand, one third to dry the forearm, and one third to dry the elbow area. Discard the towel.

3. Pick up the second towel with the dried left hand, allowing the towel to fall over the fingers and the palm of the left hand. Use the entire length of the second towel to dry the right hand and forearm.
4. Discard the second towel and don the gown.

When the hands are dried, the hands or arms should not be allowed to come in contact with each other or any other surfaces. Skin surfaces should be touched by towel only. The section of the towel used for the forearms and elbows should not be allowed to touch the hands. Each area (fingers, palm, wrist) should be dried thoroughly and in sequence; the fingers should not be redried after drying the wrist or forearm.

Gowning. Gowning should be done immediately after the hands are dried, and gloving should be done as soon as the gown has been donned and tied. Nonscrubbed personnel must be available to tie the sterile gown.

The gown is folded for packing and sterilization in such a way that the inside of the gown is outermost and the neck band is on top when the pack is opened. The neck ties should be lying loosely on top of the folded gown, not tucked inside. The inside surfaces of the gown and the ties can be touched while the gown is being donned because they will not be considered sterile once the gown is on and tied.

1. Pick up the gown by the neck ties, holding one in each hand and lifting the top portion of the gown straight up above the open pack surface. The inside surface of the gown should be facing you (Fig. 2-32, *A*).
2. When the neck ties have been lifted to chest level, hold both ties in one hand. Slide the other hand under the portion of the gown still lying on the open pack surface. Lift the gown off the surface and stand back from the counter or the table.
3. Remove the hand holding the lower portion of the gown, allowing the gown to fall open. Use this hand to again hold the neck tie. Avoid shaking the gown open; if folded properly, the gown should open sufficiently to don when held suspended by the neck ties.
4. Drop one neck tie and slide the arm into the corresponding sleeve (Fig. 2-32, *B*), using the hand still holding the tie to pull the sleeve up and over the arm (Fig. 2-32, *C*).
5. Lift the sleeved arm up to support the gown. As the unsleeved arm drops the second neck tie, slide the arm into the second sleeve. The inner surfaces of the gown in the neck and shoulder region can be touched to facilitate the placement of the gown so that the arms can be slid into the sleeves, but the outer surface should not be touched. Nonscrubbed personnel should assist to complete the gowning.
6. Standing behind the person donning the gown, pick up the neck ties and lift the shoulder portions of the gown up and onto the shoulders so that they lie comfortably. If necessary, inside portions of the gown can be touched to aid in the placement of the gown. The person donning the gown should hold the

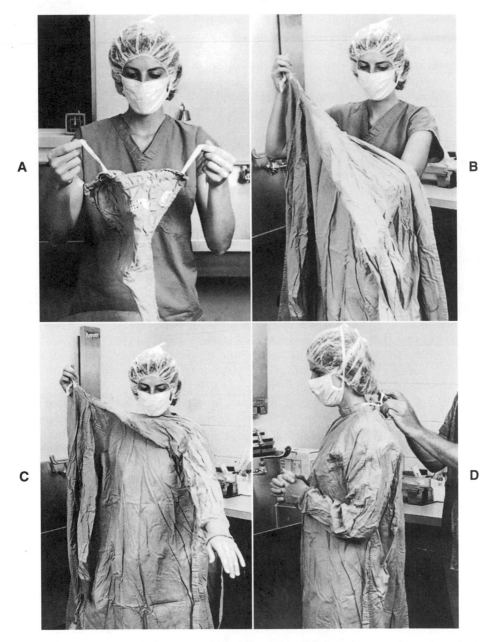

FIG. 2-32   Donning sterile gown with assistance. **A** to **E** show steps in donning and tying gown after scrubbing is complete. Once arms are in sleeves, hands are held at waist level in front of body to avoid accidental contamination. Assistant can adjust gown on shoulders before tying by grasping inner surface of gown in neck and shoulder area.

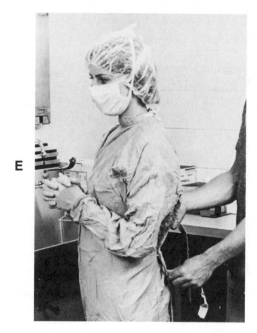

E

FIG. 2-32, cont'd   For legend see preceding page.

hands in front of the chest and above waist level while the gown is positioned and the ties are tied.
7. Tie the neck ties (Fig. 2-32, *D*).
8. Check to determine that the front, the sides, and the back sections of the gown are positioned properly.
9. Tie the waist ties so that the gown is held against the body in the waist region but not so tightly that movement is restricted (Fig. 2-32, *E*).

Gloving. Sterile surgical gloves are commercially available and disposable after each use. Every person who may have to wear gloves should be aware of the size needed to ensure the best fit. Once on the hands, the gloves should fit snugly with no wrinkles. If gloves are too loose, the glove material will slide over the skin, thus interfering with the ability to grasp and manipulate instruments. Gloves that fit well, like a "second skin," produce a slight feeling of pressure or tightness in the novice wearer, and the inexperienced technician may wish to wear a larger size. However, the feeling of tightness will pass, and with a bit of practice, properly gloved hands are capable of the same dexterity as ungloved hands. Gloves in a given size can be purchased in two finger lengths for long and short fingers. Powdered, nonpowdered, latex, and nonlatex gloves are available for those with skin sensitivities.

The outer wrap is opened by nonsterile personnel; if nonsterile personnel are not available, the outer pack wrapping should be opened before the surgical scrub is begun.

Open gloving *(Fig. 2-33)*. This technique of open gloving is *only* used when sterile gloves are worn without a gown. *Always* use closed gloving when wearing a sterile gown.

1. Open the inner wrap of the glove pack (Fig. 2-34, *A*). Gloves should be in the position shown in Fig. 2-34, *B*, with the thumb of each glove uppermost and toward the outer edge of the pack and the cuff of each glove folded toward the palm of the glove. The left glove should be on the left side, the right glove on the right side.

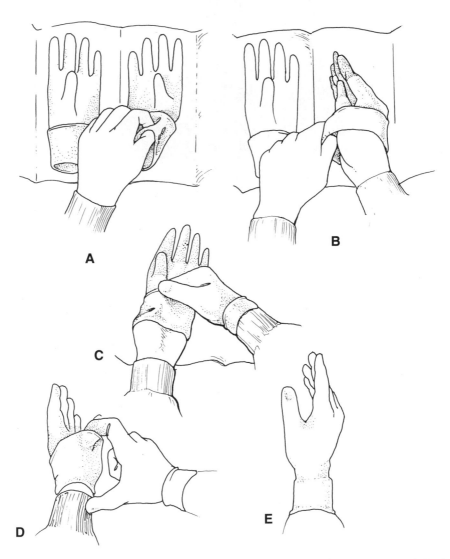

FIG. 2-33   Open gloving. **A** and **B,** Donning right glove. **C** and **D,** Donning left glove. **E,** Gloved hand.

2. Pick up the everted cuff of the right glove with the thumb and forefinger of the left hand, touching only the inner, folded-back surface of the cuff.
3. Holding the glove open with the left hand, slide the right hand into the glove (Fig. 2-34, *C*) pulling the glove over the hand, being sure the thumb of the right hand slides into the thumb of the right glove, until the tips of the fingers reach the start of the glove fingers.
4. Properly position the fingers of the hand to enter the fingers of the glove. Thrust the fingers of the hand to the ends of the glove fingers, using the left hand to pull the glove over the palm of the right hand (Fig. 2-34, *D*).

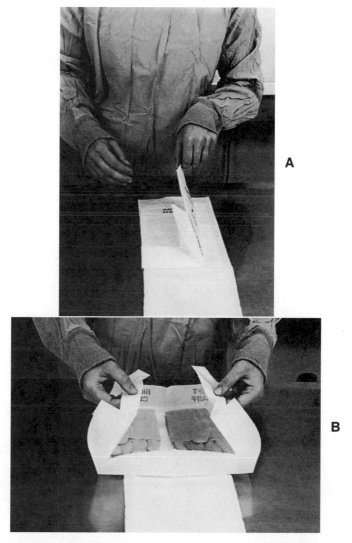

FIG. 2-34   Gloving. **A** and **B**, After donning gown, open glove pack.

Continued

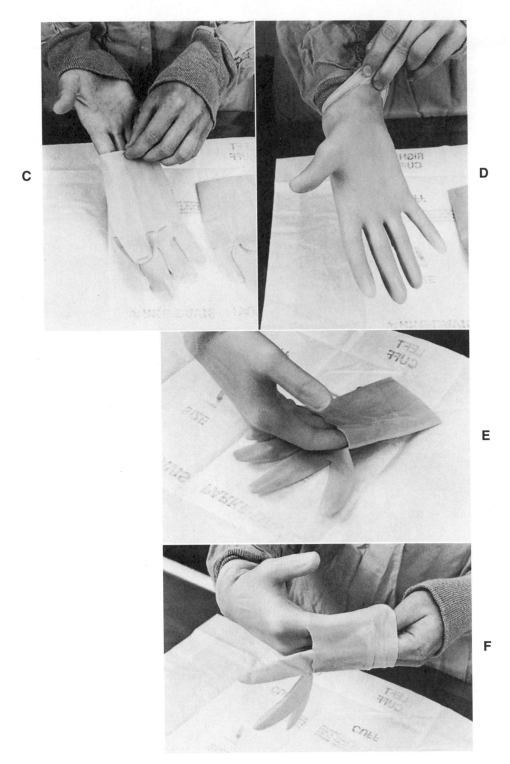

FIG. 2-34, cont'd   C and D, Glove right hand. E and F, Then glove left hand.

5. Use the gloved right hand to pick up the left glove by sliding the gloved fingers into the space between the palm of the left glove and the folded-back cuff (Fig. 2-34, *E*).
6. Lift the gloved right hand up slightly to hold the left glove open while sliding the left hand into the opened glove (Fig. 2-34, *F*).
7. After positioning the fingers and the thumb, thrust the left hand all the way into the left glove, pushing with the right hand to draw the glove over the left palm to the wrist.
8. The fingers of the right gloved hand are still under the folded cuff of the left glove. Using the right fingers, flip the left glove cuff over the left sleeve cuff of the gown to complete gloving the left hand.
9. Insert the gloved finger or fingers of the left hand between the everted cuff and the wrist area surface of the right glove. Flip the glove cuff over the right gown cuff to complete the gloving of the right hand.

NOTE: During the gloving procedure, the ungloved hand touches only the everted, unsterile, inner surface of the gloves; the gloved hand touches only the outer, sterile surface of the glove. As with gowning, be sure that it is clear before beginning the procedure what portion of the item being donned must remain sterile after donning the item and what portions will not be considered sterile after the item is donned.

Closed gloving (Fig. 2-35)

1. The gloves should be opened and placed in the same position as for open gloving. The cuffs of the gown should cover the fingers of the hands.
2. With the cuff covering the fingers and the thumb of the left hand, use the left hand to pick up the right glove by the everted cuff (Fig. 2-35, *A*).
3. Slide the thumb of the right hand (covered by the gown) between the everted cuff and the palm of the right glove (Fig. 2-35, *B*).
4. With the covered left hand, hold the cuff of the right glove while sliding the thumb and the fingers of the right hand into the right glove. As the right hand thrusts into the glove, the right cuff of the gown will be drawn back over the hand to the wrist (Fig. 2-35, *C*).
5. As the fingers of the right hand are moving into the fingers of the right glove, the covered left fingers and thumb are used to pull the cuff of the glove over the cuff of the sleeve of the gown (Fig. 2-35, *D*).
6. Use the gloved right hand to pick up the left glove by sliding the fingers into the space between the palm of the glove and the folded-back cuff.
7. As the left hand is thrust into the left glove, the left gown cuff is drawn back to the wrist of the left arm. The right hand is then used to flip the left glove cuff over the left gown cuff.

After gloving is complete, the hands should be held above the waist and in front of the chest to minimize the chances of contamination while moving to the surgical field.

Capped, masked, scrubbed, gowned, and gloved, the surgeon and/or assistant is ready for surgery. From this point on, the guidelines given later in the chapter on the maintenance of asepsis should be observed to maintain the sterile areas: the gloves and the front of the gown from the waist to the shoulder.

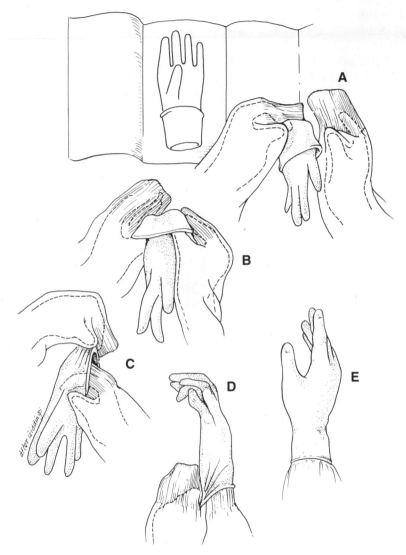

FIG. 2-35 Closed gloving. Closed gloving requires practice because hands must manipulate glove while inside sleeves of gown. **A** to **D,** Donning right glove. **E,** Gloved right hand. Use gloved right hand to pick up left glove, position hands as in **B** and use right gloved hand to aid placement of glove on left hand.

Aseptic Procedure for Personnel Between Surgical Cases

After removing and discarding all surgical attire, the surgeon and assistive personnel should perform a complete surgical scrub as previously described, including replacement with a new cap, mask, shoe covers, sterile gloves, and sterile gown before initiation of a second surgical procedure.

If a surgical procedure is incomplete and the sterile scrubbed surgeon needs to change his or her mask, unsterile assistive personnel can perform the following steps to change the surgeon's mask:

1. The scrubbed person stands away from the surgical area.
2. From behind, the nonscrubbed person unties the lower mask ties and then the upper mask ties of the mask. The mask is lifted over the head of the scrubbed person or moved over to the side and carried back over the shoulder to minimize gown contamination. Care is taken to prevent the mask or its ties from touching the front of the sterile gown.
3. If perspiration and condensed moisture have accumulated on the face, sterile sponges are used to pat the skin dry before replacing the mask.
4. The pleats of the clean mask are pulled to open the mask, and the metal strip is bent to fit over the nose. Holding the mask by the upper ties and working from behind the scrubbed person, the nonscrubbed person positions the mask in front of the face.
5. The upper ties are tied in back of the head behind the ear.
6. The lower ties are tied on the top of the head.
7. The nonscrubbed person checks with the scrubbed person to be sure the mask is positioned comfortably.

■ MAINTENANCE OF ASEPSIS

The preparation for surgery is extensive, as evidenced by the detailed information covered in this chapter. The aim of this extensive preparation is twofold: (1) to provide the surgeon with conditions that will allow for the best possible exercise of surgical skills and (2) to prevent infectious particles from invading the patient and possibly causing an infection that will complicate the patient's recovery from the surgical procedure.

Guidelines have been provided for aseptic preparation in four major areas: the surgical area, the instruments and supplies used during the surgical procedure, the patient, and the personnel directly involved with the surgical procedure. If the efforts in each of the four areas have been consistent with the guidelines, as surgery begins, the related elements will attain the ideal of asepsis as closely as possible. Insofar as possible, the microbial population of the area will have been reduced, lessening the chances of contaminating sterile items.

However, any operating room contains many items that are not sterile, and they, as well as personnel in the operating room, are a source of potentially infectious particles. Conduct in the operating room must be such that the chance of contaminating sterile items is minimized. Sterile items must be maintained in as sterile a condition as possible throughout the surgical procedure.

Rules of Asepsis

The guidelines given here, if they are adhered to, will ensure that the conduct and actions of personnel in the operating room contribute as much as possible to the maintenance of asepsis during the surgical procedure.

- All personnel must know what is sterile and what is nonsterile. Sterile personnel touch only sterile items; nonsterile personnel touch only nonsterile items.

- Sterile items should be grouped together and separated from nonsterile items to lessen the chance of contamination.
- If *any* doubt exists as to whether a specific item is sterile, it must be considered contaminated.
- If contamination occurs, it must be remedied immediately.

The following rules for conduct in the operating room will contribute to the maintenance of asepsis:

- Do not talk unless necessary. Talking increases bacterial contamination.
- Do not shake folded fabric or paper items to open. Allow the item to fall open by gravity. Any increase in air currents contributes to the risk of contamination.
- Restrict body movements to those necessary for the surgical procedure. Arm and hand gestures or any movement increases air currents.
- Do not move around the room or enter and leave the room unless necessary.
- Avoid sneezing and coughing. If a sneeze or cough cannot be avoided, turn your head away from the sterile zone.
- Keep sterile items dry. Moisture increases the risk of contamination.
- Do not leave sterile fields unattended.

The Sterile Zone

The surgical site includes the prepared area of the patient not covered by sterile drapes when surgery begins.

The sterile surgical field includes the surgical site and the sterile drapes surrounding it on the surface of the surgical table.

A sterile field is a surface that has been covered with sterile drapes and is intended to be used as a work area to hold sterile instruments and supplies. When the tray on an instrument stand is covered with sterile drapes, it becomes a sterile field. When a sterile pack is opened, the inner surface of the wrapper, with the exception of a 1-inch border around the edge, becomes a sterile field.

The sterile zone includes the surgical field; the sterile fields used to hold instruments and supplies; the sterile area of scrubbed personnel, including the front of the gown below the shoulders and above the waist and the arms and hands held in front of the gown; and the air space above the surgical and the sterile fields.

Anything below waist level or table level is considered nonsterile and cannot be touched by scrubbed personnel. Anything within the sterile zone can be touched only by scrubbed personnel. Anything outside the sterile zone can be touched only by nonscrubbed personnel.

Scrubbed Personnel and Nonscrubbed Personnel

Any member of the operating team who has completed the preoperative scrubbing, gowning, and gloving procedures is referred to as scrubbed or sterile. All others are nonscrubbed or nonsterile.

Sterile personnel touch only sterile items; nonsterile personnel touch only nonsterile items.

Scrubbed personnel. When scrubbing, gowning, and gloving are complete, the following areas are considered sterile:
- The front of the gown from the shoulders to the waist
- The hands and arms held in front of the gown above the waist and below the shoulders

To maintain asepsis in these areas, the following procedures should be observed:
- Always hold the arms above the waist, below the shoulders, and in front of the gown. Hands may be clasped, but do not fold the arms.
- Do not move around the surgical room; remain close to the surgical field.
- Remain facing the sterile zone.
- When passing a sterile person, move back to back (nonsterile area to nonsterile area).
- When passing a nonsterile person, face away from the nonsterile person to minimize the risk of contamination.
- Do not touch anything below the level of the waist or below the level of the surgical table and instrument stand.
- Do not touch anything in a nonsterile area. Do not lean over or touch a nonsterile area.
- Avoid wetting or dampening surgical attire, if possible. Dampened fabric or paper permits easier passage of contaminants from skin and/or clothing underneath gown.

Nonscrubbed personnel. Nonscrubbed personnel in the surgical room may perform various duties not directly involving the surgical field, such as the operation of monitoring devices and anesthetic equipment and passing sterile items to scrubbed personnel. All nonscrubbed personnel must wash hands thoroughly and don a cap, mask, and shoe covers before entering the operating room.

To contribute to the maintenance of asepsis, nonscrubbed personnel should do the following:
- Follow the general guidelines for conduct in the operating room.
- Stand aside to allow sterile personnel to pass.
- Pass in back of, never in front of, sterile personnel.
- Never pass between sterile personnel and the surgical field.
- Face sterile fields to lessen the risk of accidental contamination.
- Never reach over a sterile field or surgical site.
- Never lean against or lean over sterile areas; never touch sterile fields.

Contamination

Any sterile item or area within the sterile zone that comes in contact with an unsterile item is considered contaminated. Any item outside the sterile zone or a sterile field is considered contaminated. The concept of sterile/contaminated is absolute. An item or area cannot be "almost sterile" or "just a little bit contaminated." If any doubt exists as to whether an item or area is sterile, it must be considered contaminated. Any contaminated items or areas should not be used for the surgical procedure.

While preparing for surgery, if scrubbed personnel become contaminated before surgery begins, the entire process of scrubbing, gowning, and gloving should be repeated.

If pack contents are contaminated during setting up procedures, they should be discarded and replaced. For this reason backup packs should be available.

If contamination occurs during surgery and no sterile replacements are available, it will be necessary to complete surgery using contaminated items, thereby increasing the risk of subsequent infection. To avoid this, before surgery begins the technician should be sure that sufficient replacement supplies are readily accessible. Sterile replacement packs should not be opened until the need for such items occurs. If replacement items are not needed, the packs can then be used for subsequent procedures without having to rewrap and resterilize the pack.

Sterile replacement packs should include the following:
- A gown for each scrubbed person.
- Gloves for each scrubbed person.
- Drapes.
- Towels.
- Gauze sponges.
- An instrument pack duplicating those instruments being used for the surgical procedure, in case of extensive contamination.
- Individual instruments in packs that contain 1 to 4 to a pack. In case one or two items are accidentally contaminated, they can be replaced without having to open a pack containing many instruments, which would require rewrapping and resterilizing.
- A suction tip and connecting tubing for the suction apparatus.

Items such as surgical needles, scalpel blades, suture materials, catheters, needles, and syringes that may be required during surgery but are not in the instrument pack are commercially available in individual sterile packages.

To remedy contamination during surgery, the contaminated item must be removed from the sterile zone or sterile field at once. The contaminated area is then covered with fresh sterile drapes or towels. At the surgeon's discretion, a new sterile field may be created with a new pack of instruments.

Even with all possible care and attention on the part of each member of the operating team, accidental contamination will occasionally occur. If sterile items are available to replace contaminated items, the risk of subsequent infection will be significantly reduced.

AIDS and surgical nursing. The HIV virus does not infect animals other than nonhuman primates. Cautions for health care workers do not generally apply to veterinary personnel, although it is always good practice to protect oneself from direct contact with all animal body fluids. Direct exposure of animal body fluids to mucous membranes or open cuts should be reported to the facility supervisor as a means of overseeing safety practices.

Technicians have no greater risk of exposure to HIV infection than do workers in any other environment. Nonsexual, person-to-person contact does not pose a risk for HIV transmission.

Employers should be aware of the facts regarding HIV and AIDS so they can quell unfounded fears. Employees infected with virus must not be discriminated against, feared, or subjected to any limitations except those that may be imposed on them by their illness.

Sterile Personnel and Nonsterile Items

If the number of available personnel is limited, it may not always be possible to have both a scrubbed and a nonscrubbed assistant. If only one assistant is available and that assistant must scrub, it may become necessary for a scrubbed person to touch a nonsterile item. This can be done by placing a sterile towel over the gloved hand, thus permitting the adjustment of controls on monitoring devices and anesthetic equipment, the repositioning of the surgical table, or the opening of sterile packs.

Items that are dropped on the floor in the surgical area should be gently pushed under the surgical table using a foot. Kicking instruments will damage them. Instruments should not be left where they can be stepped on, which will also damage the instruments, or slipped on, causing personnel to fall. To minimize the chances of dropping instruments or supplies, items should be handled correctly.

Nonsterile Personnel and Sterile Items

Several techniques are available that permit nonscrubbed personnel to transfer items from one sterile field to another without the undue risk of contamination.

The use of these techniques permits initial preparation procedures to be done by nonscrubbed personnel, thus eliminating the necessity for scrubbed personnel to contact nonsterile areas, such as the outer surface of sterile packs. Collectively, these procedures are known as aseptic transfer techniques. For nonsterile personnel to successfully complete the aseptic transfer of an item, the sterile pack holding the item must be opened correctly.

Opening sterile packs. Single-wrap packs are opened by nonscrubbed personnel with the pack either on a flat surface or held in one hand. The inner surface of the wrap then forms a sterile field holding the sterile items. Sterile personnel can use gloved hands to pick up the sterile items from the sterile field; nonsterile personnel must use sterile transfer forceps to transfer the item from a sterile field on a flat surface to another sterile field.

When a double wrap is opened, the outer wrap is opened by a nonscrubbed technician, leaving a single-wrap sterile pack on a sterile field. The inner wrapping is opened by sterile personnel.

Wrapped sterile packs (Fig. 2-36) are opened on a flat surface in the following manner:

1. Stand away from the surface on which the pack is to be opened.
2. Place the sterile pack on a flat surface so that the wrapped edges are uppermost and facing you.
3. Remove the tape and discard it. Be sure the tape indicates that the pack has been sterilized.

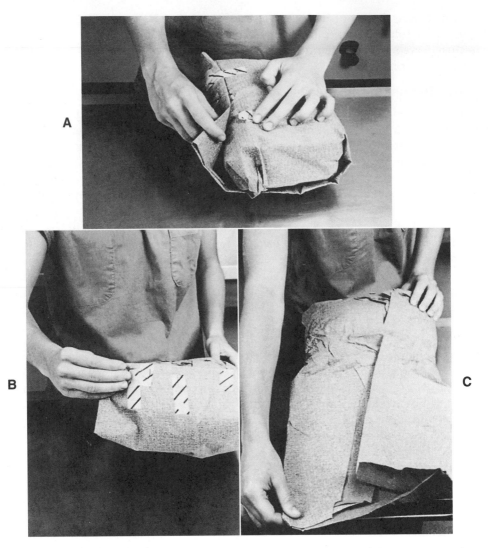

FIG. 2-36   Opening wrapped pack on flat surface. **A,** Break tape seals. **B,** Position pack so that first flap unfolded (last flap folded when pack was wrapped) will be lifted away from person opening pack. **C,** Technician must lean over pack to complete unfolding first flap, but sterile contents are protected by right and left flaps.

4. Open the distal flap first so that your arm will not have to pass over the sterile contents of the pack.
5. Open the right and left flaps, picking up the flaps by the folded-back corners.
6. Open the proximal flap last, lifting by the folded-back corner and drawing the flap toward you.

If the pack is double wrapped, the inner wrap is opened by a scrubbed person.

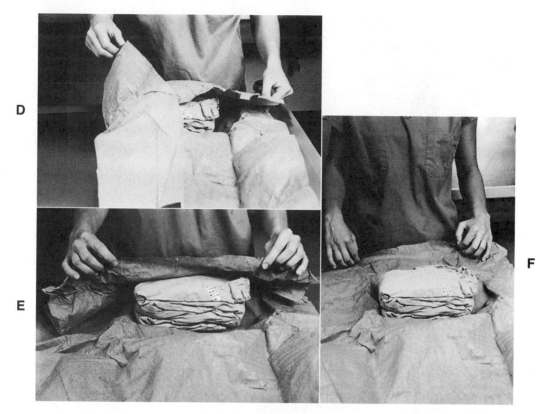

FIG. 2-36, cont'd   D, Open right and left flaps. **E,** Open proximal flap. **F,** Pack contents are exposed, and inner surface of wrap forms sterile field. From this point on, do not lean over field.

Peel-back packs (Fig. 2-37) are opened on a flat surface by using the following procedure:

1. Stand away from the surface on which the pack is to be opened.
2. Place the peel-back pack flat on the surface with the long side of the pack parallel to the surface edge.
3. At one end of the pack, the upper and bottom layers will be separated. Place the fingers of one hand on the inner surface of the exposed bottom paper to hold the pack in place on the surface.
4. Use the fingers of the other hand to peel back the upper wrap in such a way that the hand does not pass over the sterile contents. The inner surface of the bottom wrap forms a sterile field, allowing gloved personnel to pick up items or, for sterile transfer, allowing the forceps to be used to transfer items to the sterile field.

Sterile wrapped packs held in the hand while being opened are held away from the body. The technician should not lean over the sterile pack when opening it.

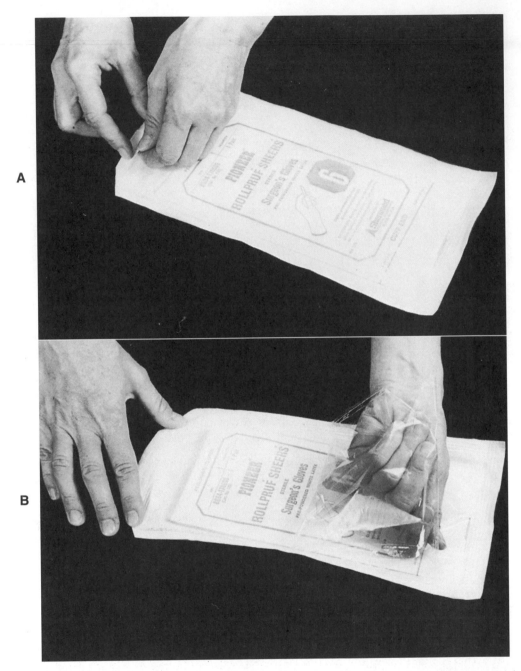

FIG. 2-37   Opening peel-back pack on flat surface. **A,** Hold pack to surface as shown. **B,** Peel back upper layer of wrap as shown.

1. Hold the pack in one hand.
2. Use the other hand to remove the tape from the package, checking to be sure the tape indicates the pack was processed.
3. Use the other hand to lift the first flap back over the arm, allowing the flap to fall on the arm.
4. Use the other hand to open the left and right flaps, allowing the flaps to drape on either side of the hand. Avoid passing the hand over the sterile pack contents.
5. With the first hand grasping the contents of the pack through the wrapping, use the other hand to lift the last flap away from the pack (and your body) and downward. The hand holding the sterile item through the pack wrapping will now be covered by the wrapping of the pack. Once a pack is opened, the sterility indicator strip should be checked for color change, indicating exposure to autoclave steam. If the indicator strip does not indicate exposure to autoclave steam, the instruments should be considered contaminated and not used. Otherwise, the sterile item will be exposed, allowing gloved personnel to lift the item from the sterile inner surface of the wrap (Fig. 2-38).

Peel-back packs (Fig. 2-39) held in the hand while being opened are opened by using the following procedure:

1. Grasp the pack between both hands, holding the pack so that each edge of the peel-back strip at one end of the package is held between the thumb and forefinger of one hand.

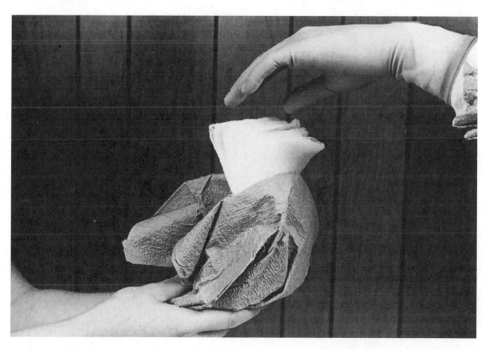

FIG. 2-38   Open pack and hold as shown. Contents can be picked up by gloved hand or dropped on sterile field.

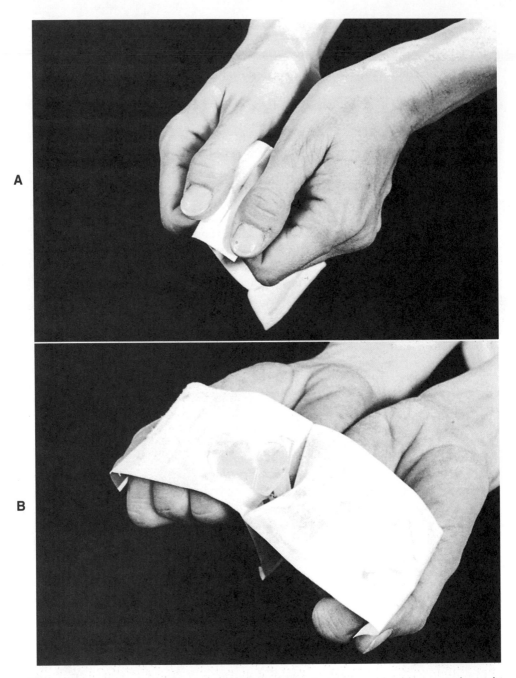

FIG. 2-39   Opening peel-back pack while holding. **A,** Hold peel-back strips as shown between thumb and forefinger of each hand. Item in pack is held between fingers. **B,** Open hands as shown and pack will peel open. Pack contents are held in place by little fingers.

2. Turn the hands outward and downward to peel apart the sealed edges of the package. Do not touch the inner surface of the wrap. Retain your hold on the peel-back strip as the package is opened so that the hands are covered (touching the outer nonsterile surface of the wrap) as the package is opened.

3. Maintain your hold on the item by applying pressure on the wrap material between the edges of the palms and the little fingers, while exposing enough of the item so that it can be easily grasped and withdrawn from the pack by a gloved hand.

Either of the above techniques can be used if the sterile item is to be placed on a sterile field instead of handed to a sterile person.

When the wrapped pack is opened, the hand not holding the contents of the pack can be used to draw the edges of the wrapping up and away from the sterile field on which the sterile item is to be placed. The hand that is covered by the opened wrap and is holding the pack contents can then transfer the item to the sterile field.

Small items in peel-back packs can be placed on sterile fields by opening the pack and turning the hands to face down toward the sterile field. As the pack edges are peeled back, the sterile item is gently flipped onto the sterile field (Fig. 2-40).

Aseptic transfer. The availability of presterilized, individually wrapped disposable instruments and supplies has significantly decreased the need for aseptic trans-

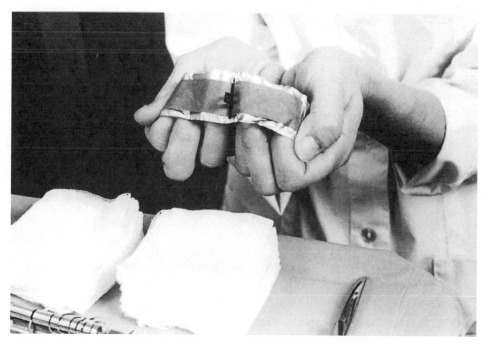

FIG. 2-40 Small items in peel-back packs can be added to the sterile field as shown here. **A,** Stand to the side of field and open pack. **B,** Separate little fingers so pack contents are not held in wrap. **C,** Flip item onto field. Avoid air space over field as much as possible.

Continued

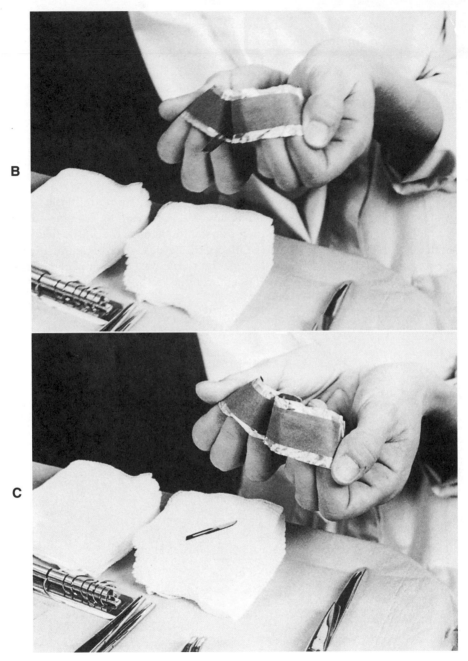

FIG. 2-40, cont'd   For legend see p. 147.

fer within the sterile field. If items from several small packs must be assembled in a particular order on a sterile field by a nonsterile person, the following procedure can be used:

1. Open all packs (including a pack of sterile gloves).
2. Wash and dry hands.
3. Don sterile gloves.
4. Transfer the items to the sterile field.
5. Remove and discard the gloves.

Pouring sterile solutions. Nonsterile personnel pour sterile solutions used during surgery because the caps and outside of the containers are nonsterile and cannot be touched by sterile personnel. Sterile solutions used during surgery should be prepared or purchased in small units. After the bottle is opened and solution is poured from it, the bottle and any remaining contents should be considered nonsterile (Fig. 2-41).

1. Assemble a wrapped sterile basin and the designated sterile solution.
2. Unwrap the sterile basin and hand it to the sterile person, or place it on the sterile field if the scrubbed person is not free to accept it, using the techniques described for opening the sterile pack while holding the pack.
3. The sterile person will hold the basin to one side and level with the sterile field, not over the sterile field.

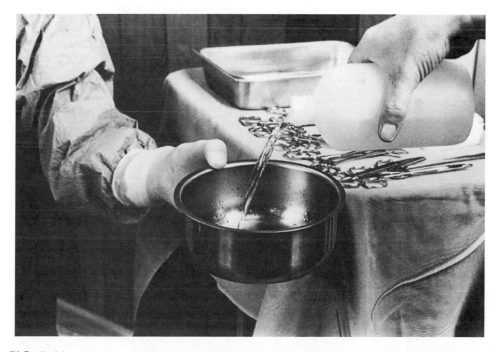

FIG. 2-41   Pouring sterile solutions. Sterile personnel holds bowl to one side of and level with sterile field. Do not allow bottle to touch bowl, but do not hold so high that liquid splashes.

4. Remove the cap from the sterile bottle and retain it in one hand, holding the bottle in the other hand.
5. Pour a small amount of sterile solution into a waste container to clean the rim of the bottle.
6. Hold the mouth of the sterile bottle over the sterile basin. Do not allow the bottle to touch the basin, but do not hold the bottle so high above the basin that splashing occurs when the solution is poured.
7. Pour the designated amount of sterile solution into the sterile basin. Remove the bottle.
8. The sterile person will place the basin of sterile solution in the instrument basin or on the tray in the sterile field so that if the solution splashes or drips as it is used, the drape of the sterile field will not become moistened.

■ THE SURGICAL TEAM: RELATED DUTIES

The surgical team consists of those individuals who have contact with the patient just before surgery, during surgery, and immediately after surgery. The number of team members will vary depending on the size of the practice and the volume of surgery performed. It is rarely practical for a small hospital to employ technicians who will "scrub in" on all routine surgical cases. For this reason, four-handed surgery is the exception in veterinary medicine rather than the rule.

Regardless of the number of members on the surgical team, there are five basic areas of responsibility for every surgical procedure, and the representative duties of each area must be apportioned and performed correctly and efficiently. These basic areas are (1) the preparation of sterile packs and supplies, (2) the induction and monitoring of anesthesia, (3) the surgical preparation of the patient, (4) the preparation and conduct of sterile personnel, and (5) immediate postsurgical care.

The following is a delineation of the duties and responsibilities of the surgical technician for each basic area.

Preparation of sterile packs and supplies
1. Follow the proper procedures of aseptic technique, especially those concerning surgical supplies and instrument care.
2. Clean the instruments and check for any defects.
3. Assemble, wrap, and identify the instrument trays and supply packs.
4. Sterilize the instruments and supplies.
5. Conduct routine tests to verify the proper functioning of the autoclave.
6. Maintain a stock of sterile instruments and supplies and monitor sterilization dates.
7. Check and restock supplies as necessary.
8. Maintain a clean and orderly supply cabinet.
9. Obtain additional instruments and supplies for the surgeon and observe the principles of aseptic technique in handling and passing supplies.

Induction and monitoring of anesthesia
1. Identify the patient and verify the operative procedure.
2. Secure all examination and test results.

3. Know the operation and the functions of the anesthetic machine and monitoring devices.
4. Select and prepare the equipment and the supplies for endotracheal intubation.
5. Recognize and report any unsafe condition of the equipment.
6. Assist with or perform the preanesthetic examination of the patient.
7. Administer preanesthetic drugs as ordered (Fig. 2-42).
8. Restrain the patient for the administration of intravenous anesthetic.
9. Assist with or perform the endotracheal intubation.
10. Attach the animal to the anesthesia machine and regulate gas flows as ordered.
11. Attach the monitoring devices to the patient.
12. Remain with the patient and monitor its condition from induction to emersion.
    a. Record and report vital signs.
    b. Test reflexes to determine the depth of anesthesia.
    c. Check the airway and ensure proper respiratory function.
    d. Extubate the patient when the gag reflex returns.
    e. Report adverse changes in the patient's condition and implement emergency measures as necessary.
13. Confirm the proper function of the intravenous lines and adjust flows as ordered.
14. Clean and restock anesthetic equipment and supplies.
15. Maintain an adequate stock of anesthesia supplies.

Surgical preparation of the patient
1. Select and prepare the equipment and supplies necessary for the presurgical preparation of the patient.
2. Confirm that the patient's urinary bladder and lower bowel are empty.

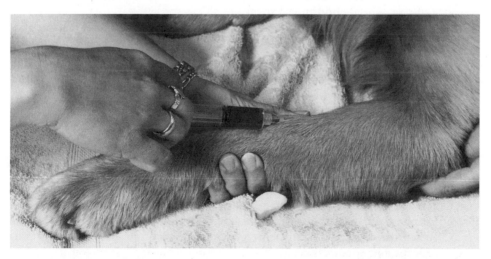

FIG. 2-42   Proper technique for administering intravenous preoperative medications.

3. Perform the presurgical preparation of the skin in accordance with correct practice.
4. Administer intravenous fluids as ordered.
5. Assist with the transfer of the patient to the operating room.
6. Help to position the patient for surgery.
   a. Know the positioning requirements for specific surgical procedures.
   b. Know the use of the operating table and positioning aids.

Preparation and conduct of sterile personnel

1. Have a thorough understanding of the surgical procedure.
2. Identify various instruments, sutures, and needles.
3. Assemble all equipment and supplies necessary for the procedure.
4. Check the order and cleanliness of the operating room. Know and enforce the principles of aseptic technique.
5. Assist in gowning and gloving the surgeon.
6. Perform a surgical scrub of the hands and arms.
7. Correctly don the cap, mask, shoe covers, gown, and gloves.
8. Assist the surgeon with draping.
9. Set up for the surgical procedure.
   a. Prepare linen for draping.
   b. Set up the instrument stand.
   c. Prepare the scalpel, needles, and suture material.
   d. Have a standard sponge count within a surgical pack to facilitate sponge counting after a surgical procedure.
10. Anticipate the surgeon's needs throughout the procedure.
    a. Pass the instruments.
    b. Cut the sutures.
    c. Hold the retractors.
    d. Apply the instruments as ordered.
    e. Sponge or suction the surgical site.
11. Recognize and report any emergency situations and initiate correct action.
12. Save all specimens as ordered.
13. At the end of each procedure, care for all used and unused instruments, supplies, and equipment.
14. Assist with cleaning and preparing the operating room for the next procedure.

Immediate postsurgical care

1. Take the animal to the recovery area and place it in suitable confinement.
2. Monitor and chart vital signs until the recovery period ends.
3. Attach, monitor, and remove intravenous lines, monitoring devices, or oxygen as ordered.
4. Extubate the patient as soon as the gag reflex returns.
5. Recognize and report any emergency states and be prepared to initiate prompt, remedial action.
6. Apply dressings as ordered.

7. Check dressings, casts, and splints and change or adjust as necessary or as ordered.
8. Turn unconscious patients every 10 to 15 minutes to prevent hypostatic congestion.
9. Administer medications as ordered.
10. Check incisions for abnormal drainage or dehiscence.
11. Closely monitor all direct external sources of heat.
12. Keep cages and patients clean and dry.
13. Remove the animal to the medical ward as soon as its condition warrants.
14. Direct the maintenance of the recovery area.
15. Check all equipment for proper functioning and replace stocks of supplies.

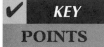

KEY POINTS

1. The adequate maintenance of asepsis in the environment depends on the frequent repetition of cleaning procedures.
2. The operating room should be cleaned daily. Anyone entering the operating room should wear a cap, a mask, shoe covers, and a clean smock or observation gown.
3. One hour before surgery is scheduled to begin, wipe the flat surfaces of furnishings and lights where dust may have settled overnight. A cloth dampened with a disinfectant solution should be used.
4. Between surgeries, put used instruments in cool water and detergent, place all waste materials and soiled linens in the proper containers, and spot clean the floor and surfaces with a disinfectant or alcohol.
5. After a surgical session is completed, follow a set routine for cleaning the operating room and the preparation room.
6. Recovery room maintenance includes two areas of concern, the routine maintenance of the room itself and the routine maintenance of the cages and animals.
7. *Concurrent* (or *continuous*) *disinfection* includes procedures for maintaining a low level of microbes while the animal is in the cage. Terminal disinfection refers to procedures that eliminate residual microbes after the patient has left the facility. It is important to follow procedures labeled for both.
8. Animals that have undergone surgery are more susceptible to infection; animals in the recovery phase may produce copious amounts of extraneous organic material that can be used by opportunists.
9. The treatment room will be subjected to more contamination than other areas.
10. In addition to the daily cleaning, the rooms in the surgical area should be thoroughly cleaned on a weekly basis using specific guidelines.
11. Maintain all equipment according to the manufacturer's instructions and check frequently for deterioration. A file of maintenance manuals should be kept, and a checklist should be established for all equipment.

Continued

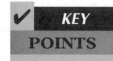
KEY POINTS

12. Factors to be considered when establishing a system for preparing sterile packs include patient safety; the cost, volume, and availability of materials; the availability of staff; and personal preference.

13. The technician preparing sterile packs assumes a twofold responsibility: (1) to follow recommended guidelines and (2) to inspect each item before it is sterilized.

14. A procedure manual for the preparation of packs should be developed and updated as necessary.

15. The ideal wrap should have the following qualities: selective permeability, resistance, flexibility, and memory.

16. Cotton muslin and other cottons can be used as wraps if correct guidelines are followed.

17. Mending textile wraps is not recommended, but a torn or worn wrap can be ripped to a smaller size and the raw edge can be hemmed.

18. Always follow prescribed guidelines in the preparation of packs for sterilization, soaking of instruments, wrapping of items for sterilization, sterilizing fluids, using an autoclave, and storing sterilized items.

19. A sterile pack is considered contaminated if any of the following conditions apply: dampness, broken or loose tape seal, illegible date, punctures or rips, contact with the floor. In the absence of these conditions, sterile packs can be considered sterile for 6 weeks. Storage on open shelves will reduce the safe shelf life to 3 weeks. Items infrequently used should be double wrapped.

20. In remote areas or during times of a natural disaster, if an emergency occurs, use sanitized items whenever possible. Instruments should be washed and rinsed in clean water, if available, and boiled for 20 to 30 minutes or soaked in 70% alcohol for 1 hour if possible.

21. Adhere to these strict guidelines before preparing the patient for surgery, verifying the following: patient's identity, intended procedure, completion of presurgical instructions and examination, any preexisting conditions, current state of vaccine record, risk factors, and the existence of a surgical release form or contract. On completion of examination, the technician will administer preanesthetic drugs.

22. It is the responsibility of the technician to prepare the skin of the surgical site, following prescribed guidelines.

23. Positions for surgery include the dorsal position, the modified dorsal position, the modified reverse dorsal position, the sternal position, and the lateral position.

24. The purpose of draping the patient is to create a sterile area around the surgical site. In veterinary medicine, the surgeon generally drapes the patient.

25. There are two types of draping procedures customarily used in small animal practice: the fenestrated sterile drape and the four-corner drape.

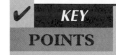

✔ **KEY POINTS**

26. Proper limb draping is essential in orthopedic surgery in which the likelihood of contamination must be kept as minimal as possible.

27. Adhere to the following guidelines for surgical procedures: observe routine hygienic measures and remove all jewelry; use the general handwashing procedures; dispose of waste material as it is produced; minimize traffic to and from the different areas of the surgical suite and keep doors closed; and wear a cap, mask, and shoe covers whenever entering the surgical room, even if surgery is not in progress.

28. Observe the variations of surgical scrubs that require approximately 3, 7, 10 and 15 minutes, as well as specific procedures for using one or two towels to dry the hands.

29. When donning sterile gloves, the outer wrap is opened either by nonsterile personnel or before the surgical scrub is begun. Either open gloving or closed gloving procedures are observed, depending on whether or not a surgical gown is worn.

30. Between surgical cases, scrubbed personnel will remove and discard the mask, gloves, and gowns; perform a short scrub; and don a clean mask and sterile gown and gloves. One must observe the proper changing procedure to maintain asepsis.

31. The aim of the extensive preparation for surgery is twofold: (1) to provide the surgeon with conditions that will allow the best possible exercise of surgical skills and (2) to prevent infectious particles from invading the patient and complicating recovery.

32. Rules of asepsis include the following: knowing what is and is not sterile; grouping sterile items together, keeping them separate from nonsterile items; considering an item contaminated if there are any doubts about its sterility; and remedying contamination immediately.

33. Observe rules contributing to the maintenance of asepsis as they apply to the sterile zone and to scrubbed and nonscrubbed personnel.

34. Observe the correct procedures for opening sterile packs and pouring sterile solutions.

35. Describe the procedure for donning the sterile surgical gown.

36. Five basic areas of responsibility for every surgical procedure are (1) the preparation of sterile packs and supplies, (2) the induction and monitoring of anesthesia, (3) the surgical preparation of the patient, (4) the preparation and conduct of sterile personnel, and (5) immediate postsurgical care.

▼ **REVIEW QUESTIONS**

1. Is mopping just as effective as wet vacuuming? What are the guidelines for cleaning with a mop?

2. In its simplest terms, what are the most basic guidelines for daily maintenance and use of the operating room?

3. What presurgical preparations are done to the clean operating room?

4. What is done to clean the operating room between surgeries?

5. Describe routine cleaning of the operating room after a surgical session.

6. After sterilization of packs and supplies has been completed for the day, what kind of maintenance is done to the pack room?

7. What are two areas of concern in recovery room maintenance?

8. What is the difference between concurrent (or continuous) disinfection and terminal disinfection?

9. Since no surgery takes place in the treatment room, does it require less intense cleaning?

10. Describe weekly cleaning of the surgical room.

▼ REVIEW QUESTIONS—cont'd

11. Describe weekly cleaning of other rooms in the surgical area.

12. What twofold responsibility does the technician assume in preparing sterile packs?

13. Describe the ideal wrap.

14. What basic care is needed for cloth wraps?

15. Identify qualities to keep in mind in selecting material for wraps or drapes.

16. Can textile wraps be mended?

17. Is it all right to use masking tape when sealing paper-wrapped packages?

18. Describe guidelines for the preparation of packs for sterilization.

19. Describe guidelines for soaking instruments.

20. Describe guidelines for wrapping fabric or paper items.

21. When is a sterile pack considered contaminated?

Continued

▼ REVIEW QUESTIONS—cont'd

22. Describe the process of preparing a patient for surgery.

23. How is the patient's skin at the intended surgical site prepared for surgery?

24. What are general rules to remember in positioning surgical patients?

25. What are the most common positions for surgery and when is each used?

26. What is the purpose of draping the patient? What are the two types of draping procedures?

27. Discuss the pros and cons of paper drapes and linen drapes.

28. Describe proper limb draping.

29. What are some overall, general guidelines for personnel in surgical procedures?

30. Describe the general handwashing procedure.

31. Who scrubs in two-handed surgery? in four-handed surgery?

32. What is the required sequence for preparation of surgical personnel?

33. Describe the procedure for donning the sterile surgical gown.

34. What are the minimal rules for scrubbed personnel changing between surgical cases?

35. What is the aim of the extensive preparation for surgery?

36. What are the basic rules of asepsis?

37. When is a sterile item considered contaminated?

38. Name five basic areas of responsibility for every surgical procedure.

ANSWERS FOR CHAPTER 2

1. Wet vacuuming is preferred over mopping for surgical areas; if a mop is used, it should be laundered and dried daily and disinfected between uses if it must be used more than once per day, and a double-bucket technique should be used.

2. The operating room should be cleaned daily. Anyone entering the operating room should wear a cap, mask, and clean smock or observation gown.

3. One hour before surgery is scheduled to begin, wipe the flat surfaces of furnishings and lights where dust may have settled overnight. A cloth dampened with a disinfectant solution should be used.

4. Between surgeries, put used instruments in cool water and detergent, place all waste materials and soiled linens in the proper containers, and spot clean floor and surfaces with a disinfectant or alcohol.

5. After a surgical session is completed, follow a set routine for cleaning the operating room: Put used instruments in cool water and detergent. Place all waste materials and soiled linens in separate bags near the door. Clean waste receptacles and all exposed surfaces with a disinfectant; line receptacles with plastic bags; spot clean as needed. Perform routine maintenance of individual pieces of equipment and check supplies. Roll wheeled equipment through disinfectant. Wet vacuum the floor, after collecting and placing all cleaning supplies near the door. Open the doors and remove the waste bags and cleaning supplies from the room. Wipe light switch and door with disinfectant. Mop floor immediately adjacent to the door and close the doors. Discard cap and mask; dispose of waste bags and soiled linen. Empty and disinfect buckets; clean the mop head.

6. After sterilization of packs and supplies has been completed for the day, the following procedures are accomplished in the pack room. Remove all waste, disinfect the receptacles, and line them with plastic bags; replace materials; collect used scrub basins and trays and scrub with a detergent/disinfectant solution. Clean equipment according to the manufacturer's instructions. Spot clean floor and room surfaces and restock supplies, if necessary. Clean and disinfect the mop head and bucket. Return the cleaning supplies to the storage area.

7. Recovery room maintenance includes two areas of concern, the routine maintenance of the room itself and the routine maintenance of the cages and animals. Only those procedures that directly concern the animals should be performed while the animals are in the room.

8. Concurrent (or continuous) disinfection includes procedures for maintaining a low level of microbes while the animal is in the cage. Terminal disinfection refers to procedures that eliminate residual microbes after the patient has left the facility. It is important to follow procedures labeled for both.

9. The treatment room will be subjected to more contamination than other areas, and the same measures used to clean the other rooms in the surgical area should be used here.

10. In addition to the daily cleaning, the surgical room should be thoroughly cleaned on a weekly basis using the following guidelines: wipe and disinfect the ceiling; dry and wet vacuum; sponge mop the walls; remove outdated sterile packs; change the filters in the ventilation systems; and scrub and disinfect the floors.

11. Weekly cleaning of other rooms in the surgical area should include the following steps: Spot clean the ceilings, disinfect walls, and check supplies. Disinfect shelves, clean refrigerators, and defrost them if needed. Scrub the floors.

12. The technician preparing sterile packs assumes a twofold responsibility: (1) to follow recommended guidelines and (2) to inspect each item before it is sterilized to ensure that the item will function as intended at the time of use.

13. The ideal wrap should have the following qualities: selective permeability, resistance, flexibility, and memory.

14. Cotton muslin and other cottons can be used today as wraps if guidelines are followed. When woven textiles are used, more layers of wrap must be used than when paper wraps are used. Textile wraps must be prepared in predetermined sizes; paper wraps can be cut to the most convenient size for each pack. Each textile wrap must be washed, dried, and inspected for damage before it can be reused.

15. Qualities to keep in mind when selecting material for wraps or drapes are the specific advantages of (a) cottons or crepe-type papers, (b) medium tones of green, gray, or blue, and (c) various thread counts.

16. Mending textile wraps is not recommended.

17. When sealing paper-wrapped packages, do not use ordinary masking tape instead of indicator tape because the adhesive on masking tape will not adhere adequately during steam sterilization.

18. The following guidelines should be followed in the preparation of packs for sterilization: All items to be sterilized must be clean and in good repair. Wrap material and pack sizes must be suitable. For textile wraps, double wraps must be used. Soft items should be folded using the accordion pleat technique. All packs should be wrapped by one method, and the outer wrap should be sealed with tape, labeled, and dated. Sterilization indicator strips and tape must be used.

19. Instruments should be soaked by using the following general guidelines: Open box locks and unlock ratchets as each instrument is gently placed in warm water and detergent. Wash all surfaces with a brush and rinse in clean water twice. With locks and ratchets open, place instruments flat on an absorbent surface to drain. If using instrument milk, follow instructions. Cover the draining instruments with lint-free, absorbent material and blot dry. Check each instrument for its general condition and set aside if repair or replacement is needed. Separate large numbers of instruments into specific types. Place instruments in a covered, dust-free storage area.

20. Fabric or paper items should be wrapped using the following guidelines. All items to be wrapped should be clean, dry, and in good repair. All folding should follow the accordion pleat method. No pack should touch the sides or the top of the autoclave chamber. Items used one at a time should be packaged singly; gauze sponges should be packaged in standardized quantities. The outside of the pack is secured with tape and labeled.

21. A sterile pack is considered contaminated if any of the following conditions apply: dampness, broken or loose tape seal, illegible date, punctures or rips, contact with the floor. In the absence of these conditions, sterile packs can be considered sterile for 6 weeks. Storage on open shelves will reduce the safe shelf life to 3 weeks. Items infrequently used should be double wrapped. If the item is commercially prepared and sterilized, the expiration date set by the manufacturer can be used if the item is stored properly.

22. Before preparing the patient for surgery, verify the following: patient's identity, intended procedure, completion of presurgical instructions and examinations, any preexisting conditions, current state of vaccine record, risk factors, and the existence of a surgical release form or contract. On completion of examination, the technician will administer preanesthetic drugs before the veterinarian gives the general anesthetic. When the animal has been anesthetized, the trachea is intubated, and the animal is secured to the preparation table. Intravenous fluid administration is begun, and monitoring devices are attached before the preparation of the skin.

23. The skin of the surgical site is prepared by using the following steps: Verify the sex of the animal, if applicable, and express the bladder. Clip all hair from prescribed areas and scrub with a surgical scrub preparation with gauze sponges. Apply a germicidal degreasing agent with a sterile sponge in the circular or linear stroke pattern. Transfer the animal to the surgical theater. When the animal has been secured to the operating table, paint the surgical site in a circular or linear stroke pattern with a germicidal agent using a sterile gauze sponge.

24. Surgical patients are positioned only after the anesthetic has been stabilized. Maintain the airway and support the head and neck. The surgical position must allow for the following conditions: maintenance of adequate respiratory function and circulation; exposure and visibility of the operative field; access for the administration and monitoring of anesthetics; and noninterference with monitoring devices and intravenous lines.

25. Positions for surgery include the dorsal position, the modified dorsal position, the modified reverse dorsal position, the sternal position, and the lateral position. The modified reverse dorsal position is used in neck surgery or upper abdominal surgery in large dogs. The sternal position is used for surgery on the dorsal aspect of the body. The lateral position is sometimes used for procedures involving the kidneys, lungs, hips, and extremities.

26. The purpose of draping the patient is to create a sterile area around the surgical site. In veterinary medicine, the surgeon generally drapes the patient. There are two types of draping procedures customarily used in small animal practice. One is the use of a fenestrated sterile drape placed over the entire operating site and secured with towel clips. The second type is the four-corner drape in which four drapes are applied one by one in a clockwise or counterclockwise manner and secured to the patient with towel clips.

27. Disposable materials reduce the possibility of contamination and are cheaper to use because linen drapes must be laundered and sterilized. Many surgeons prefer linen drapes because they are more absorbent, are easier to handle, and conform to the patient's body better than paper drapes.

28. Proper limb draping is essential in orthopedic surgery in which the likelihood of contamination must be kept as minimal as possible. The surgically prepared limb is held or suspended upward by clipping a hemostat or towel clamp to a piece of tape or gauze that has been secured to the foot. A drape is then placed under the suspended leg and secured. The leg is now lowered onto the sterile drape below, and three additional drapes are applied around the limb. As an added precaution, some surgeons apply a sterile stockinette to the entire leg and cut the stockinette at the proposed incision site. The incision is made directly through the drape.

29. Adhere to the following guidelines for surgical procedures: Observe routine hygienic measures and remove all jewelry. Use the general handwashing procedures. Dispose of waste material as it is produced. Minimize traffic to and from the different areas of the surgical suite and keep doors closed. Wear a cap, mask, and shoe covers whenever entering the surgical room, even if surgery is not in progress.

30. The general handwashing procedure should last between 1 and 2 minutes and adhere to the following guidelines: Hold the hands under a stream of warm water in a downward position; clean the nails and apply a cleansing agent to the hands, spreading it from the wrist to the fingertips. Rub the hands together vigorously. Interlace the fingers and move them back and forth. Do not omit the backs of the hands. Rinse, allowing the water to drain from the fingertips. Wash and dry hands twice. Do not allow the hands to touch the faucets. Discard towels after use. Apply a lotion and work in thoroughly.

31. In two-handed surgery, only the surgeon will scrub; in four-handed surgery, the surgeon and an assistant will scrub. The surgeon and the assistant are then referred to as scrubbed or sterile personnel.

32. Follow this sequence during the preparation of surgical personnel: Remove jewelry and change clothing. Don headgear and perform the surgical scrub. Follow the correct procedure for handling masks and eyeglasses. Don a sterile gown and gloves.

33. Ideally, after donning the cap and mask and performing the surgical scrub, the surgical team member enters the surgical room. Nonsterile personnel will have removed the outer wraps of gown and glove packs. The surgical team members will open the inner wrap and don the gown and gloves. If less than ideal conditions exist, this may not be practical. If it is not, the gown and glove packs are opened close to the scrub sink. Scrubbed personnel don the gown and gloves and move immediately to the surgical room or the area of the room where surgery is performed. For a detailed description of the process for donning a gown, see the text, pages 129 to 131. After the gown is tied, gloves should be donned immediately.

34. Ideally, between surgical cases, scrubbed personnel will remove and discard the mask, gloves, and gowns; perform a short scrub; and don a clean mask and sterile gown and gloves. If this is not possible, then at least masks and gloves should be changed between cases. Observe the proper changing procedure.

35. The aim of the extensive preparation for surgery is twofold: (1) to provide the surgeon with conditions that will allow for the best possible exercise of surgical skills and (2) to prevent infectious particles from invading the patient and complicating recovery.

36. Rules of asepsis include the following: knowing what is and is not sterile; grouping sterile items together, separate from nonsterile items; considering an item contaminated if there are any doubts about its sterility; and remedying contamination immediately.

37. Any sterile item or area within the sterile zone that comes in contact with an unsterile item is considered contaminated.

38. Five basic areas of responsibility for every surgical procedure are (1) the preparation of sterile packs and supplies, (2) the induction and monitoring of anesthesia, (3) the surgical preparation of the patient, (4) the preparation and conduct of sterile personnel, and (5) immediate postsurgical care.

SELECTED READINGS

Davey JG: Discovering nursing students' understandings about aseptic technique, *International Journal of Nursing Practice*, 105(6), 1997.

DeLaune SC, Ladner PK: *Fundamentals of nursing standards & practice,* Boston, 1998, Delmar Publishing Co.

Doebbeling BN, Stanley GL: Comparative efficacy of alternative hand-washing agents in reducing nosocomial infections in intensive care units, *New England Journal of Medicine,* 88(6), 1992.

Fox NJ: Space, sterility and surgery: circuits of hygiene in the operating theatre, *Social Science and Medicine,* 649(9), 1997.

Kozier B, Erb G, Blais K, Wilkinson JM: *Fundamentals of nursing: concepts, process, and practices,* Reading, Pa, 1995, Addison-Wesley.

Maki DG, Ringer M: Prospective randomised trial of povidone-iodine, alcohol, and chlorhexidine for prevention of infection associated with central venous and arterial catheters, *Lancet,* (339)5, 1991.

O'Neale M: Clinical issues: sterile sleeves; weight and size of surgical instrument sets; aseptic technique; product evaluation committees, *AORN Journal,* 242, 245, 1998.

Rahn R, Schneider S: Preventing post-treatment bacteremia: comparing topical povidone-iodine and chlorhexidine, *Journal of the American Dental Association,* 1145(3), 1995.

Skin disinfection methods compared, *Australian Nursing Journal,* 19, 1996.

Smeltzer SC, Bare BG: *Medical surgical nursing,* New York, 1992, JB Lippincott Co.

Stein P: Aseptic technique: covering all the bases . . . an inservice in our operating room, *Nursing Management,* 64F, 1994.

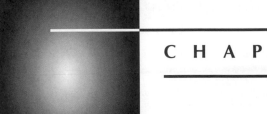

C H A P T E R **3**

The Surgical Area
Design, Equipment, and Instrumentation

PERFORMANCE OBJECTIVES

After completion of this chapter the student will:

Discuss how the design and maintenance of a surgical area ensures patient safety by preventing cross-contamination.

Name the basic equipment used in each room of the surgical area.

List the guidelines for conduct to be observed in the operating room to prevent fire and explosion.

Identify selected surgical instruments.

Describe the function of selected surgical instruments, equipment, and supplies.

Recognize several types and sizes of absorbable and nonabsorbable sutures.

Select instruments for inclusion in basic instrument packs.

Apply the knowledge of the care and handling of surgical instruments and supplies to the performance of the duties of a surgical technician.

◼ PHYSICAL DESIGN OF SURGICAL AREA AND BASIC EQUIPMENT

The size and complexity of the surgical area in the small animal hospital are determined by the existing available space and the volume of surgery performed in the practice. Ideally, the surgical area includes a preparation room, a pack room, a recovery room, a treatment room, and an operating room. If space and personnel are limited, it may be impossible to designate separate rooms for each of these functions. Nevertheless, the design of the surgical area should be such that patient safety is ensured by preventing cross-contamination during surgical procedures. In addition, the layout of the surgical area must allow for the ease of sanitation and the efficient functioning of surgical personnel.

Preparation Room (Fig. 3-1)

The preparation room should be separate from the operating room and should house the equipment and supplies required to prepare the surgeon, the surgical as-

164

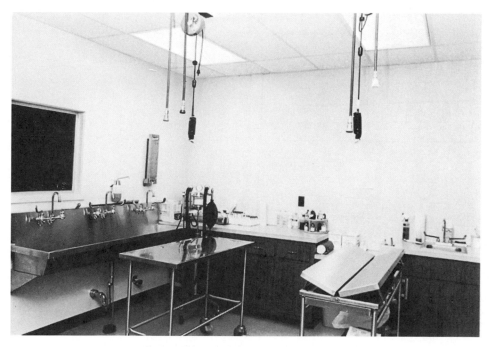

FIG. 3-1   Surgical preparation area.

sistants, and the patient. It may be correctly argued that the proper surgical preparation of the surgeon and the patient should take place in separate areas. Because of space considerations this is rarely practical, and the following description assumes that both functions are carried out apart from one another but in the same location.

Basic equipment

Surgeon's scrub sink. A deep sink fitted with elbow-, knee-, or foot-operated hot and cold water flow. Over or near the sink is a foot-operated surgical scrub solution dispenser and a timer to ensure an adequate scrub time.

Patient preparation surface. A table, a mobile preparation cart, or a preparation tub fitted with a rack used to prepare the patient for surgery (Fig. 3-2).

Wet/dry vacuum cleaner. Used to remove hair as it is clipped from the patient during the presurgical preparation.

Small animal clipper fitted with no. 40 surgical preparation blade. Used as part of the surgical preparation of the patient for the removal of hair. It is convenient to have the clipper retract into a reel that is secured to the ceiling over the preparation area. The use of the clipper reel reduces the possibility of dropping the implement, which could fracture the case and the blade teeth. Broken teeth cause abrasions and small cuts on the skin of the surgical site that may become heavily colonized with bacteria, adversely affecting the healing process.

Refrigerator. Used to store biologicals and fluids that may be required before and during the procedure.

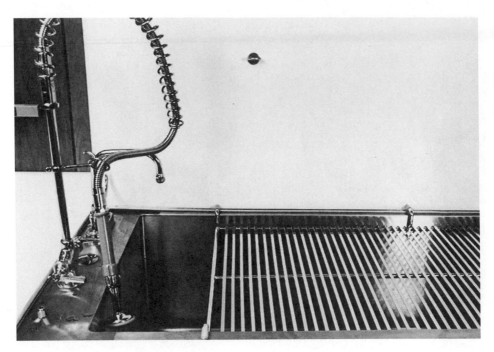

FIG. 3-2   Surgical preparation tub with rack.

Supply locker (Fig. 3-3). Used to store extra gloves, gowns, instruments, drugs, and surgical supplies. An open locker provides an instant visual display of items, which is essential in an emergency and useful in taking an inventory.

Anesthesia machine. Anesthetic induction usually takes place in the preparation area. Some hospitals maintain a machine in the preparation room and another in the operating room so that a patient can be anesthetized and prepared while a surgical procedure is being performed. Also, traffic flow is minimized if the technicians are not required to push machines in and out of the operating room.

Endotracheal intubation equipment. Tracheal tubes, laryngoscopes, and all other intubation equipment should be stored in one convenient, uniform location in the preparation room. It is the responsibility of the surgical technician to maintain intubation equipment and to verify that tubes are clean and free of holes and that laryngoscopes are functioning.

Intravenous fluid administration equipment. Some hospitals administer intravenous fluids routinely to all surgical patients, and some reserve this treatment for cases in which the animal's condition is poor or when the surgical procedure will be lengthy. In any case, the intravenous poles, needles, catheters, administration sets, and fluids, including whole blood and plasma, should be stored as close to the operating room as possible. The preparation room is convenient because the routine administration of fluids can be accomplished as soon as the patient is anesthetized. During an emergency, the surgical team must receive a prompt response to an order for fluids or blood.

Large waste receptacle with liner.

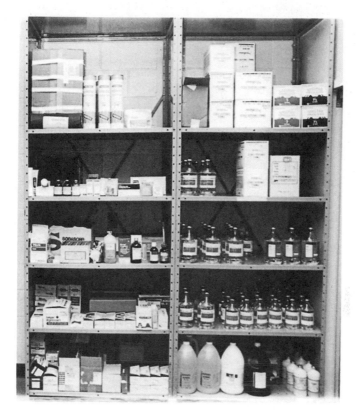

FIG. 3-3   Surgical supply locker.

Pack Room (Fig. 3-4)

The pack room contains the equipment and supplies necessary to clean, assemble, wrap, and sterilize surgical instruments and supplies.

Basic equipment
Sterilizing unit (moist heat or gas)
Washer and dryer
Ultrasonic instrument cleaner
Sink
Counter space or large table for folding linens
Linen receptacle
Sterile and nonsterile supply closets
Waste receptacle with liner

Patient Recovery Room (Fig. 3-5)

The recovery area should be a warm, quiet room conveniently located to ensure that recovering animals receive adequate attention. The length of time patients will remain in recovery is determined by their level of consciousness and the adequate stabilization of their vital signs.

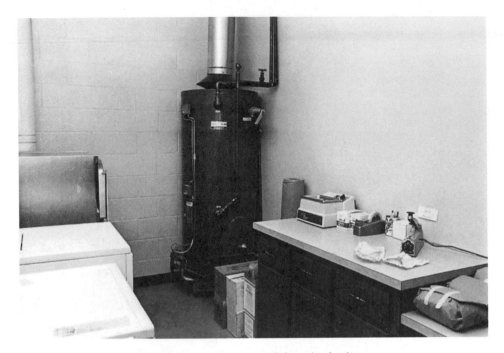

FIG. 3-4   Pack room with laundry facilities.

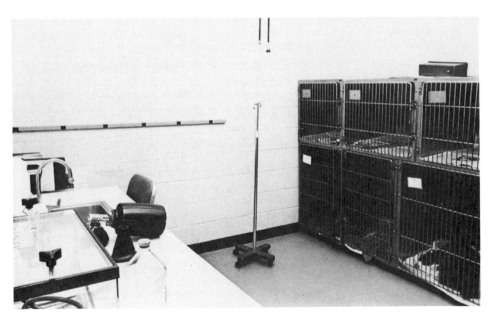

FIG. 3-5   Postsurgical recovery area.

Basic equipment

Recovery cages (padded to prevent injury if the recovery is stormy)
Monitoring equipment (Fig. 3-6)
Therapeutic oxygen administration equipment (Fig. 3-7)
Emergency drug closet and/or crash kit (Fig. 3-8)
Intravenous fluid administration supplies (Fig. 3-9)

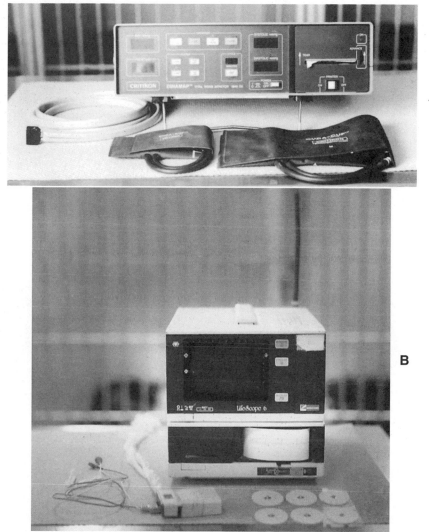

A

B

FIG. 3-6   Monitors used to record vital signs, such as systolic and diastolic blood pressure, mean arterial pressure, and heart rate rhythm and character. (Courtesy Angell Memorial Animal Hospital.)

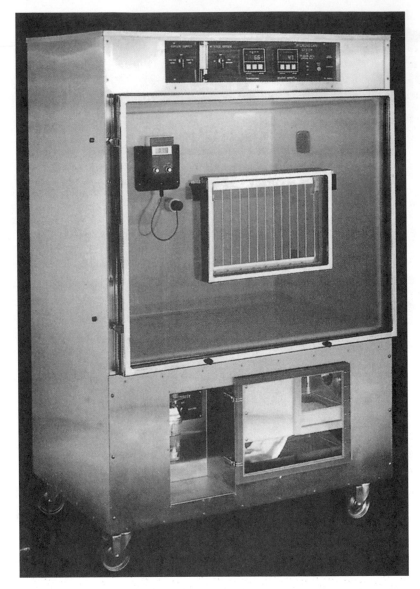

FIG. 3-7   A self-contained life-support system that regulates temperature, humidity, and oxygen levels.

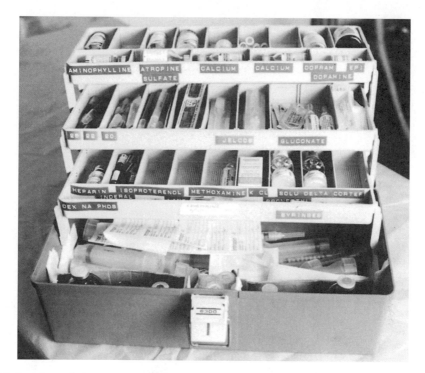

FIG. 3-8   A crash kit containing drugs and supplies for emergency use. (Courtesy Angell Memorial Animal Hospital.)

Rewarming pads and supplies (Fig. 3-10)
Incubator (for young or tiny animals)
Supply closet (for dressings, towels, and blankets)
Waste receptacle with liner

Treatment Room (Fig. 3-11)

The treatment room is reserved for noninvasive surgical procedures such as dental procedures, and the care of minor lacerations and abscesses. More severe lacerations may require sterile surgery.

Basic equipment

Treatment table
Anesthesia machine and monitoring devices
Electrosurgical unit (uses a spark gap between a metal point and tissue to "burn" off certain types of growths)
Ultrasonic dental scaler and manual dental instruments (Fig. 3-12; see also Figs. 3-74 to 3-77)
Supply locker
Small refrigerator
Radiograph viewer

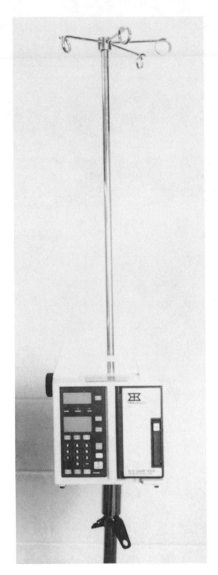

FIG. 3-9   A microprocessor-controlled, volumetric (ml/hr), peristaltic infusion pump. This unit will drip all fluids including blood. (Courtesy Angell Memorial Animal Hospital.)

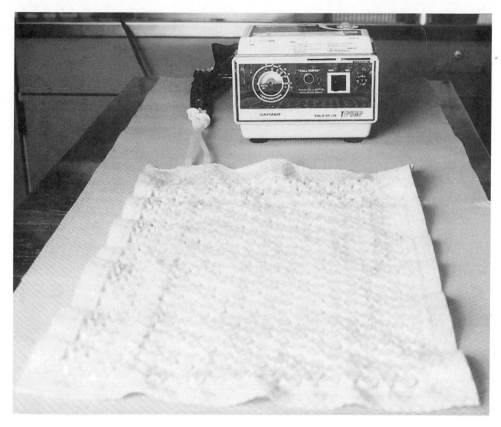

FIG. 3-10   A surgical warming pad, which uses water at a preset temperature. (Courtesy Angell Memorial Animal Hospital.)

Clipper and reel
Large sink
Cold sterilization trays
Collections of assorted instruments
Endoscopy unit (fiber optics scope) (Figs. 3-13 and 3-14)

Veterinary ultrasonography. Ultrasonography employs a special function called the Doppler effect, which is described as the relationship of the apparent frequency of sound, light, or radio waves to the relative motion of the source of the waves and the observer. The frequency increases as the two approach each other and decreases as they move apart. This effect can be experienced when a car horn makes a continuous sound as it approaches and falls in pitch as it passes by.

Diagnostic ultrasound equipment uses high-frequency sound waves to give information about the position, shape, and internal texture of body tissues. The information gained is unique and unlike that obtained by radiography. Radiographs

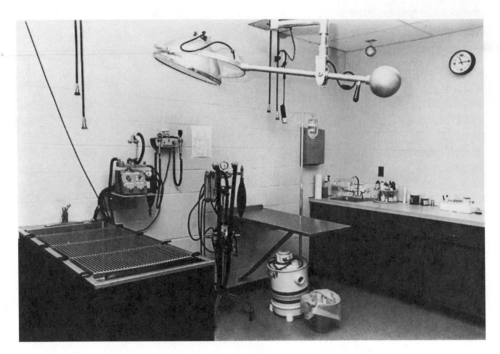

FIG. 3-11   Treatment room for nonsterile procedures.

cannot distinguish between fluid and soft tissue and cannot distinguish textures of soft tissue organs. Ultrasonography allows differentiation of solid from cystic structures (e.g., renal cyst from tumor) and recognition of fine textural abnormalities within an organ (e.g., metastatic neoplasia). Real-time ultrasound enables us to evaluate motion, such as in cardiac motility and fetal viability studies. With a specialized ultrasound function called Doppler ultrasonography, the rate and quality of blood flow to detect vascular stenoses, flow turbulence, and cardiac valvular dysfunction can be evaluated. This is particularly important in cardiovascular studies and in evaluation of renal blood flow in transplant patients. The latest ultrasound technology includes color Doppler ultrasonography, which consists of overlaying standard Doppler information in a color map, over a real-time gray-scale image (Fig. 3-15).

The major benefits of ultrasonography over other imaging modalities are speed, safety, cost, versatility, and acquisition of unique patient information. Ultrasound (US) examinations are safe because no ionizing radiation is used; veterinary patients are usually awake or only slightly sedated; and (with the exception of US-guided biopsy) the procedure is noninvasive. This makes ultrasonography particularly attractive to veterinary clients. Compared with an abdominal exploratory surgery or selective cardiac angiography, a US examination is not only safer and faster, but also significantly less costly to the client.

Many large facilities now use computed axial tomography (CAT) scans, which use radiation to produce an image as a diagnostic tool. (See Fig. 3-17).

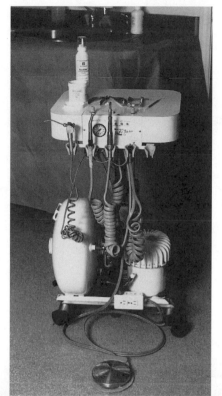

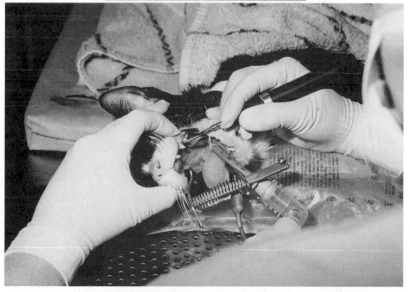

FIG. 3-12   A, A veterinary dentistry unit. **B,** Technician uses scaler to remove tartar from a cat's teeth. Note placement of mouth speculum.

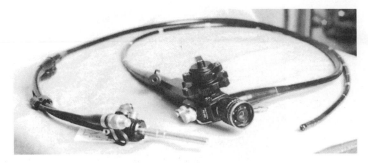

FIG. 3-13   A fiber optics scope enables the practitioner to visualize and treat patient structures in a less invasive and traumatic manner than conventional surgery. (Courtesy Angell Memorial Animal Hospital.)

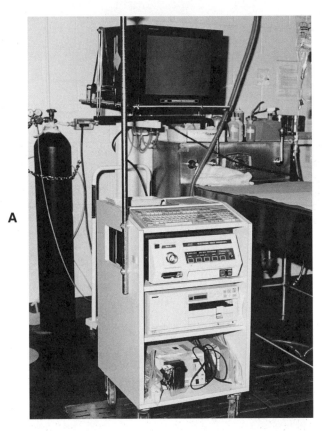

FIG. 3-14   **A,** An endoscopy unit.

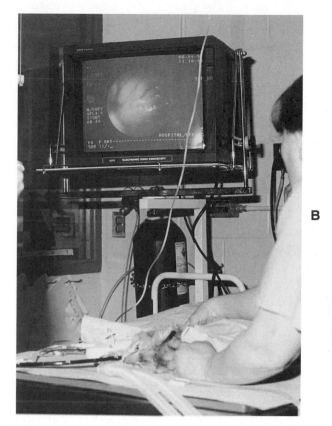

B

FIG. 3-14, cont'd   B, In this case a fiber optics scope (Fig. 3-13) has been passed into the esophagus of a cat suspected of having a foreign body. The architecture of the stomach is projected and enlarged onto a screen for diagnostic viewing.

Operating Room (Fig. 3-16)

To ensure patient safety, the operating room is separated from other hospital functions. The following regulations are observed in the design and use of an operating theater:

- All materials used in the construction of exposed surfaces are nonporous and impervious to harsh cleaning agents.
- There is a maximum of two doors leading into the operating room. Two-way swinging doors allow the free passage of sterile personnel without the use of hands and arms. Doors are opened and closed as infrequently as possible to reduce air currents.
- Air pressure in the operating room is maintained at a higher level than in adjacent rooms to reduce the movement of airborne bacteria. The room ventilators are equipped with air filters to remove bacteria from the air.
- Maintenance equipment used to clean the operating room is not used in other areas of the hospital.

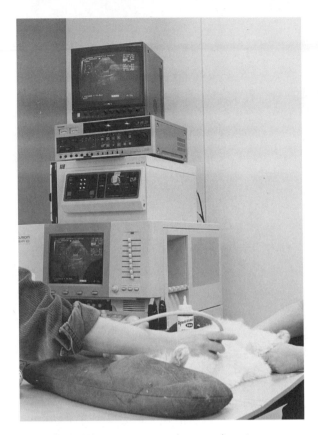

FIG. 3-15   Diagnostic ultrasound equipment.

- When entering the operating room at any time, all personnel wear a cap, a mask, shoe covers, and a freshly laundered uniform or scrub suit. Street clothes are unacceptable.
- Surgical personnel must know sterile and nonsterile boundaries and adhere to the principles of aseptic technique.

Fire hazards in the operating room. Although most anesthetics used in veterinary surgery are nonflammable and nonexplosive, the technician should be aware of the present dangers of fire, explosion, and electrical hazards. Fires and explosions can occur if a flammable agent exists in the presence of oxygen and is ignited by a source such as static electricity or an electrical spark. The following considerations regarding fire hazards govern conduct in the operating room:

- All anesthetics are considered dangerous even if they are nonflammable and nonexplosive. They are stored and used at least 3 feet away from electrical equipment.
- Operating room flooring, castors, and wheels are made of material that is conductive, that is, capable of dispersing static electricity.

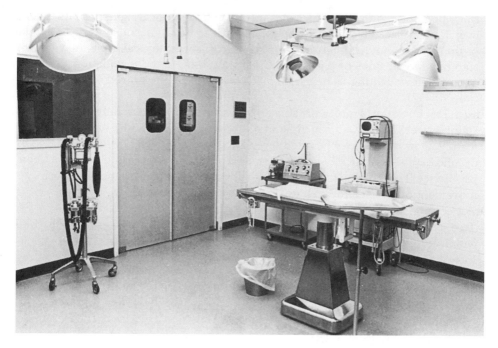

FIG. 3-16   Operating room.

- Operating room clothing is made of cotton or some other antistatic material. Wool, nylon, and most synthetic fabrics generate static electricity.
- Hair and fur produce static electricity and are covered with drapes, towels, or caps.
- Fire extinguishers are readily available and in working order.
- All electrical equipment is routinely checked, and any pieces that are defective or have frayed cords are removed. Electrical devices are always turned off before being plugged in to prevent contact sparking. Grounding is essential for electrocautery and defibrillator units.
- Most plastics are highly flammable and are not used in the operating room without special precautions.
- Explosive or flammable cleaning agents are not used in the operating room.
- Smoking is not allowed in or near the operating room.
- Humidity in the operating room is maintained at 50% or above to reduce static electricity.

Basic equipment
Surgical spotlights. Surgical lights are designed to provide intense illumination of a relatively small area while expending a minimum amount of heat. The type and size of the lighting unit are determined by the kind and amount of surgery performed, the size of the room, and the personal preference of the surgeon. Caution

must be exercised in the choice and installation of surgical lights. Lights that are oversized or placed too near the operating site can cause thermal burns on the skin of the patient and overheat the surgical instruments. Surgical lights may be free-standing mobile units or permanent floor or wall-mounted installations. Intensity controls allow lighting to be varied, and the lights can be moved in several directions.

Surgical table. Surgical tables suitable for veterinary use are generally constructed of stainless steel and have a tilt-top and a foot-operated hydraulic base. The tilt-top feature allows the table to be tilted several degrees vertically. The foot-operated hydraulic base allows the tabletop to be raised or lowered according to the surgeon's preference. The tabletop is fixed to the base with a screw bolt that allows horizontal movement of the tabletop in a full circle when the bolt is released.

Other equipment

Temperature-controlled heating pad to aid in body heat retention (see Fig. 3-10)

Monitoring devices (see Fig. 3-6)

Intravenous drip stand (see Fig. 3-9)

Instrument tray (instrument stand) (see Fig. 3-99)

Back table or counter

Suction equipment to remove fluid accumulations from the surgical site (see Fig. 3-108)

Defibrillator unit (Fig. 3-18)

Radiograph viewer

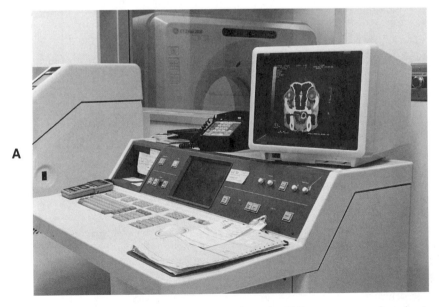

FIG. 3-17   **A,** A computerized axial tomography unit. CAT scans are produced using radiation in which a three-dimensional image of a body structure is constructed by a computer from a series of plane cross-sectional images made along an axis.

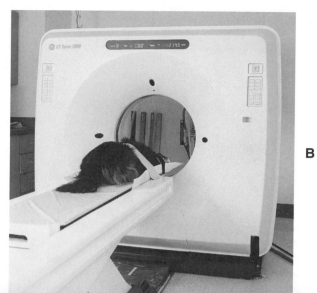

B

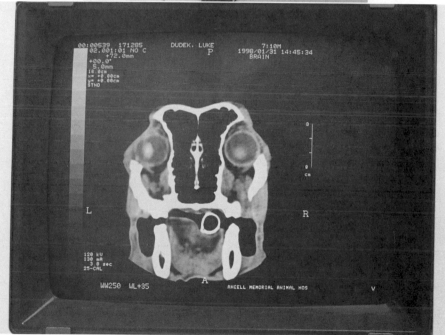

C

FIG. 3-17, cont'd   B, The patient is sedated and restrained on the bed of the unit. The operator controls the process from the computer station in **A. C,** Close-up of the three-dimensional image of the dog's skull projected onto the monitor.

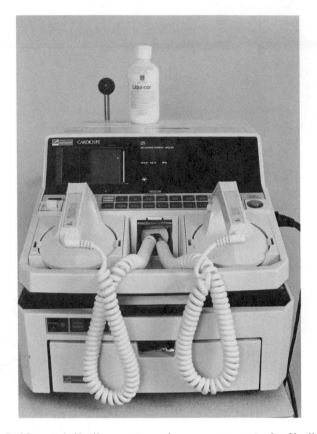

FIG. 3-18   A defibrillator unit used to convert ventricular fibrillation.

Anesthetic machine
Electrosurgical and coagulation unit (Fig. 3-19, *B*)
Table lift and scale (Fig. 3-20)
Positioning devices
Waste receptacle with liner
Wall clock

■ SURGICAL INSTRUMENTS

Early surgical instruments were borrowed or fashioned from the tools of butchers, carpenters, tailors, and blacksmiths. The development of reliable anesthetic agents for use in human and animal surgery provided an impetus for the advancement of the surgical art. As surgical procedures were expanded and refined, instrument design evolved to accommodate the differences in tissues and the demands of specific procedures. There are thousands of different surgical instruments currently available. The instruments illustrated in this chapter are some that are commonly encountered in veterinary practice.

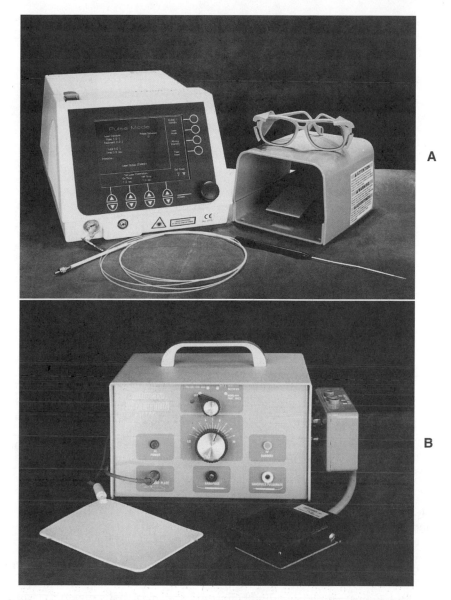

FIG. 3-19 **A,** A surgical unit that uses a laser beam to excise tissue. **B,** An electrosurgery unit.

Instrument Manufacture

The manufacture of surgical instruments begins with the selection of the metal. The most commonly used material is stainless steel, which is an alloy of iron, chromium, silicon, manganese, nickel, molybdenum, sulfur, phosphorus, and titanium. There are two basic compound types: martensitic and austenitic. The former is generally referred to as hardenable stainless steel and has a high-carbon and low-

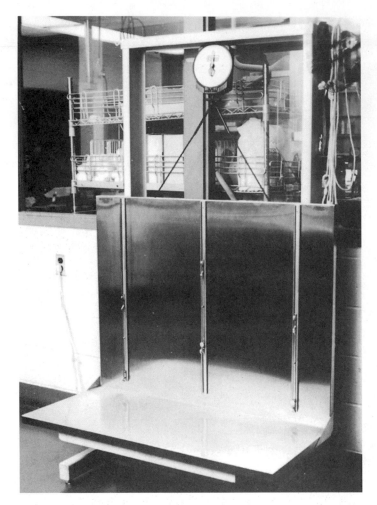

FIG. 3-20   An automatic table lift and scale make surgical preparation easier on the technician and patient. (Courtesy Angell Memorial Animal Hospital.)

chromium content, rendering it very strong, highly magnetic, and susceptible to corrosion.

Martensitic instruments are highly finished and are usually plated to reduce corrosion. Thumb forceps, hemostats, retractors, cutting edge instruments, needle holders, and some orthopedic instruments are examples of instruments made of this type of stainless steel. The technician must be aware of its tendency to corrode if not correctly cleaned, dried, and sterilized.

Austenitic stainless steel is compounded mainly of chromium and nickel. This steel has high tensile strength (the resistance of a material to longitudinal stress) and is very resistant to corrosion. Surgical implants, pans, bowls, handles, and trays are examples of this type of stainless steel. The degree of hardness is achieved by subjecting the alloy to varying degrees of heat.

The next step is the polishing of the metal to a dull finish that will reduce the light reflection from the surgical lamps. The final step in the manufacturing process is passivation, which consists of bathing the instrument in a nitric acid bath. This process clears the metal of foreign matter and debris, aids in the formation of chromium oxides, and produces a corrosion-resistant "skin." The protective quality of the surface can be seriously altered by scrubbing or scraping the instruments with abrasive cleaners, steel wool, or hard objects.

Cutting Instruments

Scalpel blades and handles. To be of value for surgical application, a scalpel blade must be sterile, extremely sharp, and available in several sizes and shapes. To satisfy these requirements, most surgeons prefer to use presterilized, disposable scalpel blades that are affixed to a handle, which may be made of disposable plastic or reusable stainless steel. In small animal surgery, the no. 3 and, less often, the no. 4 handles are used. Some surgeons prefer a one-piece hard-backed blade and handle unit. This scalpel is less frequently encountered because the blade must be expertly sharpened and different blade sizes cannot be interchanged. Ophthalmic surgery and microsurgery demand a long, thin, tapered or rounded handle fitted with small disposable blades. Also used in ophthalmic surgery is a microsurgical device that uses a laser for cataract extractions (Fig. 3-19, *A*).

Scalpel blades are made of carbon steel or stainless steel and are used for incising the skin and transecting tissue. The scalpel is held by the fingers and thumb, and the index finger is extended along the top of the instrument (Fig. 3-21).

The following list indicates the uses for selected blades and handles:

Instrument	Use
Scalpel handles (Fig. 3-22, *A*)	
No. 3	Small animal surgery
No. 4	Large animal surgery
Beaver handles	Ophthalmic surgery
Scalpel blades (Fig. 3-22, *B*)	
No. 10	Incising skin, used with no. 3 handle
No. 11	Severing ligaments, used with no. 3 handle
No. 12	Lancing abscesses, used with no. 3 handle
No. 15	Small, precise, or curved incisions, used with no. 3 handle
Nos. 20 to 23	Surgical applications with no. 4 handle
Beaver blades	Ophthalmic surgery and microsurgery

Electrosurgery unit (Fig. 3-19, *B*). The electroscalpel converts electric energy by adapting currents through cutting and coagulation tips. A skin incision is made by the passage of an electric current through a small contact point on the tissue, which causes the microcoagulation of tissue proteins. The advantages of the electroscalpel are the minimizing of surgical hemorrhage and the prevention of the growth of undesirable cells by contact destruction. However, because more tissue is involved in the contact of an electroscalpel or a coagulator tip, healing may be extended several days beyond the time required for surgery that is performed with a conventional scalpel.

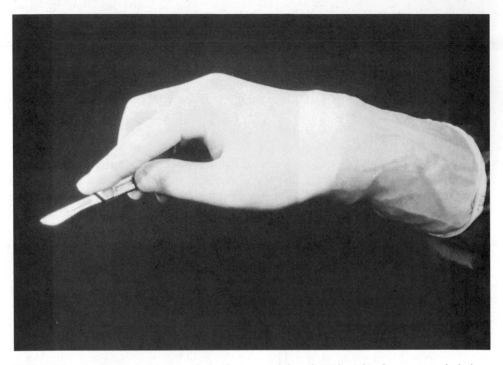

FIG. 3-21   Scalpel is held securely by fingers and thumb with index finger extended along top of instrument.

Surgical scissors. Operating scissors are available in many lengths and weights. They are generally classified by the type of points (blunt/blunt, sharp/blunt, sharp/sharp), the shape of the blades (straight or curved), and the cutting edge of the blades (plain or serrated).

Operating scissors are used in four ways: to cut through or snip tissue, to separate tissue by inserting the tips into the tissue and spreading the points, to separate tissue by exerting a steady force of the tips against the tissue until separation is adequate, and to cut suture material. Only wire scissors are used for cutting wire sutures. The use of other scissors will irreparably damage the cutting edges.

Surgical scissors and their uses are shown below:

Instrument	Use
Operating scissors (Fig. 3-23)	Cutting sutures and paper drape material
Mayo dissecting scissors (Fig. 3-24)	Cutting tough tissue, fascia
Doyen abdominal scissors (Fig. 3-25)	Cutting tough tissue
Straight Metzenbaum scissors (Fig. 3-26)	Cutting delicate tissue
Iris scissors (Fig. 3-27)	Intraocular tissue
Stitch scissors (Fig. 3-28)	Removing sutures
Wire-cutting scissors (Fig. 3-29)	Cutting wire sutures
Bandage scissors (Fig. 3-30)	Cutting dressing material

Text continued on p. 192

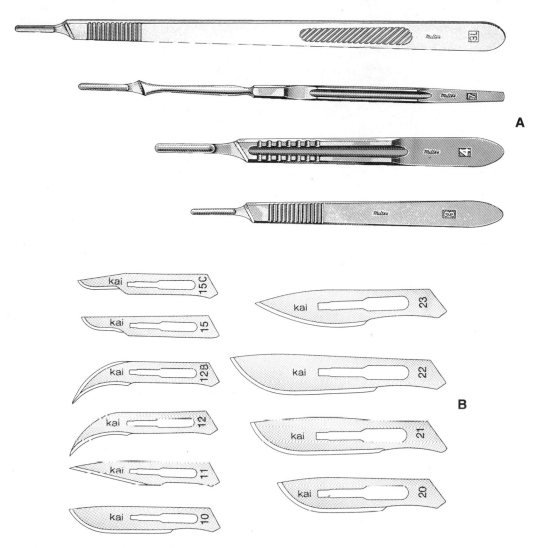

FIG. 3-22   A, Scalpel handles. Bottom two handles are most commonly used. Longer handles are used in ophthalmic surgery or in other special procedures. **B,** Scalpel blades. No. 20 blade is used with no. 4 handle, and smaller no. 10 blade is used with no. 3 handle. Nos. 11, 12, and 15 blades are used with no. 3 handle. (Courtesy Miltex.)

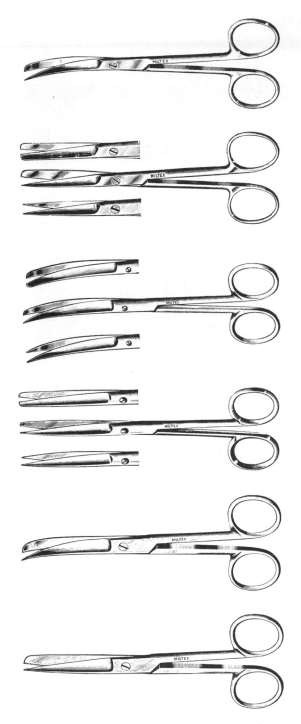

FIG. 3-23   Operating scissors. (Courtesy Miltex.)

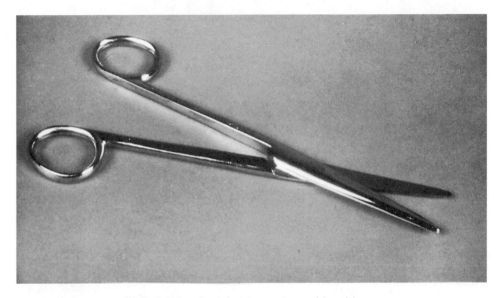

FIG. 3-24   Straight Mayo scissors, blunt/blunt.

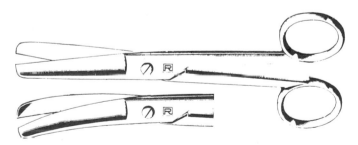

FIG. 3-25   Doyen abdominal scissors. (Courtesy Richards Manufacturing.)

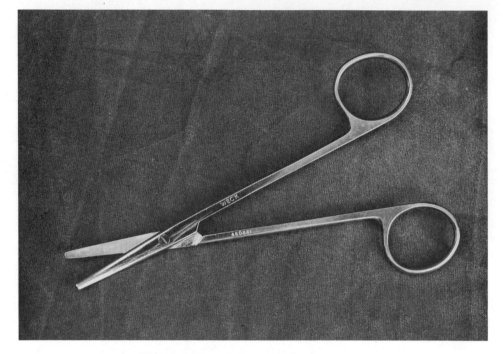

FIG. 3-26   Straight Metzenbaum scissors.

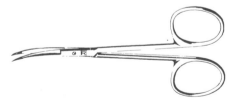

FIG. 3-27   Iris scissors. (Courtesy Richards Manufacturing.)

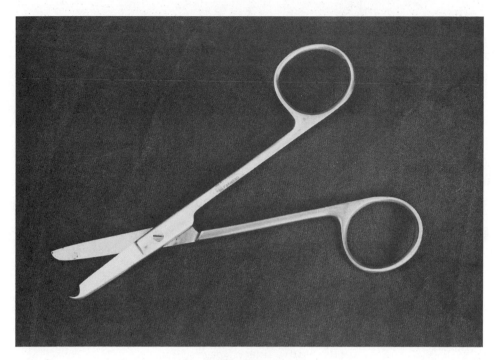

FIG. 3-28   Stitch scissors.

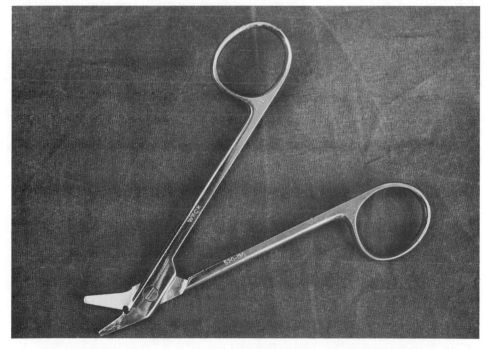

FIG. 3-29   Wire-cutting scissors have short, thick jaws with serrated edges.

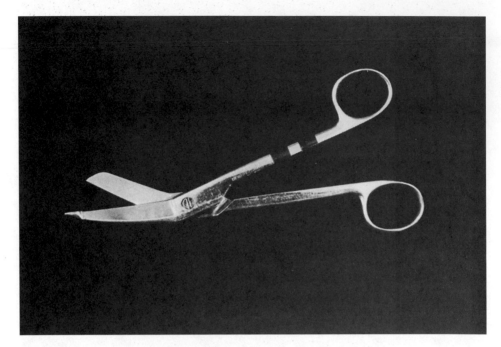

FIG. 3-30   Lister bandage scissors.

Forceps

Thumb forceps. Thumb forceps are used to grasp tissue or dressing material. Depending on the style, they are capable of holding tissue firmly, either horizontally or vertically, and produce minimal tissue damage. Thumb forceps are constructed like tweezers, having two tines bonded together at the proximal end, which allow the grasping ends to spring open or be squeezed shut. The lateral sides of each tine are often grooved or indented to facilitate handling the forceps with the thumb and fingers in a modified pencil grip. The tips may be pointed, flattened, or rounded, and the grasping surface may have small teeth or large teeth (rat tooth). Tooth configuration may be 1 : 2, 2 : 3, 3 : 4, or 4 : 5. The grasping surface may be serrated or smooth. Length varies depending on the tasks for which they were designed. In general, thumb forceps with teeth are not used on easily traumatized tissue, such as lung, intestine, or blood vessel.

Thumb forceps and their uses are listed below:

Instrument	Use

Dressing forceps
  Bayonet
  Adson (Fig. 3-31, *A*)
  Cushing (Fig. 3-31, *B*)
	Handling dressing material (have serrations, but no teeth on the jaws)

Tissue forceps (Fig. 3-31)
  Brown Adson (Fig. 3-31, *E*)
  Stille
  Carmody
	Grasping and holding tissue (may have serrations or teeth)

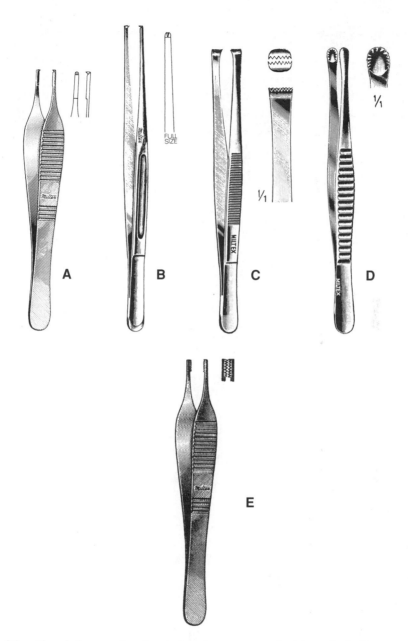

FULL
SIZE

$1/1$

$1/1$

A   B   C   D

E

FIG. 3-31   Thumb forceps showing various jaw patterns. **A,** Adson. **B,** Cushing. **C,** Martin. **D,** Russian. **E,** Brown Adson. (Courtesy Miltex.)

Hemostatic and tissue forceps. Hemostatic and tissue forceps are used to clamp, hold, or retract blood vessels, tissues, and tissue bundles. They are characterized by having a ratchet device at the ring end, which holds the instrument closed, and a boxlock, which bonds the two shanks together (Fig. 3-32). The boxlock is created by one shank passing through a slot in the other shank of the pair. At the central point at which one shank passes through the other, the instrument is riveted together so that when the instrument is held closed, the ratchet halves and the tips of the jaws match exactly.

Hemostatic and tissue forceps may have straight or curved jaws and several types of grasping surface patterns (Fig. 3-33). Transverse serrations will crush tissue more than longitudinal serrations. The smaller-sized forceps have transverse serrations, and the larger-sized forceps are designed with a number of jaw patterns.

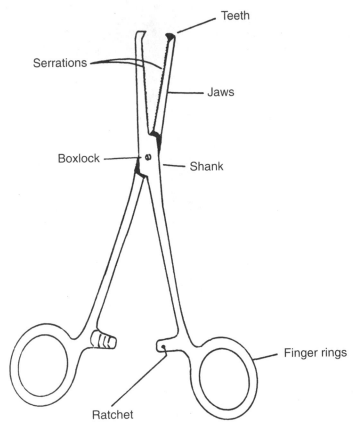

FIG. 3-32   Parts of surgical instrument. (Courtesy Ohio State University.)

Hemostatic and tissue forceps and their uses are listed below:

Instrument	Use
Allis tissue forceps (Fig. 3-34)	Tissue grasping and blunt dissection
Babcock forceps (Fig. 3-35)	Intestinal surgery and blunt dissection
Kelly/Crile forceps (Fig. 3-36)	General surgery, hemostasis, and blunt dissection and tissue retraction
Doyen intestinal forceps (Fig. 3-37)	Intestinal surgery and blunt dissection
Ferguson angiotribe (straight or curved) (Fig. 3-38)	Abdominal surgery, tough tissue bundles, and blunt dissection
Halsted mosquito forceps (straight or curved) (Fig. 3-39)	General surgery, hemostasis, and blunt dissection tissue retraction
Kocher forceps (Fig. 3-40)	General surgery, hemostasis, and blunt dissection
Mixter forceps (Fig. 3-41)	General surgery, hemostasis, and blunt dissection
Rochester-Pean forceps (Fig. 3-42)	General surgery, arterial hemostasis, and blunt dissection
Rochester-Carmalt forceps (Fig. 3-43)	General surgery, arterial hemostasis, and blunt dissection
Allen intestinal clamp (Fig. 3-44)	Intestinal surgery and blunt dissection

Retractors

Retractors are used to pull apart the edges of incised surgical sites so that the surgeon is provided with a better visual exposure of the body cavity and a free access to tissues and organs. Retractors may be hand-held or self-retaining. The use of hand-held retractors requires that a scrubbed surgical technician place the hook, hoe, or rake grasping ends of each retractor on either edge of the incision and pull the edges away from the midline of the incision. In veterinary surgery, the use of hand-held retractors has two major disadvantages. First, it is rarely practical for a scrubbed as-

Text continued on p. 203.

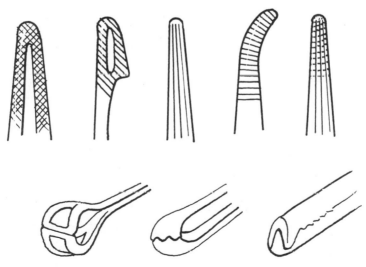

FIG. 3-33   Jaw patterns of surgical instruments.

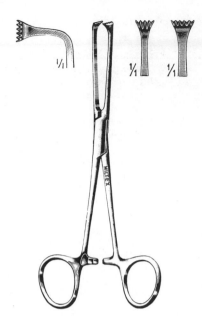

FIG. 3-34   Allis tissue forceps. (Courtesy Miltex.)

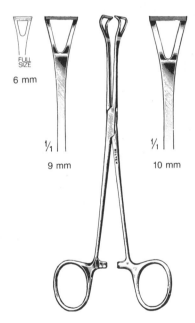

FIG. 3-35   Babcock intestinal forceps. (Courtesy Miltex.)

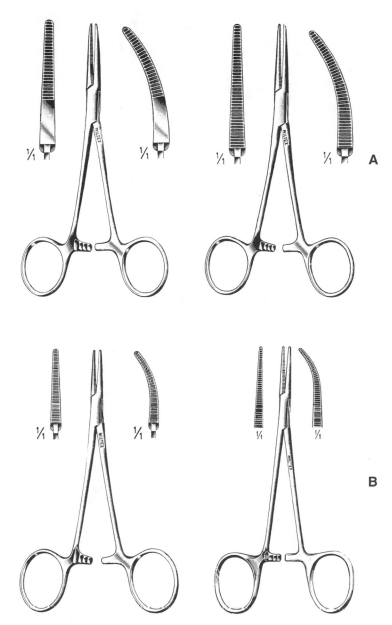

FIG. 3-36   **A,** Kelly and, **B,** Crile hemostatic forceps. (Courtesy Miltex.)

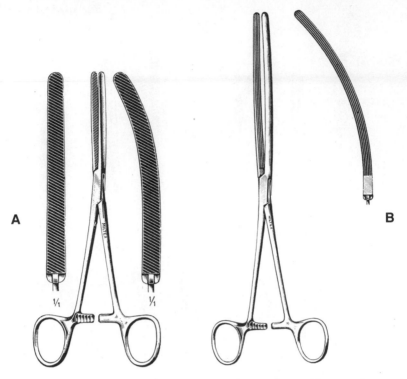

FIG. 3-37 **A,** Doyen intestinal forceps. **B,** Doyen forceps have oblique or longitudinal serrations along entire length of jaw. Instrument is used to occlude bowel to prevent spillage of its contents. (Courtesy Miltex.)

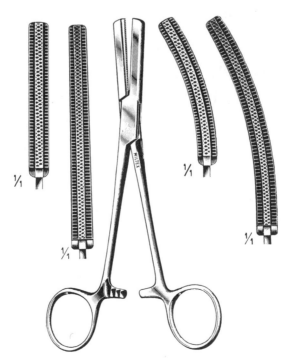

FIG. 3-38 Ferguson angiotribe. (Courtesy Miltex.)

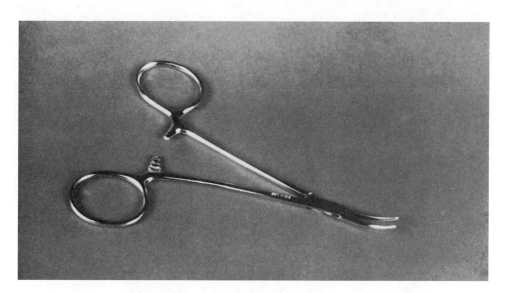

FIG. 3-39   Halsted mosquito forceps, curved.

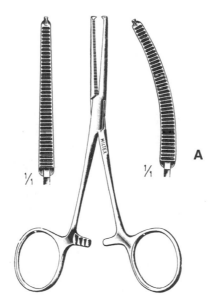

FIG. 3-40   **A,** Kocher forceps. (Courtesy Miltex.)
Continued

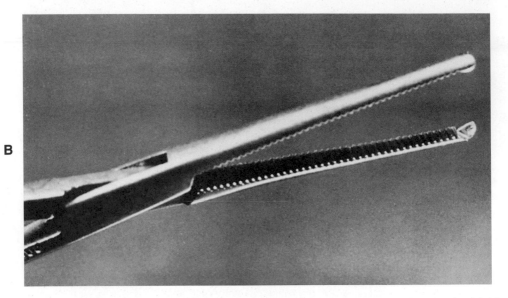

FIG. 3-40, cont'd   B, Kocher forceps have deep, transverse serrations along entire length of jaw with interlocking teeth at tips. (Courtesy Miltex.)

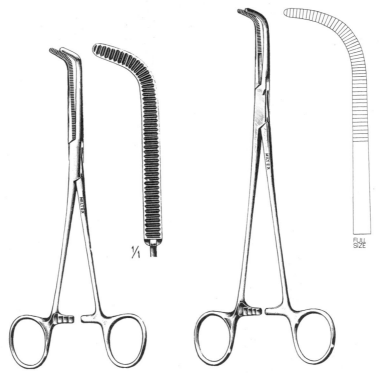

FIG. 3-41   Mixter hemostatic forceps, curved. (Courtesy Miltex.)

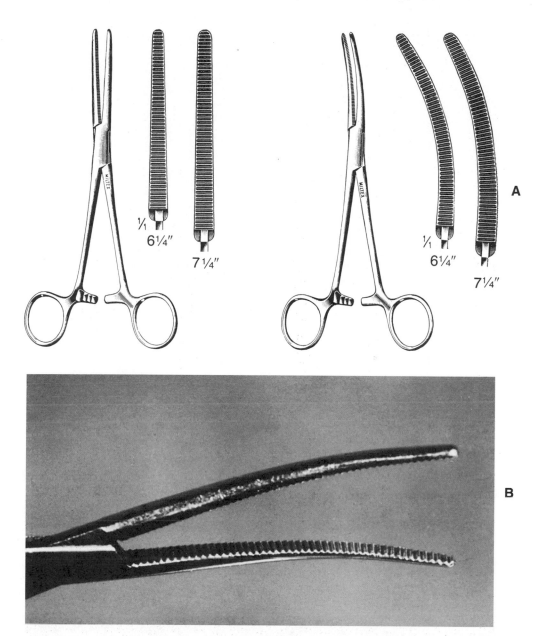

FIG. 3-42   A, Rochester-Pean hemostatic forceps, curved and straight. **B,** Rochester-Pean forceps have transverse serrations along entire length of jaw. (Courtesy Miltex.)

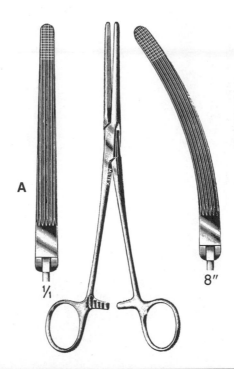

A

¹⁄₁

8″

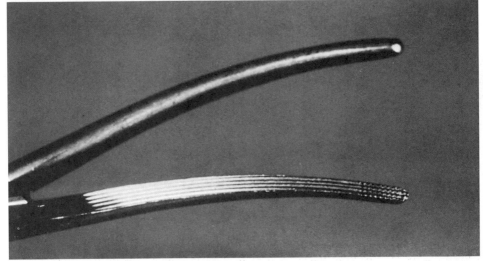

B

FIG. 3-43   **A,** Rochester-Carmalt forceps. **B,** Rochester-Carmalt forceps have longitudinal serrations and cross-hatched pattern at tips of each jaw. (Courtesy Miltex.)

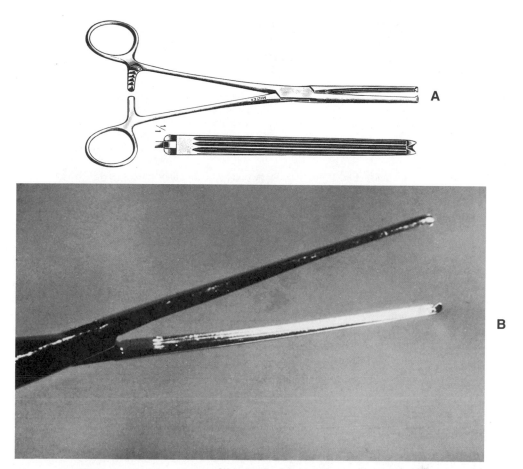

FIG. 3-44 **A,** Allen intestinal clamp. **B,** Allen clamp has long thin jaws with longitudinal serrations along its length and interdigitating teeth at tips. (Courtesy Miltex.)

sistant to be present throughout routine procedures; second, if the patient is small, the close proximity of another pair of hands and arms may physically interfere with the surgeon's free access to the operative site.

Manual or self-retaining retractors are designed with the grasping arms or blades attached to a grooved slide bar or ratchet. The retractor is placed in the proper position in the incision, and the arms are moved apart until the correct degree of retraction is attained. Manual retractors have a locking device such as a set-screw, which, when applied, maintains the arms or blades in the desired position, eliminating the need for an assistant.

Standard full-sized (human) abdominal and thoracic retractors have serious limitations for veterinary surgery. They are too heavy and the blades are too long for the average small animal surgical procedure.

Retractors and their use are listed below:

Instrument	Example of use
Wilson rib spreader (self-retaining) (Fig. 3-45)	Thoracic surgery, medium to large surgiical site
Gelpi retractor (self-retaining) (Fig. 3-46)	Medium- to large-sized operative site, perineal area, or spinal muscle
Army-Navy retractor (hand-held) (Fig. 3-47)	Small- to medium-sized operative site, orthopedic surgery
Volkmann retractor (hand-held) (Fig. 3-48)	Superficial procedures on tiny animals (fascia or muscle)
Senn retractor (hand-held) (Fig. 3-49)	Retracting tissue (fascia or muscle)
Weitlaner retractor (self-retaining) (Fig. 3-50)	Medium- to large-sized operative site (primarily spinal muscle retraction)
Frazier laminectomy retractor (Fig. 3-51)	Spinal muscle retraction

Needle Holders

Needle holders are used to grasp and hold the suture needle, and some have the capacity to cut the suture as well. Differences in the size and weight of the instrument and variations in the jaw patterns are adaptations to the size and shape of the suture needle. Straight suture needles are driven by hand because using a needle holder to drive a straight needle may bend or fracture the needle. Curved needles are driven with a needle holder because it allows the needle to pass quickly and cleanly through tissue in an arc that conforms to the curve of the needle.

A combination holding and cutting instrument is popular among veterinary surgeons who work alone because the suture may be tied and cut with the same instrument, eliminating the need for an assistant or for picking up and putting down a pair

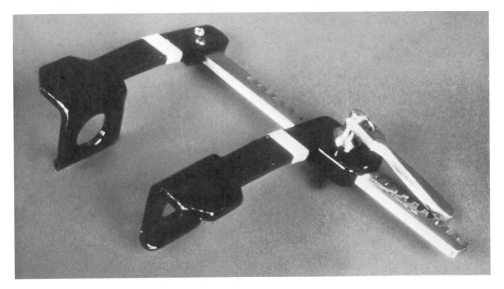

FIG. 3-45   Wilson rib spreaders. (Courtesy Ohio State University.)

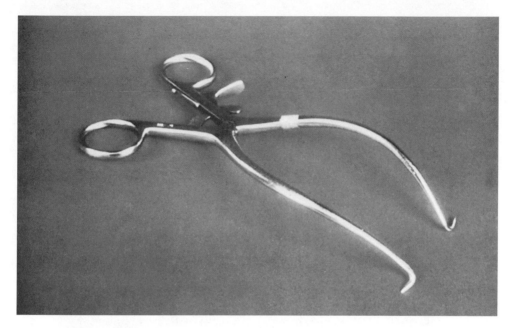

FIG. 3-46   Gelpi perineal retractor. (Courtesy Ohio State University.)

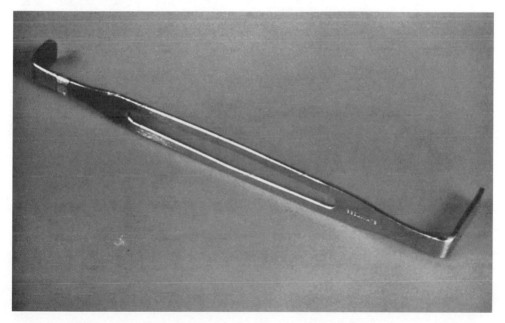

FIG. 3-47   Army-Navy retractor. (Courtesy Ohio State University.)

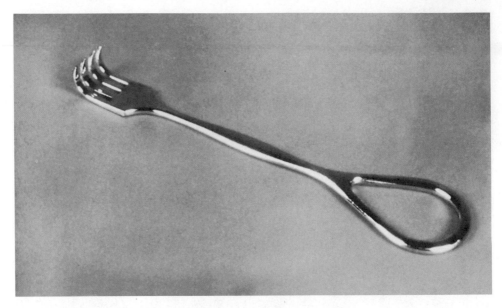

FIG. 3-48   Volkmann rake retractor. (Courtesy Ohio State University.)

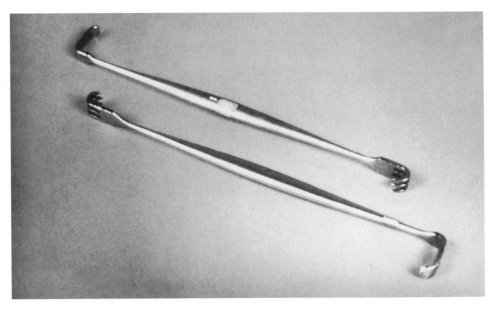

FIG. 3-49   Senn double-ended retractor. (Courtesy Ohio State University.)

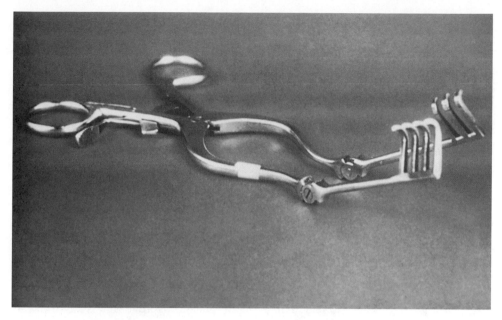

FIG. 3-50   Weitlaner retractor. (Courtesy Ohio State University.)

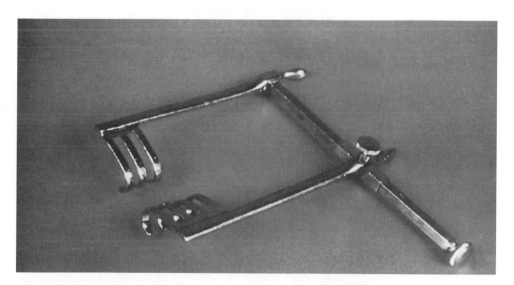

FIG. 3-51   Frazier laminectomy retractor. (Courtesy Ohio State University.)

of scissors to cut each suture. Those who dislike the instrument do so because of its tendency to snip the suture material unintentionally while the knot is being tied.

Needle holders and their uses are listed below:

Instrument	Use
Gillies-Sheehan needle holder (Fig. 3-52)	General surgery, cuts and ties, holds medium to coarse needles
Mayo-Hegar needle holder (Fig. 3-53)	General surgery, ties, and holds medium to coarse needles
Olsen-Hegar needle holder (Fig. 3-54)	General surgery, cuts and ties, holds medium to coarse needles
Sarot needle holder (Fig. 3-55)	Thoracic surgery, holds medium to fine needles
Crile-Wood needle holder (Fig. 3-56)	General surgery, holds medium to fine needles

Orthopedic Instruments

In 1958, orthopedics made a great advance when the Swiss Association for the Study of Internal Fixation (AO/ASIF) defined the biochemical principles for successful internal fixation of fractures and used these axioms to create an entire system of stainless steel implants and instruments. The theme of this system is the rapid return of function after fracture treatment. This is accomplished by anatomic reduction, stable internal fixation with implants, preservation or enhancement of blood supply to

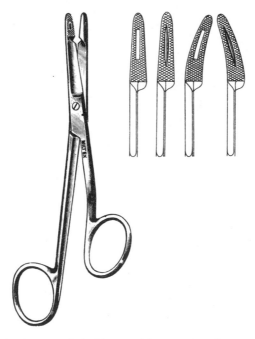

FIG. 3-52   Gillies-Sheehan needle holder combines suture scissor, one fenestrated saw, and one angled finger ring. (Courtesy Miltex.)

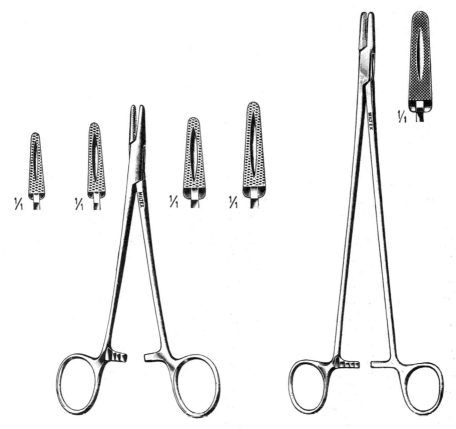

FIG. 3-53   Mayo-Hegar needle holder. (Courtesy Miltex.)

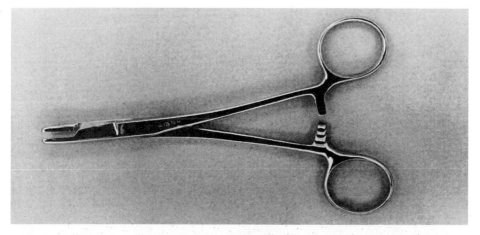

FIG. 3-54   Olsen-Hegar needle holder holds needle and has scissors for cutting suture material.

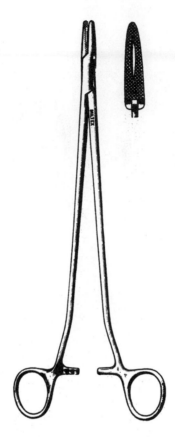

FIG. 3-55   Sarot needle holder, 10½ inch. (Courtesy Miltex.)

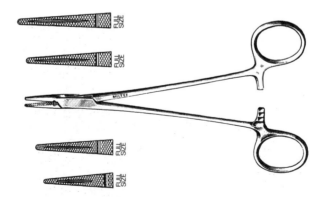

FIG. 3-56   Crile-Wood needle holder. (Courtesy Miltex.)

the fracture zone, strict preoperative planning and aseptic technique, and atraumatic handling of the bone and surrounding tissues* (Fig. 3-57).

Orthopedic instruments and appliances are among the most specialized and expensive of all surgical instruments. Most bone instruments and implantation devices are made of stainless steel or a cobalt-chromium alloy (Vitallium). These alloys are used because they are inert, that is, not easily changed by chemical reactions within the body after implantation. One of the most valuable instruments in veterinary orthopedic surgery is the power drill. This instrument is available in different sizes, and its use is dictated by the surgeon and the intended use. Power to the drill is supplied through a rubber hose connected to a tank of compressed nitrogen. Some uses of power drills include shaving away bone, such as in back surgery or hip surgery, securing bone plates with screws, or cutting bone. Power drills can be steam sterilized

*Courtesy Synthes Co.

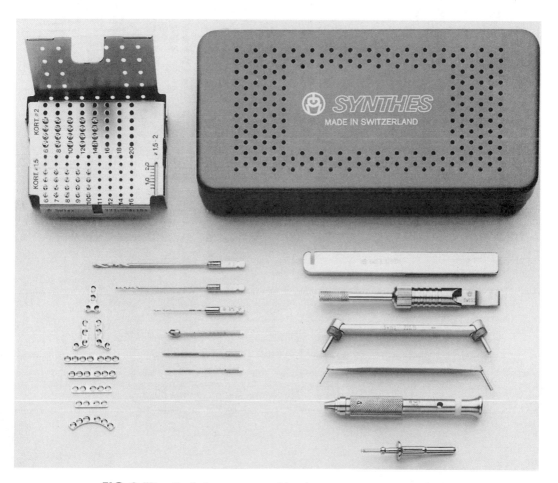

FIG. 3-57   Basic instrument and implant sets. (Courtesy Synthes.)

Continued

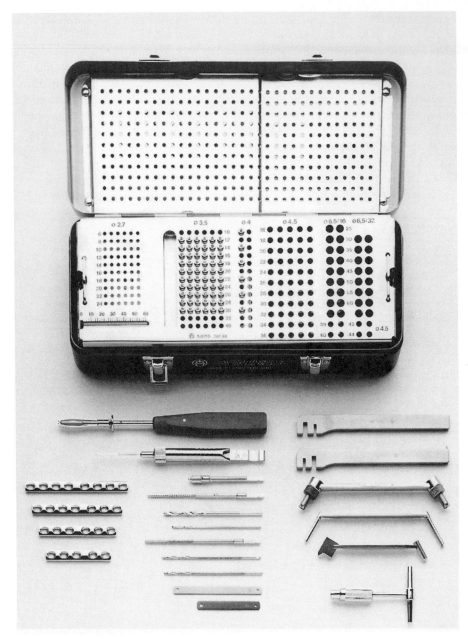

FIG. 3-57, cont'd   For legend see preceding page.

with other instruments. They cannot, however, be immersed in water. They need to be wiped clean of any blood and debris and then wrapped and sterilized (see Figs. 3-71 to 3-73).

This text does not offer a complete discussion of orthopedic instruments; however, some basic examples are illustrated, and the function of each is listed below:

Instrument	Use
Cutting and shaping instruments	Orthopedic surgery, to cut, shape, or scrape bone
Bone-cutting forceps (Fig. 3-58)	To cut bone
Osteotomes and mallet (Fig. 3-59)	To cut and shape bone
Gigli wire saw (Fig. 3-60)	To saw bone
Saterlee bone saw (Fig. 3-61)	To saw bone
Bone gouge (Fig. 3-62)	To cut or break bone
Bone rasp (Fig. 3-63)	To smooth rough bone edges
Trephine (Fig. 3-64)	To drill out a cylinder of bone
Bone curette (Fig. 3-65)	To scrape foreign matter
Rongeurs (Fig. 3-66)	To remove or break up bone particles
Joseph periosteal elevator (Fig. 3-67)	To raise fractured bone ends

Text continued on p. 216

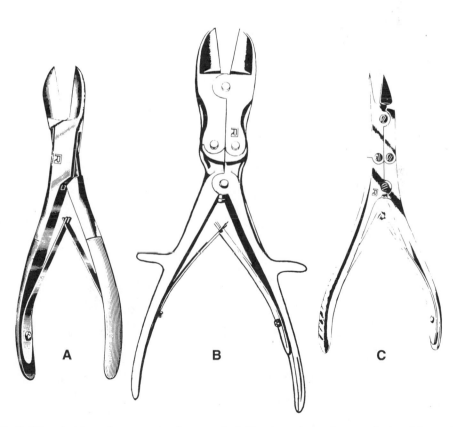

FIG. 3-58   **A,** Liston bone-cutting forceps. **B,** Stille-Liston bone forceps. **C,** Small bone forceps. (Courtesy Richards Manufacturing.)

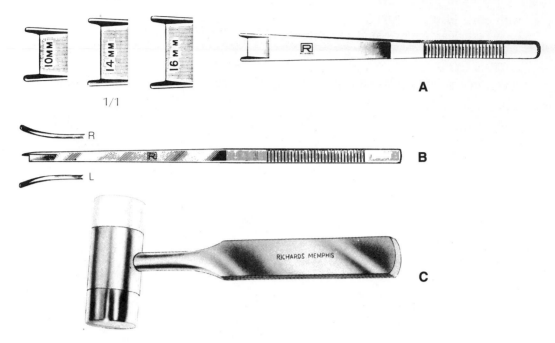

1/1

FIG. 3-59   **A,** Cinelli osteotome. **B,** Anderson-Neivert osteotome. **C,** Richards combination bone mallet. (Courtesy Richards Manufacturing.)

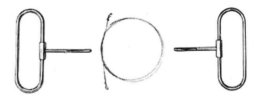

FIG. 3-60   Gigli wire saw. (Courtesy Richards Manufacturing.)

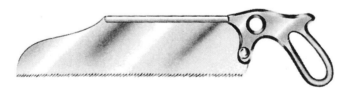

FIG. 3-61   Saterlee bone saw. (Courtesy Richards Manufacturing.)

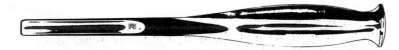

FIG. 3-62   Smith-Petersen bone gouge. (Courtesy Richards Manufacturing.)

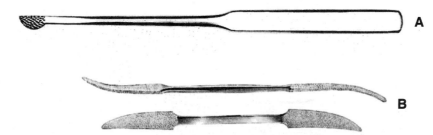

A

B

FIG. 3-63   **A,** Facet rasp. **B,** Putti bone rasp. (Courtesy Richards Manufacturing.)

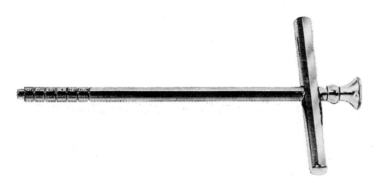

FIG. 3-64   Michelle trephine. (Courtesy Richards Manufacturing.)

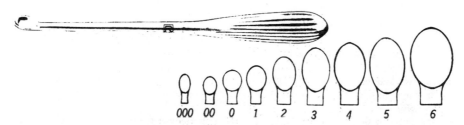

FIG. 3-65   Brun bone curette. (Courtesy Richards Manufacturing.)

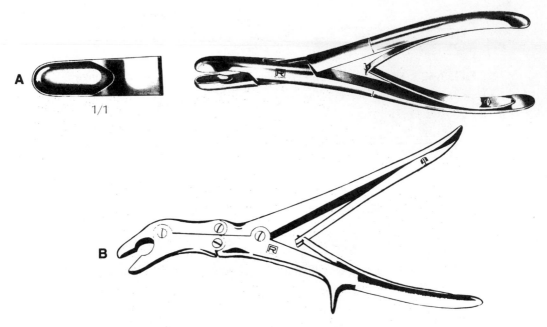

A

1/1

B

FIG. 3-66   **A,** Adson rongeur. **B,** Angular rongeur. (Courtesy Richards Manufacturing.)

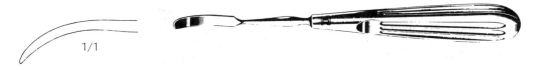

1/1

FIG. 3-67   Joseph periosteal elevator. (Courtesy Richards Manufacturing.)

Bone-holding instruments
  Bone-holding forceps and clamps
    (Fig. 3-68)
Internal fixation and implantation
  devices
  Intramedullary pins (Fig. 3-69)
  Bone chuck (Fig. 3-70)
  Plates, screws, and screwdriver
  Bone drill and bits (Fig. 3-71)
  Pin cutter (Fig. 3-72)
External fixation devices
  Mason meta (spoon) splints (Fig. 3-73)

Orthopedic surgery, to hold bone firmly to
  avoid bruising the periosteum and to prevent
  further damage to tissue and bone ends
To maintain fractured bone ends in apposition

To aid in implanting intramedullary pins

To immobilize the fractured limb, used alone or
  with internal fixation

Text continued on p. 220

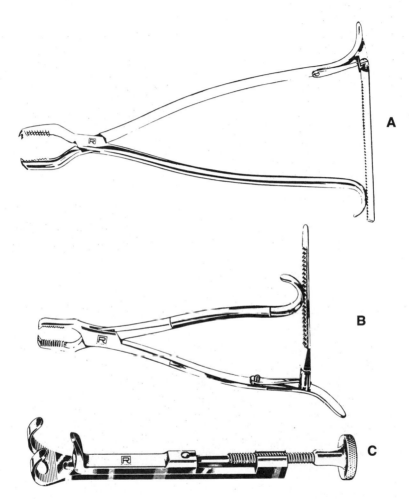

FIG. 3-68   **A,** Lane bone-holding forceps. **B,** Baby Lane bone-holding forceps. **C,** Lowman bone clamp. (Courtesy Richards Manufacturing.)

A

<table>
<tr><th colspan="5">Plain</th></tr>
<tr><th colspan="5">Description</th></tr>
<tr><th colspan="2">Length</th><th rowspan="2">End view</th><th rowspan="2">Tip</th><th rowspan="2">Opposite end</th></tr>
<tr><th>Inch</th><th>mm</th></tr>
<tr><td>9</td><td>228.6</td><td></td><td>Trocar</td><td>Trocar</td></tr>
<tr><td>9</td><td>228.6</td><td></td><td>Trocar</td><td>Chuck</td></tr>
<tr><td>9</td><td>228.6</td><td></td><td>Diamond</td><td>Chuck</td></tr>
<tr><td>9</td><td>228.6</td><td></td><td>Trocar</td><td>Round</td></tr>
<tr><td>9</td><td>228.6</td><td></td><td>Diamond</td><td>Round</td></tr>
<tr><td>9</td><td>228.6</td><td></td><td>Diamond</td><td>Diamond</td></tr>
</table>

<table>
<tr><th colspan="5">Threaded</th></tr>
<tr><th colspan="5">Description</th></tr>
<tr><th colspan="2">Length</th><th rowspan="2">End view</th><th rowspan="2">Tip</th><th rowspan="2">Opposite end</th></tr>
<tr><th>Inch</th><th>mm</th></tr>
<tr><td>9</td><td>228.6</td><td></td><td>Trocar</td><td>Trocar</td></tr>
<tr><td>9</td><td>228.6</td><td></td><td>Trocar</td><td>Round</td></tr>
<tr><td>9</td><td>228.6</td><td></td><td>Diamond</td><td>Round</td></tr>
<tr><td>9</td><td>228.6</td><td></td><td>Diamond</td><td>Diamond</td></tr>
</table>

Diameter						
5/64″ (1.9 mm)	3/32″ (2.3 mm)	7/64″ (2.7 mm)	1/8″ (3.1 mm)	9/64″ (3.5 mm)	5/32″ (3.9 mm)	3/16″ (4.7 mm)

B

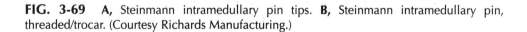

FIG. 3-69 A, Steinmann intramedullary pin tips. **B,** Steinmann intramedullary pin, threaded/trocar. (Courtesy Richards Manufacturing.)

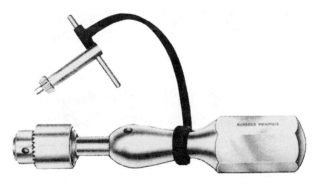

FIG. 3-70   Jacobs bone chuck. (Courtesy Richards Manufacturing.)

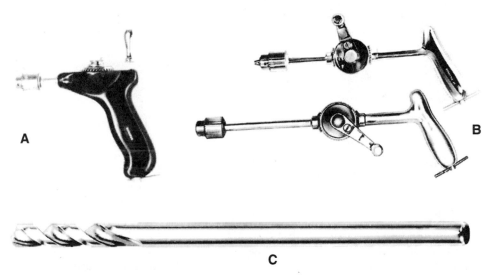

A

B

C

FIG. 3-71   **A,** Richards pistol-grip bone drill. **B,** Richards-Lovejoy bone drill. **C,** Twist drill bit. (Courtesy Richards Manufacturing.)

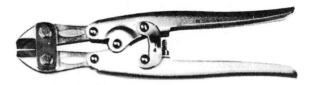

FIG. 3-72   Spring-action pin cutter. (Courtesy Richards Manufacturing.)

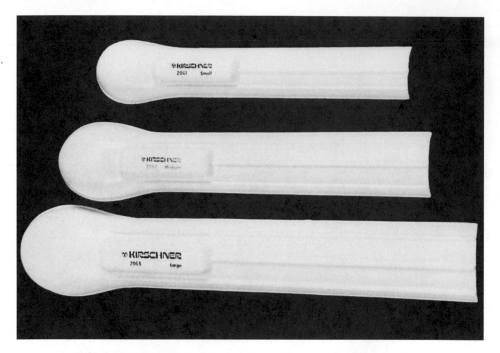

FIG. 3-73   Small, medium, and large Mason meta (spoon) splints.

Dental Instruments

In small animal medicine, routine dentistry is generally limited to extractions and tartar removal. Veterinary dentistry has changed dramatically over the past decade. In small animal medicine, "routine" dentistry is still generally limited to cleaning/polishing and tooth extractions. However, nonroutine procedures now performed include root canals, fillings, and capping teeth. Most dental extractions, although performed by a qualified technician, are overseen by a veterinarian. Ultrasonic scalers and high-speed dental machines have supplanted manual methods for tartar removal, but the technician should be familiar with the use of nonmechanical scaling tools. Although dentistry may be considered a medical procedure, the instruments are included in this volume because it always requires the use of a general anesthetic.

Dental instruments and their uses are listed below:

Instrument	Use
Molar extractors (Fig. 3-74)	As pliers to extract teeth from the jaw, sometimes to crack large tartar accumulations
Root elevators (Fig. 3-75)	To loosen the tooth root as an aid in extraction
Manual tartar remover (Figs. 3-12, 3-76, and 3-77) or ultrasonic dental scaler (Fig. 3-77)	To remove tartar accumulations; ultrasonic devices employ water-cooled, oscillating tips
Mouth speculum (Fig. 3-78)	To prop open the mouth to afford maximum display of tooth surfaces
Dental prophy angles (Fig. 3-79)	To hold burs or polishing cups

Text continued on p. 225

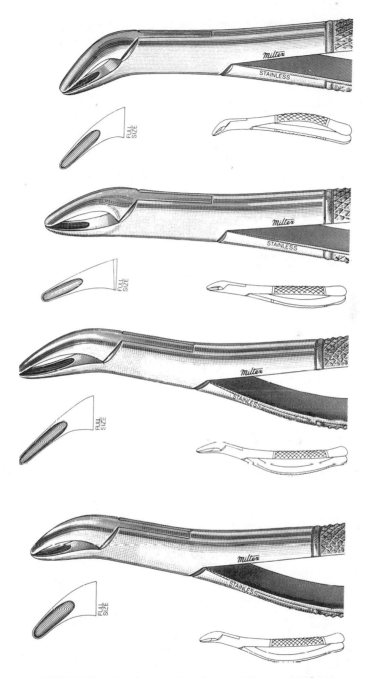

FIG. 3-74   Tooth extraction forceps. (Courtesy Miltex.)

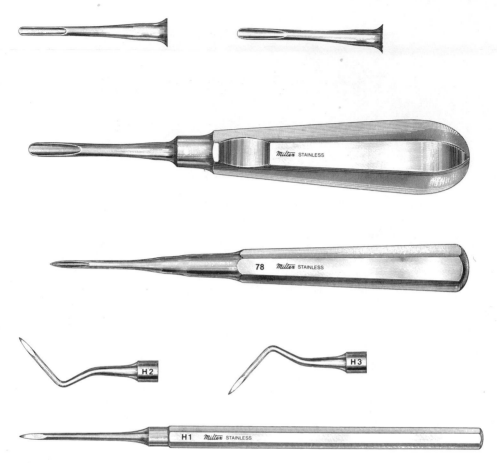

FIG. 3-75   Root elevators are used to loosen roots from sockets before tooth extraction. (Courtesy Miltex.)

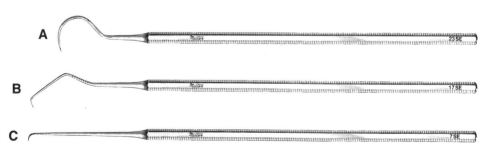

FIG. 3-76   **A** to **C,** Dental explorers. (Courtesy Miltex.)

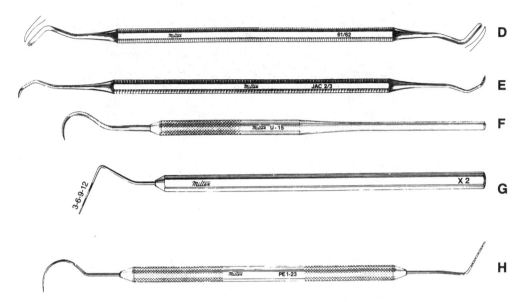

FIG. 3-76, cont'd   **D,** Excavator. **E** and **F,** Used to remove scale. **G** and **H,** Dental probes. (Courtesy Miltex.)

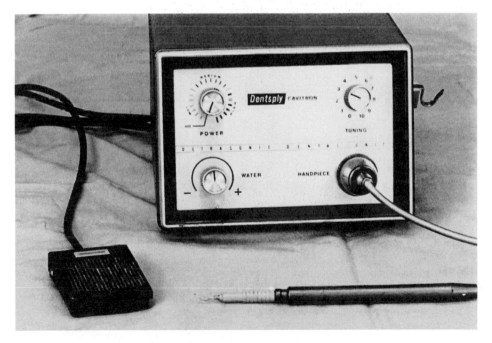

FIG. 3-77   Ultrasonic dental scaler.

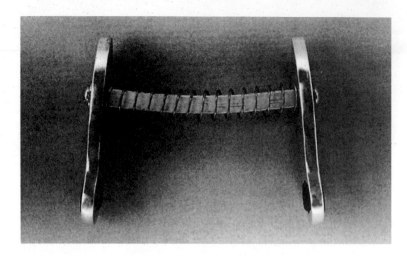

FIG. 3-78   Mouth speculum.

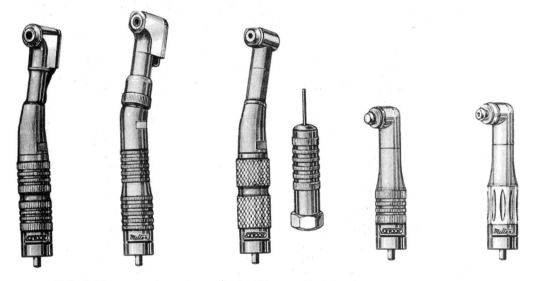

FIG. 3-79   Dental prophy angles hold burrs of polishing cups. (Courtesy Miltex.)

Miscellaneous Surgical Instruments

Miscellaneous surgical instruments and their uses are listed below:

Instrument	Use
Spay hook (Fig. 3-80)	In ovariohysterectomy to retrieve each uterine horn
Sponge forceps (straight or curved) (Fig. 3-81)	To apply final paint to the surgical site and for sterile dressing material
Tongue-grasping forceps (Fig. 3-82)	To pull the tongue forward to achieve a maximum display of the mouth and throat
Towel clips (Fig. 3-83)	To hold the surgical drapes in place
Biopsy punch (Fig. 3-84)	To punch or core out pieces of tissue for histologic examination
Instrument clip (Fig. 3-85)	To hold ringed instruments in the sterilization pack

Surgical Instrument Sets

No concrete rules govern the inclusion of specific instruments in surgical packs. Each hospital has an established collection, and each surgeon selects the tools preferred and required for the procedure to be performed. The preparation of surgical packs almost always is the responsibility of the technician, and it is impossible to correctly arrange instrument sets without a thorough knowledge of the names and functions of each item and an understanding of the surgical procedure for which the pack is intended.

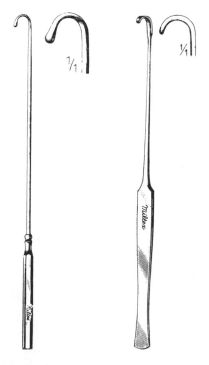

FIG. 3-80   Spay hook. (Courtesy Miltex.)

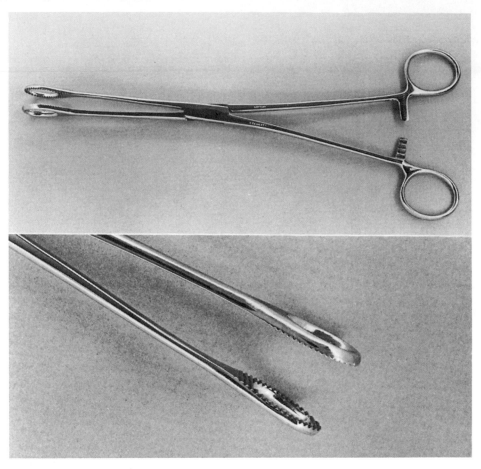

FIG. 3-81   Sponge forceps.

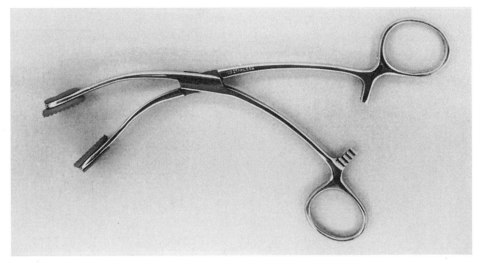

FIG. 3-82   Tongue-grasping forceps.

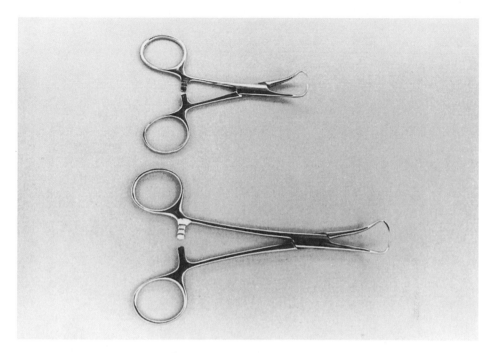

FIG. 3-83   Backhaus towel clips.

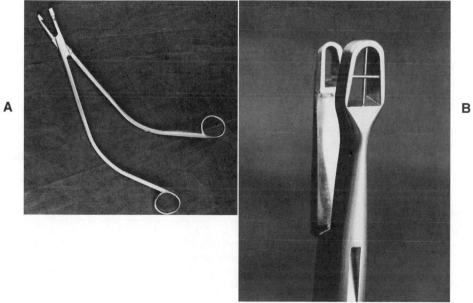

FIG. 3-84   **A,** Biopsy punch. **B,** Close-up of jaw configuration of biopsy punch.

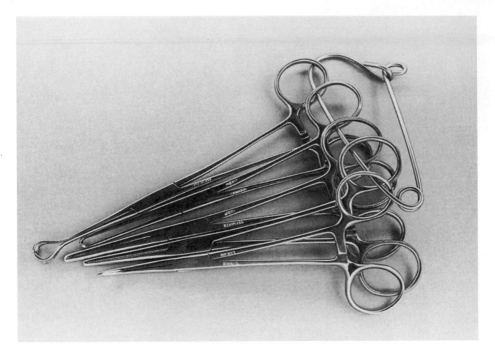

FIG. 3-85   Ringed instrument clip.

The composition of the surgical pack is determined by surgeon preference, the type of procedure, and in some cases the size of the patient. The physical size of the pack will be limited by the dimensions of the sterilization chamber. This must be considered before purchasing large instruments or sterilization trays. In special cases, the surgeon will communicate unique or unusual aspects of the procedure so that specific items can be prepared separately or included in the pack. In any case, the technician must prepare an adequate number of each major instrument grouping to avert the undesirable circumstance in which a sterile instrument is desperately required but not available.

Basic abdominal set (Fig. 3-86)

Instrument	Number to include
Cutting instruments	
Scalpel blades	Presterilized, disposable blades are not included in the pack. For most routine procedures, a no. 10 blade is aseptically dropped onto the instrument tray when required.
Operating scissors for cutting suture and drape	1 or 2 pairs
Scalpel handle	1 no. 3 handle
Mayo scissors	1 sharp/blunt; 1 blunt/blunt
Metzenbaum scissors	1

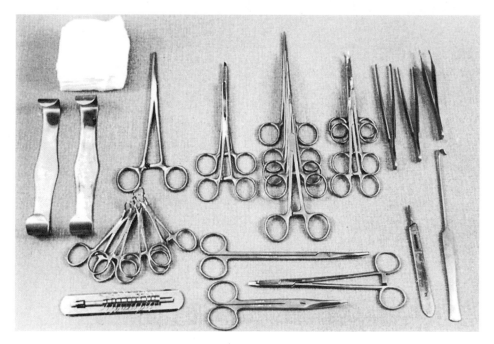

FIG. 3-86   Basic abdominal set.

Forceps	
Thumb forceps	2 or 3 preferred types
Hemostatic forceps	8 to 12 preferred types and sizes
Tissue forceps	5 or 6 preferred types and sizes
Needle holders	1 or 2 preferred types
Sutures and needles	
Suture material	Presterilized surgical suture is not included in the pack. For most small animal procedures, sizes 0 through 4-0 are aseptically dropped onto the instrument tray. Synthetic or wire suture is available in individual sterile packets.
Miscellaneous	
Spay hook	1
Towel clips	4 to 8 preferred types
Stainless steel solution bowl	1

Cardiovascular thoracotomy set

Instrument	Number to include
Basic abdominal pack	
Rib retractors	2 to 4 preferred types
Bone cutting forceps	1
Satinsky vena cava clamp	1
Wagensteen patent ductus clamp	1
Kapp-Beck-Thompson bronchus clamp	1
Sarot needle holder	1
Artery clamps	2
Suction pump, tubing	1 unit

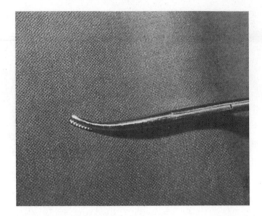

FIG. 3-87   Misalignment of the tips of mosquito forceps. This instrument will not pick up tissue in surgery.

Basic orthopedic set

Instrument	Number to include
Bone chuck and drill	1 each
Bone holding forceps	2 to 3 required types
Rongeurs	3 to 4 preferred types
Bone cutting forceps	1 to 2 preferred types
Gelpi retractor	1
Volkmann rake retractor	2
Intramedullary pins	Several, various sizes and points
Pin cutter	1
Orthopedic wire	As directed
Wire cutting scissors	1
Power tools	As directed

Care and Handling of Surgical Instruments

- Instruments should be used only for the purposes for which they were intended. Veterinarians must purchase all their own instruments, equipment, and supplies, and the costs are enormous and continually increasing.
- Instruments should be *placed* on surfaces, never dropped or thrown. Rough handling of some instruments can cause misalignment of the jaws and/or ratchets, rendering the piece useless for surgery (Figs. 3-87 to 3-89).
- Grease or oil should never be used to lubricate instruments because this will inhibit steam penetration during sterilization. Instrument milk is recommended for lubrication.
- Instruments should never be cleaned with abrasive materials or cleansers, because this will disturb the protective skin and promote corrosion and pitting of the metal.
- Instruments should be dried thoroughly after washing to prevent rust formation.
- If instruments are to be left in cold sterilization, an antirust additive (a mixture of sodium carbonate and sodium nitrite, which comes in tablet form and can be obtained from any pharmacy or pharmaceutical supplier) must be added to the solution.

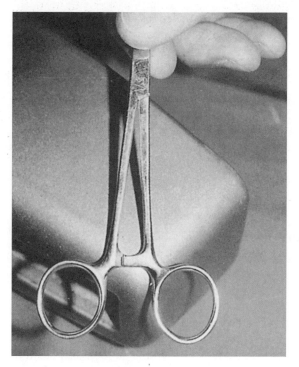

FIG. 3-88   The ratchet of forceps should be checked by engaging the ratchet on the first tooth and tapping the shanks on a solid object.

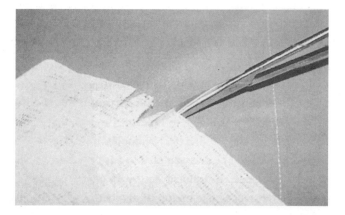

FIG. 3-89   Scissors should smoothly cut four layers of surgical gauze at the tips.

- The safest way to attach and remove scalpel blades is with a hemostat or needle holder. After use, blades should be placed in a covered container and discarded, according to law, when the container is full. Even old, worn blades can inflict serious lacerations. Clean, used blades can be saved and used for skin scrapings.

- Moist heat sterilization will dull the edges of cutting instruments. On a routine basis, these implements should be sharpened by the manufacturer or another qualified expert.
- Metal etching and engraving devices should never be used to identify surgical instruments.
- When an ultrasonic instrument cleaner is used, different kinds of metals should not be mixed. Electrolysis may occur, and the instrument surfaces may be damaged.
- The instruments used in sterile surgery must not be used for nonsterile procedures. They must be identified and kept separate.
- Periodically, surgical scissors must be professionally sharpened by someone who specializes in the craft.

■ SUTURE MATERIAL AND NEEDLES
Suture Material

The surgeon's choice of suture material is usually based on personal preference; however, because mechanical properties as well as biologic interactions must be considered, certain principles must be observed in advance. There is an enormous variety of suture material available, and the surgeon must choose a suture that most closely approaches the ideal for each particular procedure.

The purpose of any suture is to hold the wound edges in apposition until the wound can endure normal stress without the support of the sutures. To achieve this, a suture need only be mechanically sound; but, because the suture must pass through tissue, biologic interaction, type and location of the tissue, and the presence of infection or drainage must be considered.

There are two major classes of suture material: absorbable and nonabsorbable. Absorbable sutures (manufactured from animal and synthetic sources) are digested and assimilated by the body during the healing process and do not require removal. During the healing process, absorbable sutures are replaced by healthy tissue as a result of an inflammatory reaction. Therefore all absorbable sutures may be expected to produce some degree of tissue reaction. Absorbable material is used when sutures must be buried (applied within a body cavity) or when it is desirable or necessary for the body to remove the suture by absorption.

Absorbable sutures (Fig. 3-90)

Polyglactin 910. Polyglactin 910 is a braided synthetic fiber that is much like PGA suture in that it retains strength for approximately 21 days. Polyglactin 910 is relatively easy to handle, stable for use in contaminated wounds, and causes minimal tissue reaction.

Poldioxanone (PDS). PDS is available as a monofilament suture in varying sizes. It has greater flexibility than either PGA or Polyglactin 910. The tensile strength of this suture is greater than PGA or Polyglactin 910, with absorption being complete 182 days after implantation.

Surgical gut (catgut). Surgical gut is produced from the submucosal layer of sheep or hog intestine. Surgical gut may be plain (unmodified) or chromicized. Chromic gut is treated with chromic acid salts to prolong absorption time and to decrease soft

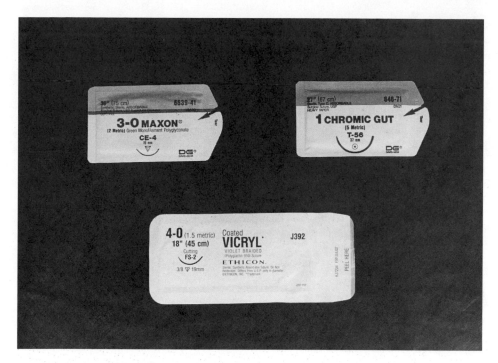

FIG. 3-90   Examples of absorbable suture materials.

tissue reaction. Plain gut will be absorbed by the body in 3 to 5 days, and chromic gut will be absorbed in 10 to 15 days. Surgical gut is elastic, is easy to handle, and will not shrink and strangulate tissues. However, it causes inflammatory tissue reactions and harbors bacterial growth. In addition, it absorbs water and swells, often resulting in a loosening of the surgical knots.

Nonabsorbable sutures (Fig. 3-91) Nonabsorbable sutures are so called because they are not absorbed or digested by tissues. They remain in the tissues until removed. If they are buried, they usually become encysted.

Nylon. Nylon suture is available as both a monofilament and a multifilament material. This suture material causes minimal tissue reaction and loses its strength completely after 6 months in tissue. The major disadvantage of this type of suture is its handling characteristics and knot security. The "memory" of this material is high, causing a tendency to revert to its natural configuration.

Polyester fibers. Polyester is a braided multifilament available in plain and coated forms. Coatings for this suture include Teflon and silicone and add a lubricated quality to the suture. This is one of the strongest nonmetallic sutures available (with little or no loss of strength after implantation), yet also the one that causes the most tissue reaction because of the shedding of the coating. The other disadvantages of this material are its poor knot security and tissue reactivity. It is recommended that other synthetic material be used in contaminated wounds.

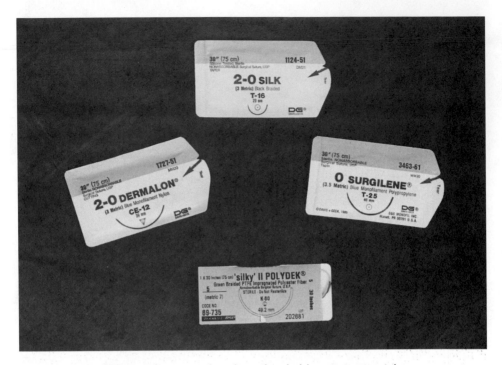

FIG. 3-91   Examples of nonabsorbable suture materials.

Silk. Silk sutures are prepared from threads spun by the silk worm. The threads are either twisted or braided to make the suture. Most surgeons prefer braided silk because it is stronger and has better handling qualities. Silk is inexpensive, is readily available, and will retain its strength. However, it will support bacterial growth and cause more tissue inflammation than cotton, synthetics, or metals. Silk is generally used in ophthalmic, cardiovascular, and gastrointestinal surgery and for vessel ligation.

Wire. Wire sutures are made from high-grade stainless steel and are available in both monofilament and braided forms. Wire is noncorrosive in vivo, is inert, will not support bacterial growth, and has a high tensile strength. Its major disadvantage is difficulty in handling. It lacks elasticity and produces large, bulky knots. The cut ends of wire suture may injure or lacerate tissue. Wire adapts to tissue less effectively than other monofilaments, resulting in small, open holes between the tissue and the wire. The larger sizes of wire suture must be twisted rather than tied. This is advantageous when suturing bone because the suture can be twisted to any desired degree of tension. In suturing tissue, however, the twisting of the wire may cause tissue strangulation.

Metal clips and staples (Fig. 3-92). Metal clips and staples are used to ligate small blood vessels, pull wound edges together, and secure material to incised skin. They are made of noncorrosive metals that are inert. Clips and staples are easy to handle and apply. Because they can be safely and effectively sterilized, they can be applied

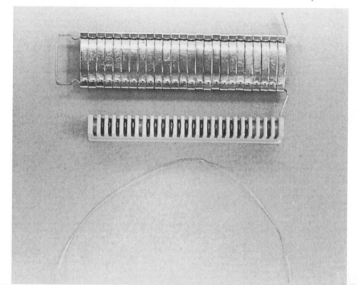

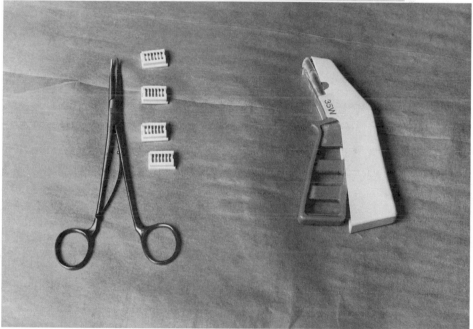

FIG. 3-92   Large and small hemostatic clips.

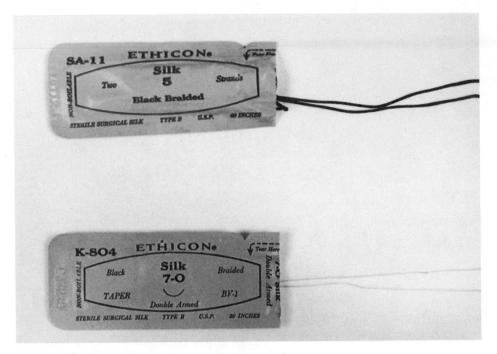

FIG. 3-93   Contrast of size 5 silk suture and size 7-0 silk suture.

to infected wounds. The major disadvantages include serious scarring of tissues, unless the clips are removed early, and the need for special and expensive devices for their application and removal.

Choice of suture material. The cardinal rule in choosing a suture material is that the strength of the material need be no greater than the strength of the tissue on which it is used. Oversized material causes tissue trauma and increases inflammatory reaction. Under most circumstances the surgeon will request the type and size of suture for each procedure. Generally, absorbable material is used when prolonged strength is not required or when infection is present or anticipated. Nonabsorbable suture is indicated when tissue reaction must be minimized, when endurance beyond 2 to 3 weeks is desirable, or when the suture can ultimately be removed. Nonabsorbable suture is selected for skin closure and absorbable suture for subcutaneous tissue closure.

After the basic principles have been observed, the choice of material is a matter of personal preference.

Suture sizes (Fig. 3-93) The customary method of sizing suture material is awkward and confusing but is well established and not likely to be revised in the near future.

The largest suture available is no. 5 and is approximately the size of ordinary string. The sizes progress downward in number and size to no. 1, which is still a very

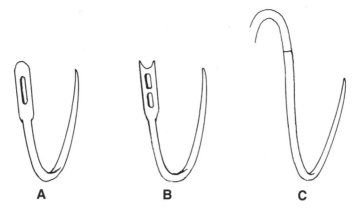

FIG. 3-94   Suture attachments. **A,** Square eye. **B,** French eye. **C,** Swaged needle.

heavy, thick suture. Below no. 1, sizes begin with 0 (ought) and again progress downward in size: 00 (double ought), 000 (three or triple ought), 4-0, 5-0, to 10-0, which is the smallest size. In routine small animal surgery, sizes 0 through 4-0 are standard. Sizes 5-0 through 7-0 are used for delicate vascular work and sizes 8-0 through 10-0 for ophthalmic surgery. The larger sizes are used in fascial repair, bone and tendon work, and postmortem suturing.

Wire suture is sized by gauge and varies from 18 gauge (coarse) to 40 gauge (very fine).

Suture Needles

There are no universal standards for the size and shape of suture needles; manufacturers are free to design their own. As a result, there are literally hundreds of different needles available. Basically all suture needles are identified by five characteristics: the type of suture attachment, the shape of the body of the needle, the point, the cross section, and the size.

Suture attachment (Fig. 3-94). *Eyed needles* are frequently encountered because they are reusable and can be used with almost any type of suture material. Eyed needles may be either straight or curved and have any type of point or cross section. The major disadvantage of eyed needles is that the suture must be threaded through the eye, creating a bulky bundle that must pass through the tissue, which will create a hole larger than the suture material. For this reason, eyed needles are avoided for use on easily damaged tissues, such as bowel or blood vessels. Eyed needles have a round, oval, square, or French eye.

The alternative to the eyed needle is the *swaged needle,* which has the suture attached to it during manufacture and therefore has no eye. The hole created is no larger than the size of the suture and is preferred for cardiovascular and intestinal surgery. Swaged needles are useful with nylon and polypropylene sutures, which are difficult to thread into an eyed needle. Because this type of needle can be used with only one length of suture, it retains its sharpness throughout the procedure and is

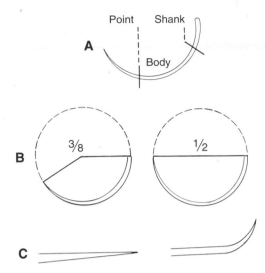

FIG. 3-95   **A,** Parts of suture needle. **B,** Three-quarter circle and half circle needles. **C,** Straight and half-curved needles.

then discarded. For the same reason swaged needles are also very expensive.

The *loosely swaged needle* is constructed in such a way that a sharp tug will remove the needle from the suture. This is an advantage when it is desirable to separate the needle and the suture quickly and easily.

Configuration of needle body (Fig. 3-95). The configuration of the needle body may be straight or curved. Straight needles are driven through tissue by hand, whereas curved needles require a needle holder. The ½ circle is preferred for coarse to medium-sized needles, and the ⅜ and ⅝ circle represent the shape of the fine needles used in ophthalmic surgery and skin closure. Needles are also available in S-shaped and half-curved configurations.

Point and cross section (Fig. 3-96). The point and cross section of the needle to be used are determined by the type of tissue to be sutured. For soft tissues, a round cross section needle with a point that is tapered (atraumatic) is preferred because it will not leave small cuts in the tissue along the suture line. Standard cutting needles (traumatic) have three cutting edges that form a triangle and incise the tissue in the direction of the pull of the suture. Reverse cutting needles have the apex of the triangle on the back of the needle and a flat edge in the direction of the pull. This configuration prevents further damage to the cut edges of the tissue. Cutting and reverse cutting needles, having spear, spatula, or trocar points, are used for skin closure or other tough tissue that will resist the advancement of round, taper-point needles.

Size. Although there are no universal standards, the general rule for needle size is the lower the number, the larger the needle; nos. 0, 1, and 2 are coarse needles, and nos. 17, 18, and 20 are fine needles (Fig. 3-97).

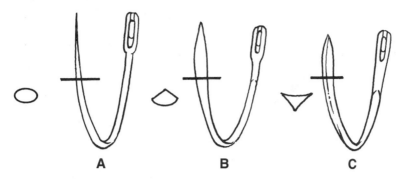

FIG. 3-96   Suture needle cross sections. **A,** Round or taper point, **B,** Cutting point. **C,** Reverse cutting point.

Care and Handling of Suture Materials and Needles

- Because of its derivation, surgical gut is damaged by drying and is supplied in presterilized wetpacks. Suture material should remain unopened until needed. Surgical gut cannot be subjected to dry or moist heat sterilization.
- Suture needles are essentially cutting instruments and are dulled by heat sterilization and routine use. When needles are cleaned, each one should be checked for crimped or weakened bodies and shanks and for burred tips. Worn needles should be discarded.
- Needles to be sterilized should be organized by size in a spring-type needle retainer. Each surgical pack should include several needles of varying types and sizes.
- Suture materials, needles, and other small packages of surgical supplies should be organized and stored in such a way that they can be readily obtained and inventoried.

■ INTRAOPERATIVE HANDLING OF SURGICAL INSTRUMENTS AND SUPPLIES

When necessary, the technician will be asked to "scrub in" on sterile procedures to assist the surgeon. Technical assistance during surgery may include preparing and arranging the instrument tray, passing instruments or other sterile items, applying and/or holding instruments as directed, cutting sutures, and sponging off or suctioning the surgical site.

Preparing and Arranging the Instrument Tray

An unscrubbed assistant places the sterilized instrument pack on the tray, untapes the outer wrap, and allows the outer wrap to cover the tray. The inner wrap may now be opened with gloved hands and allowed to create a second layer over the tray. If the drapes are sterilized with the instruments, they will appear first as the pack is opened. If sterilized separately, the drapes are opened and passed to the surgeon using a sterile transfer method. The drapes are opened by allowing them to unfold, never by shaking them out. The accordion fold method of preparation facilitates unfolding. While the surgeon is placing the drapes, the sterile towel clips

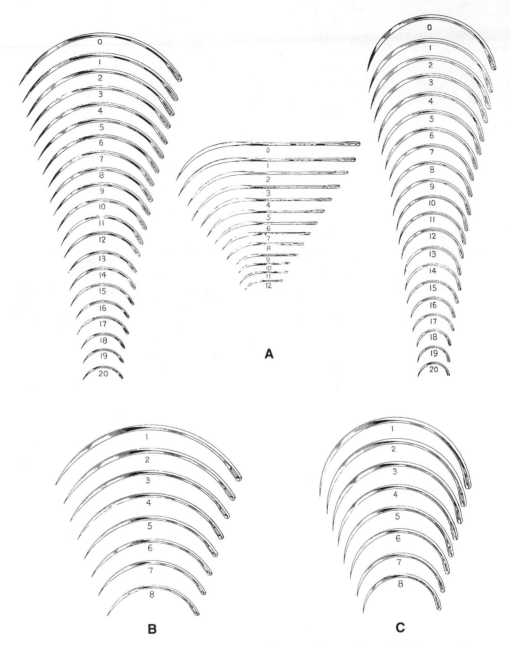

A

B

C

FIG. 3-97 Examples of surgeon's suture needles. **A,** Half-curved, cutting edge, regular eye. **B,** Three-eighth circle, cutting edge, regular eye. **C,** Half circle, cutting edge, regular eye.

are removed from the pack and handed to the surgeon one at a time. When drap-ing is completed, the technician will call for the scalpel blade to be dropped onto the tray. The scalpel handle is removed by the surgeon or technician from the in-strument pack, and the blade is attached with a hemostat (Fig. 3-98). The remain-ing instruments are removed and arranged on the tray. Instrument arrangement is largely a matter of personal preference, but generally instruments are grouped by type and function and arranged in the order in which they will be used (Fig. 3-99). Because the size of the tray is limited, extra or oversized instruments and sponge packs are kept in a cabinet or on a back table and called for as needed. The tray should not be overcrowded because this increases the risk of instruments being knocked off. During the course of the procedure anything that is no longer needed should be promptly removed. When the instruments are arranged, sterile suture material is called for and aseptically dropped onto the tray. The reels are removed and set aside, and the package is discarded. Patient safety requires that the opera-tive procedure be completed as quickly as possible. The tray should be ready as soon as the draping is complete.

Passing Instruments

When passing any instrument, the technician gently but firmly slaps it into the wait-ing palm of the surgeon. This method is used to avoid dropping the instrument and

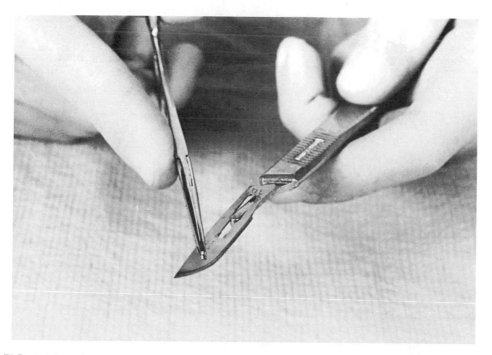

FIG. 3-98 The safest way to attach and remove scalpel blades is with an instrument—not with fingers.

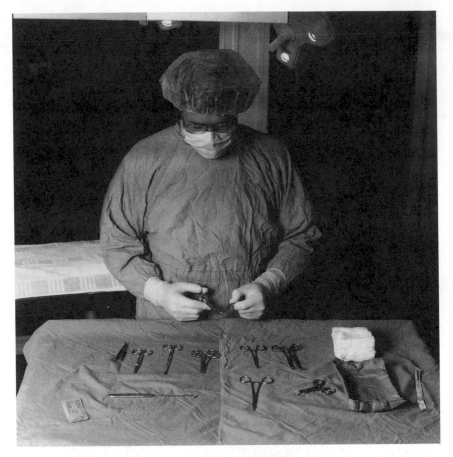

FIG. 3-99   The surgeon will arrange the instrument stand in his or her preferred manner.

allows the surgeon to receive it without looking up each time. Instrument ratchets or jaws should always be closed before being passed. Instruments with finger rings are always passed rings first (Fig. 3-100).

Thumb forceps are slapped into the palm with the tines pointing downward. Scalpels are passed so that the technician and the surgeon are protected from the blade (Fig. 3-101).

Applying and/or Holding Instruments

Curved instruments are passed and applied with the concave side up (Fig. 3-102). Finger ring instruments are held by placing the thumb and ring finger through the rings and extending the index finger along the shank (Fig. 3-103). The tissue or vessel is grasped with the tip of the jaws and the ratchet is locked.

Self-retaining retractors are fitted into the incision and spread, and the retaining device is locked in place. Hand-held retractors require an assistant to spread and

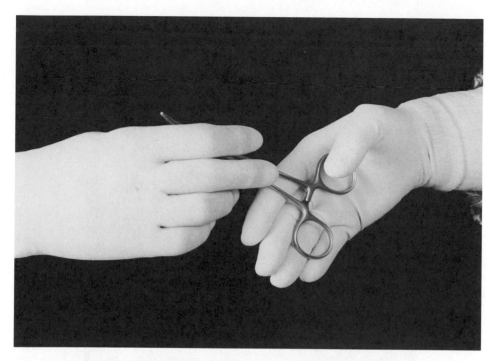

FIG. 3-100   Passing ringed instruments.

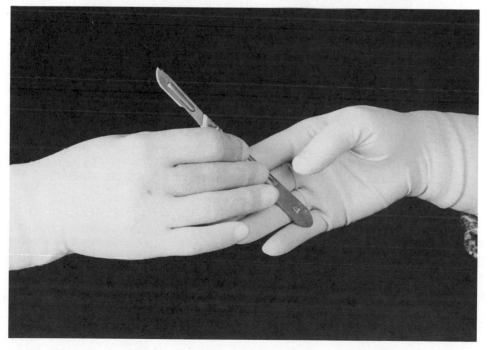

FIG. 3-101   Correct way to pass scalpel.

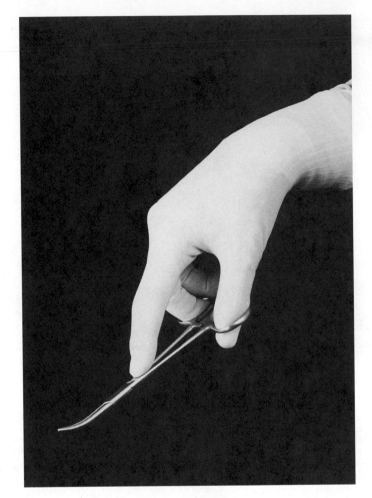

FIG. 3-102   Curved instruments are applied to tissues with the concave side up.

hold the incision open until the work is complete. Retractors are applied with great care because careless or prolonged retraction will seriously damage tissues.

Thumb forceps are held in a pencil grip (Fig. 3-104).

Cutting Sutures

When suture material is to be cut, the scissors are brought to the surgical site with the blades closed (Fig. 3-105). The jaws are then opened slightly, and only the tips are used to cut the suture. The surgeon will indicate how far above the knot the suture should be cut.

Sponging Off or Suctioning the Surgical Site

The technician may be expected to watch for and sponge blood accumulations from the surgical site. Sponging is accomplished by blotting rather than wiping the blood.

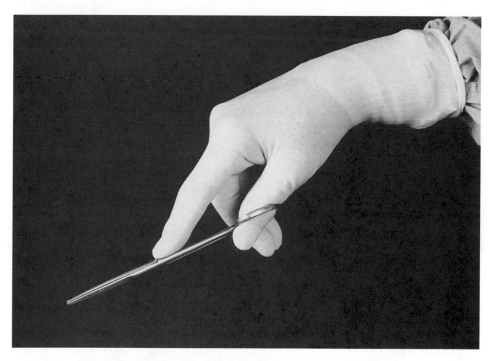

FIG. 3-103   Correct way to hold ringed instruments.

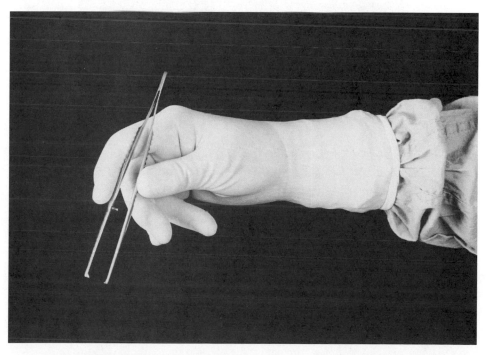

FIG. 3-104   Thumb forceps held in modified pencil grip.

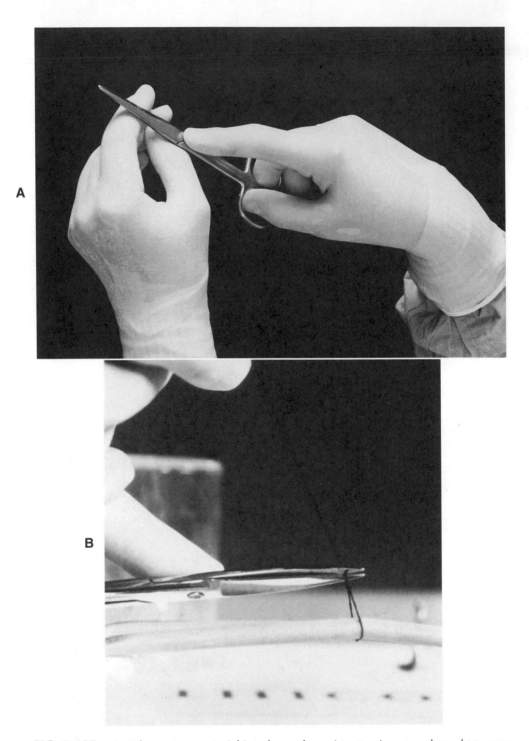

FIG. 3-105   **A,** When suture material is to be cut by assistant, scissors are brought to operative site with jaws closed. **B,** Jaws are parted slightly, and suture is cut with tips only.

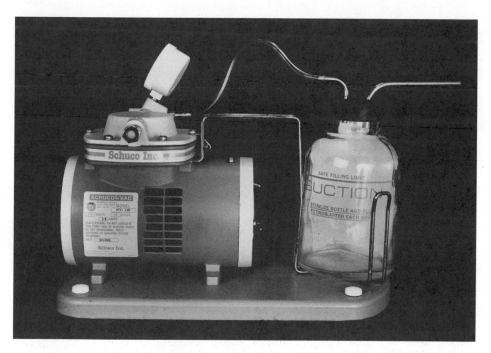

FIG. 3-106   Mechanical suction device.

Rubbing the sponge across the site will promote bleeding, and blotting will staunch it. Wet sponges absorb better than dry ones, so sponges should be moistened with sterile saline before use. Moistened sponges are also less irritating to tissues than dry ones.

For routine procedures, sponges are sterilized in packs of 10 or 20. This not only prevents waste but also allows the surgical technician to count the exact number of sponges used during a procedure. All used sponges are dropped into one receptacle and counted before the incision is closed to be certain none have been retained in the body.

Another way of removing fluids from the operative site is with a mechanical suction device (Fig. 3-106).

Each surgeon works differently; therefore real efficiency occurs only after the technician learns the surgeon's method of operation. To be of value as a surgical assistant requires a thorough knowledge of surgical instrumentation and the sequence of events that comprise the procedure so that the surgeon's needs can always be anticipated.

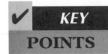

KEY POINTS

1. Ideally the surgical area includes a preparation room, a pack room, a recovery room, a treatment room, and an operating room. The layout of the surgical area must allow for the ease of sanitation and the efficient functioning of surgical personnel.

2. The preparation room should be separate from the operating room and should house the equipment and supplies required to prepare the surgeon, the surgical assistants, and the patient.

3. Basic equipment in a preparation room includes surgeon's scrub sink, patient preparation surface, wet/dry vacuum cleaner, small animal clipper with no. 40 surgical preparation blade, refrigerator, supply locker, anesthesia machine, endotracheal intubation equipment, intravenous fluid administration equipment, and a large waste receptacle with liner.

4. The pack room contains the equipment and supplies necessary to clean, assemble, wrap, and sterilize surgical instruments and supplies.

5. The recovery area should be a warm, quiet room conveniently located to ensure that recovering animals receive adequate attention. The length of time patients will remain in recovery is determined by their level of consciousness and the adequate stabilization of their vital signs.

6. The treatment room is reserved for nonsterile surgical procedures, such as dentistry, cat castrations, and the care of lacerations and abscesses.

7. Ultrasonography allows differentiation of solid from cystic structures and recognition of fine textural abnormalities within an organ.

8. Although most anesthetics are nonflammable and nonexplosive, the technician should be aware of the present dangers of fire, explosion, and electrical hazards.

9. The most commonly used material in surgical instruments is stainless steel, polished to a dull finish to reduce light reflection and bathed in a nitric acid bath.

10. Scalpel blades must be sterile, extremely sharp, and available in several sizes and shapes. Scalpel blades are made of carbon steel or stainless steel and are used for incising the skin and transecting tissue.

11. Surgical scissors are classified by the type of points (blunt/blunt, sharp/blunt, sharp/sharp), the shape of the blades (straight or curved), and the cutting edge of the blades (plain or serrated).

12. Operating scissors are used in four ways: to cut through or snip tissue, to separate tissue by inserting the tips into the tissue and spreading the points, to separate tissue by exerting a steady force of the tips against the tissue, and to cut suture material.

13. Thumb forceps are used to grasp tissue or dressing material; hemostatic and tissue forceps are used to clamp, hold, or retract blood vessels, tissues, and tissue bundles.

14. Retractors are used to pull apart the edges of incised surgical sites so that the surgeon is provided with a better visual exposure of the body cavity and a free access to tissues and organs.

15. Orthopedic instruments and appliances are among the most specialized and expensive of all surgical instruments.

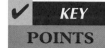

KEY POINTS

16. In small animal medicine, routine dentistry is generally limited to extractions and tartar removal.
17. Because mechanical properties as well as biologic interactions must be considered, certain principles must be observed in the surgeon's choice of suture material. There is no perfect suture material.
18. The purpose of any suture is to hold the wound edges in apposition until the wound can endure normal stress without the support of the sutures.
19. There are two major classes of suture material, absorbable and nonabsorbable. Absorbable sutures are digested and assimilated by the body during healing and do not require removal. Absorbable materials are manufactured from animal and synthetic sources.
20. Metal clips and staples are used to ligate small blood vessels, pull wound edges together, and secure material to incised skin.
21. The cardinal rule in choosing a suture material is that the strength of the material need be no greater than the strength of the tissue on which it is used.
22. Basically, all suture needles are identified by five characteristics: the type of suture attachment, the shape of the body of the needle, the point, the cross section, and the size.
23. The configuration of the needle body may be straight or curved. Straight needles are driven through tissue by hand, whereas curved needles require a needle holder. Needles are also available in S-shaped and half-curved configurations.
24. The point and cross section of the needle to be used are determined by the type of tissue to be sutured.
25. Although there are no universal standards, the general rule for needle size is the lower the number, the larger the needle.
26. The technician's assistance during surgery may include preparing and arranging the instrument tray, passing instruments or other sterile items, applying and/or holding instruments as directed, cutting sutures, and sponging off or suctioning the surgical site.

▼ REVIEW QUESTIONS

1. What rooms does the ideal surgical area provide?

2. What basic equipment should be found in a preparation room?

Continued

▼ REVIEW QUESTIONS—cont'd

3. Identify basic equipment for a pack room.

4. Identify basic equipment for the recovery room.

5. What function does the treatment room serve?

6. How does the information provided by ultrasonography differ from that seen in conventional radiography?

7. What basic equipment is needed in the treatment room?

8. Review the regulations observed in the design and use of an operating theater.

9. Discuss considerations regarding fire hazards that affect conduct in the operating room.

10. What basic equipment is found in the operating room?

11. Discuss the qualities needed in a scalpel for small animal surgery in terms of condition, size, shape, and material used in its manufacture.

12. Identify uses for the following blades and handles: no. 3 and no. 4 handles, the Beaver handle, and scalpel blades no. 10, no. 11, and no. 12.

13. Discuss the function, advantages, and disadvantages of the electroscalpel.

14. How are surgical scissors classified?

15. Outline the four ways operating scissors are used.

16. Identify some of the most common surgical scissors and their uses.

17. Describe the functions of each of the following: thumb forceps, hemostatic and tissue forceps, retractors, and needle holders.

18. What type of surgery requires the most expensive instruments and appliances? Why?

19. Describe routine dentistry in small animal medicine. What is the technician expected to know?

20. Discuss general guidelines for the care and handling of surgical instruments.

21. What should influence the surgeon's choice of suture material?

22. What attributes would the perfect suture have? Is there such a suture?

23. What is the purpose of any suture?

Continued

▼ REVIEW QUESTIONS—cont'd

24. Name the two major classes of suture material.

25. Identify properties and absorption rates for each of the following suture materials: surgical gut (catgut), polyglycolic acid.

26. Identify the four groups of nonabsorbable suture materials.

27. Discuss advantages and disadvantages of each of the following suture materials: silk, cotton, braided synthetic, monofilament, and wire.

28. What are the functions, pros, and cons of metal clips and staples?

29. What is the cardinal rule in choosing a suture material?

30. Describe the five characteristics used to identify suture needles.

31. Describe the advantages and disadvantages of eyed needles, swaged needles, and loosely swaged needles.

32. Describe possible configurations of the needle body.

33. How is the appropriate point and cross section of the needle to be used determined? What are the options?

34. What is the general rule for needle sizes?

35. What, in general, may be the technician's assistance during surgery?

36. Discuss guidelines for preparing and arranging the instrument tray.

37. Discuss guidelines for passing instruments in surgery.

38. Describe the technique for cutting suture material.

39. What might the technician be expected to do about blood accumulations in the surgical site?

ANSWERS FOR CHAPTER 3

1. Ideally the surgical area includes a preparation room, a pack room, a recovery room, a treatment room, and an operating room. The layout of the surgical area must allow for the ease of sanitation and the efficient functioning of surgical personnel.

2. Basic equipment in a preparation room includes surgeon's scrub sink, patient preparation surface, wet/dry vacuum cleaner, small animal clipper with no. 40 surgical preparation blade, refrigerator, supply locker, anesthesia machine, endotracheal intubation equipment, intravenous fluid administration equipment, and a large waste receptacle with liner.

3. The pack room contains the equipment and supplies necessary to clean, assemble, wrap, and sterilize surgical instruments and supplies. Basic equipment for the pack room includes sterilizing unit (moist heat or gas), washer and dryer, ultrasonic instrument cleaner, sink, counter space or large table for folding linens, linen receptacle, sterile and nonsterile supply closets, and waste receptacle with liner.

4. Basic equipment for the recovery room includes recovery cages (padded to prevent injury, if necessary), monitoring equipment, therapeutic oxygen administration equipment, respirator, emergency drug closet, intravenous fluid administration supplies, rewarming pads and supplies, incubator, supply closet (for dressings, towels, and blankets), and waste receptacle with liner.

5. The treatment room is reserved for nonsterile surgical procedures, such as dentistry, cat castrations, and the care of lacerations and abscesses.

6. Conventional radiography cannot distinguish between fluid and soft tissue, nor between textures of soft tissue organs.

7. Basic equipment in the treatment room includes treatment table, anesthesia machine and monitoring devices, electrosurgical unit, ultrasonic dental scaler and manual dental instruments, supply locker, small refrigerator, radiograph viewer, clipper and reel, large sink, cold sterilization trays, and collections of assorted instruments.

8. In the design and use of an operating theater, the following regulations are observed: exposed surfaces are nonporous and impervious to harsh cleaning agents; a maximum of two two-way swinging doors lead into the operating room; doors are used as infrequently as possible; air pressure is at a higher level than in adjacent rooms; room ventilators are equipped with air filters; equipment used to clean the operating room is not used in other rooms at any time; all personnel in the operating room must wear a cap, a mask, and a freshly laundered uniform or scrub suit; surgical personnel must know sterile and nonsterile boundaries and adhere to the principles of aseptic technique.

9. Although most anesthetics are nonflammable and nonexplosive, the technician should be aware of the present dangers of fire, explosion, and electrical hazards. The following considerations regarding fire hazards govern conduct in the operating room: all anesthetics are considered dangerous and are stored and used at least 3 feet away from electrical equipment; several materials in the operating room can disperse static electricity; operating room clothing is made of antistatic material; hair and fur are covered to avoid static electricity; functional fire extinguishers are available; electrical equipment is routinely checked; grounding is essential for electrocautery, electrosurgical, and defibrillator units. Plastics and other flammable agents are not used without special precautions; smoking is not allowed; humidity is maintained at 50% or above.

10. Basic equipment for the operating room includes surgical spotlights, surgical table and pad, monitoring devices, intravenous drip stand, instrument stand with tray, back table or counter, suction equipment, radiograph viewer, anesthetic machine, electrosurgical and coagulation unit, positioning devices, waste receptacle with liner, wall clock, and electrosurgical unit.

11. A scalpel blade must be sterile, extremely sharp, and available in several sizes and shapes. In small animal surgery, the no. 3 and, less often, the no. 4 handles are used. Ophthalmic surgery and microsurgery demand a long, thin, tapered or rounded handle fitted with small disposable blades. Scalpel blades are made of carbon steel or stainless steel and are used for incising the skin and transecting tissue.

12. Uses for selected blades and handles are as follows:

Scalpel handles	Use
No. 3	Small animal surgery
No. 4	Large animal surgery
Beaver handles	Ophthalmic surgery

Scalpel blades

No. 10	Incising skin (use no. 3 handle)
No. 11	Severing ligaments (use no. 3 handle)
No. 12	Lancing abscesses (use no. 3 handle)

13. The electroscalpel converts electric energy by adapting currents through cutting and coagulation tips. The advantages of the electroscalpel are the minimizing of surgical hemorrhage and the prevention of the growth of undesirable cells by contact destruction. However, healing may take longer than with a conventional scalpel.

14. Surgical scissors are classified by the type of points (blunt/blunt, sharp/blunt, sharp/sharp), the shape of the blades (straight or curved), and the cutting edge of the blades (plain or serrated).

15. Operating scissors are used in four ways: to cut through or snip tissue, to separate tissue by inserting the tips into the tissue and spreading the points, to separate tissue by exerting a steady force of the tips against the tissue, and to cut suture material.

16. Surgical scissors and their uses are listed below:

Operating scissors	Dissecting tissue/cutting sutures
Mayo dissecting scissors	General operative procedures
Doyen abdominal scissors	Cutting tough tissue
Curved Metzenbaum scissors	Cutting deep, delicate tissue
Iris scissors	Intraocular tissue
Stitch scissors	Removing sutures
Wire-cutting scissors	Cutting wire sutures
Bandage scissors	Cutting dressing material

17. Thumb forceps are used to grasp tissue or dressing material. Depending on the style, they are capable of holding tissue firmly (either horizontally or vertically) and produce minimal tissue damage. Hemostatic and tissue forceps are used to clamp, hold, or retract blood vessels, tissues, and tissue bundles. Retractors are used to pull apart the edges of incised surgical sites so that the surgeon has a better visual exposure of the body cavity and free access to tissues and organs.

    Needle holders are used to grasp and hold the suture needle, and some have the capacity to cut the suture as well. A combination holding and cutting instrument is popular among veterinary surgeons who work alone because the suture may be tied and cut with the same instrument. However, some dislike the instrument because of its tendency to snip the suture material unintentionally while the knot is being tied.

18. Orthopedic instruments and appliances are among the most specialized and expensive of all surgical instruments. Most bone instruments and implantation devices are made of stainless steel or a cobalt-chromium alloy because they are inert.

19. In small animal medicine, routine dentistry is generally limited to extractions and tartar removal. Although the ultrasonic sealer has supplanted manual methods for tartar removal, the technician should be familiar with the operation of nonmechanical sealing tools.

20. Some general guidelines for the care and handling of surgical instruments include the following: Instruments should be used only for the purposes for which they were intended; they should be *placed* on surfaces, never dropped or thrown. Instrument milk—not grease or oil—is used for lubrication. Instruments should never be cleaned with abrasive materials or cleansers; they should be dried thoroughly. In cold sterilization, an antirust additive must be added to the solution. The safest way to attach and remove scalpel blades is with a hemostat. Moist heat sterilization will dull the edges of cutting instruments. Metal etching and engraving devices should never be used to identify surgical instruments. When an ultrasonic instrument cleaner is used, different kinds of metals should not be mixed. Electrolysis may occur, and the instrument surfaces may be damaged. Sterile surgical instruments must not be used for nonsterile procedures. They must be identified and kept separate.

21. Because mechanical properties as well as biologic interactions must be considered, certain principles must be observed in the surgeon's choice of suture material. Among these are strength and endurance of the suture material and the type of tissue to be sutured.

22. To achieve perfection, a suture would have to be a monofilament of a uniform small size; possess a high tensile strength; be completely absorbable, inexpensive, pliable, and easily manipulated; and would never slip when tied. There is no such material.

23. The purpose of any suture is to hold the wound edges in apposition until the wound can endure normal stress without the support of the sutures.

24. There are two major classes of suture material, absorbable and nonabsorbable. Absorbable sutures are digested and assimilated by the body during healing and do not require removal. Absorbable materials are manufactured from animal and synthetic sources. Animal-derived sutures include surgical gut.

25. Surgical gut (catgut) is produced from the submucosal layer of sheep or hog intestine. Plain gut will be absorbed by the body in 3 to 5 days, and chromic gut will be absorbed in 10 to 15 days. Polyglycolic acid (PGA) suture is manufactured from polyglycolic acid or hydroxyacetic acid, which is extruded in fine threads and then woven into suture material of different sizes. PGA sutures retain strength for 2 to 3 weeks and cause less inflammatory reaction than catgut.

26. Nonabsorbable suture materials may be divided into four groups: silk and cotton, braided synthetics, monofilament synthetics, and wire and metal.

27. Silk suture is inexpensive, is readily available, and will retain its strength. However, it will support bacterial growth and cause more tissue inflammation than cotton, synthetics, or metals. Advantages of cotton sutures include reasonable cost, pliability, ease of sterilization, and less marked tissue reaction than that caused by silk suture. However, cotton suture will support bacterial growth and therefore is not generally used for skin closure. When wet, cotton suture material is difficult to handle.

    Braided synthetic sutures are less irritating than cotton and silk, have a high tensile strength, are not inclined to shelter bacterial growth, and are easily sterilized. The major disadvantage of these materials is that they knot poorly.

    The monofilament sutures are relatively inert in tissue, do not shelter bacteria, and have a high tensile strength but are difficult to handle and tie. If the material is to be buried, it must be heat sterilized and handled aseptically.

    Wire sutures are made from high-grade stainless steel and are available in both monofilament and braided forms. They are noncorrosive in vivo, are inert, will not support bacterial growth, and have a high tensile strength, but they are difficult to handle.

28. Metal clips and staples are used to ligate small blood vessels, pull wound edges together, and secure material to incised skin. Clips and staples are easy to handle and apply. Because they can be safely and effectively sterilized, they can be applied to infected wounds. The major disadvantages include serious scarring of tissues and the need for special and expensive devices for their application and removal.

29. The cardinal rule in choosing a suture material is that the strength of the material need be no greater than the strength of the tissue on which it is used. Generally, absorbable material is used when prolonged strength is not required or when infection is present or anticipated. Nonabsorbable suture is indicated when tissue reaction must be minimized, when endurance beyond 2 to 3 weeks is desirable, or when the suture can ultimately be removed.

30. Basically, all suture needles are identified by five characteristics: the type of suture attachment, the shape of the body of the needle, the point, the cross section, and the size.

31. Eyed needles are reusable and can be used with almost any type of suture material. Eyed needles may be either straight or curved and have any type of point or cross section. The major disadvantage of eyed needles is that they will create a hole larger than the suture material.

    The swaged needle has the suture attached to it during manufacture and therefore has no eye. The hole created is no larger than the size of the suture and is preferred for cardiovascular and intestinal surgery. Swaged needles are very expensive. The loosely swaged needle is constructed in such a way that a sharp tug will remove the needle from the suture. This is an advantage when it is desirable to separate the needle and the suture quickly and easily.

32. The configuration of the needle body may be straight or curved. Straight needles are driven through tissue by hand, whereas curved needles require a needle holder. Needles are also available in S-shaped and half-curved configurations.

33. The point and cross section of the needle to be used are determined by the type of tissue to be sutured. Choices range from the round cross-section needle with a point that is tapered (atraumatic),

standard cutting needles (traumatic), reverse cutting needles, and cutting and reverse cutting needles with spear, spatula, or trocar points.

34. Although there are no universal standards, the general rule for needle size is the lower the number, the larger the needle.

35. The technician's assistance during surgery may include preparing and arranging the instrument tray, passing instruments or other sterile items, applying and/or holding instruments as directed, cutting sutures, and sponging off or suctioning the surgical site.

36. Guidelines for preparing and arranging the instrument tray include the following steps. An unscrubbed assistant places the sterilized instrument pack on the instrument tray, untapes the outer wrap, and allows the outer wrap to cover the tray. The inner wrap may now be opened with gloved hands and allowed to create a second layer over the tray. If the drapes are sterilized with the instruments, they will appear first as the pack is opened. If sterilized separately, the drapes are opened and passed to the surgeon using a sterile transfer method. The drapes are opened by allowing them to unfold. While the surgeon is placing the drapes, the sterile towel clips are removed from the pack and handed to the surgeon one at a time. When draping is completed, the scalpel handle is removed from the instrument pack and the blade is attached with a hemostat. The remaining instruments are removed and arranged on the tray. Extra or oversized instruments and sponge packs are kept in a cabinet or on a back table and called for as needed. The instrument tray should not be overcrowded. During the course of the procedure anything that is no longer needed should be promptly removed. When the instruments are arranged, sterile suture material is aseptically dropped onto the tray. The reels are removed and set aside, and the package is discarded. The tray should be ready as soon as the draping is complete.

37. When passing any instrument, the technician gently but firmly slaps it into the waiting palm of the surgeon. Instrument ratchets or jaws should always be closed before being passed. Instruments with finger rings are always passed rings first. Thumb forceps are slapped into the palm with the tines pointing downward. Scalpels are passed so that the technician and the surgeon are protected from the blade.

   Curved instruments are passed and applied with the concave side up. Finger ring instruments are held by placing the thumb and ring finger through the rings and extending the index finger along the shank. Thumb forceps are always held in a pencil grip, never as tweezers.

38. When suture material is to be cut, the scissors are brought to the surgical site with the blades closed. The jaws are then opened slightly, and only the tips are used to cut the suture. The surgeon will indicate how far above the knot the suture should be cut.

39. The technician may be expected to watch for and mop blood accumulations from the surgical site. Sponging is accomplished by blotting rather than wiping the blood. All used sponges are dropped into one receptacle and counted before the incision is closed to be certain none have been retained in the body.

   Another way of removing fluids from the operative site is with a mechanical suction device. Mechanical suction is not used routinely in veterinary surgery because its operation requires a scrubbed assistant.

SELECTED READINGS

Betts CW, Crane SW: *Manual of small animal therapeutics,* New York, 1986, Churchill Livingstone.

Bojrab MJ: *Current techniques in small animal surgery,* Baltimore, 1997, Lea & Febiger.

Bourley LM, Vassere PB: *General small animal surgery,* Philadelphia, 1985, JB Lippincott.

Cunningham: *Textbook of veterinary physiology,* Philadelphia, 1997, WB Saunders.

Hurov L: *Handbook of veterinary surgical instruments and glossary of surgical terms,* Philadelphia, 1978, WB Saunders.

Slatter D: *Textbook of small animal surgery,* ed 2, vol 1, Philadelphia, 1993, WB Saunders.

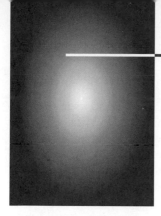

CHAPTER **4**

Small Animal Surgery

PERFORMANCE OBJECTIVES

After completion of this chapter the student will:

List the seven general functions to be performed by the technician before any surgical procedure.

List the indications for neutering dogs and cats.

List the 10 general signs to observe in the animal recovering from surgery.

Describe the difference between first intention wound healing and second intention wound healing.

The purpose of this chapter is to familiarize the technician with common veterinary surgical procedures. This knowledge is designed to allow the technician to (1) communicate more effectively with clients, veterinarians, and co-workers about surgical procedures; (2) assist in surgery; and (3) provide the essential preoperative and postoperative care for the surgical patient.

The chapter begins with a section on general surgical principles and practices; this includes generalized information on wound healing, suture removal, and electrosurgery.

Before individual operations are discussed, there is a section of general rules to be followed before, during, and after surgery. Each surgical procedure is discussed separately in the following order: indications for surgery, instruments needed for the operation, a description of the surgical procedure, and the role of the technician for the particular procedure. The technician should understand that the surgical procedures discussed are not a complete list of operations, but rather are representative examples common to the different anatomic systems. References are provided for additional information concerning surgical procedures not specifically discussed in this text.

No portion of this chapter should be assumed to provide license for technicians to perform functions that may be prohibited. The duties of individual technicians are determined by the policy of the employing veterinary hospital as well as applicable state laws.

In this chapter the term *surgeon's preference* is mentioned frequently. This is because most operations do not have specific instructions such as, "cut exactly 2 cm to the left and 3 cm distal to the xiphoid process." Because animals are of various shapes and sizes, the surgeon must exercise knowledge and expertise based on experience and preference. Surgeon's preference includes such factors as the length and location of incisions, the types of instruments used, the position of the table, the preferable side of the table from which to work during surgery, the number of layers to be sutured during closure, the use of clips versus suture materials, the choice of suture materials, the position of the surgical lights, and the degree to which surgical technicians participate in the operation.

■ GENERAL SURGICAL PRINCIPLES AND PRACTICES
Wound Healing

For the purpose of this chapter, a wound is defined as any disruption of tissue continuity. The disruption may be accidental (traumatic) or deliberate (surgical). Failure to understand how wounds heal may cause improper postoperative care, which can lead to complications. Wound healing is frequently divided into two types: first and second intention healing.

First intention wound healing. The surface of a healing wound is a granular surface, and this tissue has come to be called *granulation tissue*. First intention wound healing is the healing of a wound without infection or excessive granulation tissue. This type of wound healing is sometimes referred to as "side-to-side" healing because the wound edges are held together in apposition by sutures or some other mechanical device and can heal directly with less scar tissue formation.

When a wound is created, the blood vessels at the wound edges constrict for a brief period. Small vessels clot, but large vessels may continue to bleed. Shortly after the initial vasoconstriction, blood vessels revert to the opposite extreme, vasodilation. This enlarging of the vessels, particularly venules, stretches the blood vessel and allows plasma, proteins, and white blood cells to exude into the wounded area. The white blood cells engulf (phagocytize) any cellular debris resulting from the wound. The amount of cellular debris present varies, depending on the cause of the wound. The white blood cells also engulf the foreign material and the microorganisms present in the wound.

The significance of a debris-free wound edge cannot be overemphasized. Wounds cannot heal by first intention if a large amount of cellular debris is present.

Surgical assistants should avoid wiping the wound edges vigorously with sponges to keep them dry. Blotting tissues with a saline moistened sponge is preferred.

Sutures or some other mechanical device is used to appose the wound edges in a side-to-side fashion. The epithelial cells at the skin surface begin a rapid series of division and usually bridge the surface of the wound within 48 hours. However, the technician should keep in mind that the skin edges cover the wound several days before the deeper parts of the wound have healed. A healed skin surface does not necessarily mean that the entire wound has healed. For further information, see the suture removal section in this chapter.

In the case of a clean wound, after approximately 2 days, the skin surface is joined, a large amount of cellular debris has been eliminated by the white blood cells, and fibroblasts appear. Fibroblasts are cigar-shaped cells that produce collagen, a chemical that forms small fibers. These fibers then rapidly fill the wound and surround the capillaries. The collagen fibers first appear around the fourth or fifth day but continue to form for 4 to 5 weeks. After 1 month, the fibroblasts have almost disappeared and the wound is filled with dense collagen fibers, which form the scar. By 10 days after the initial wound, the scar is strong enough to hold most wound edges together without the aid of sutures. However, the wound does not completely gain full strength for another 2 to 4 weeks.

Soon after the fibroblasts appear, new capillary blood vessels also grow into the wound. These new blood vessels are formed by "budding" from the venules at the edges of the wound. The capillaries rapidly bridge the wound edges.

With time the scar remodels somewhat, usually by shrinking (constriction). This fact is significant only when the exact dimensions of healing tissue are critical, such as in tendons, joint capsules, or eyelids. In veterinary medicine, the cosmetic appearance of a scar is usually not an important factor unless the animal is of show quality.

Second intention wound healing. Second intention wound healing is the open healing of a wound that contains two granulating surfaces and some degree of suppuration. Suppuration is the formation of pus, which is the liquid that results from inflammation. It contains large quantities of white blood cells, cellular debris, and the tissue elements liquified by the enzymes in the white blood cells.

Wounds are allowed to heal open (second intention) for several reasons, infection being the most common. If moderate amounts of cellular debris and microorganisms are present, the wound will not heal by first intention. Infected wounds are often allowed to heal by second intention, or closure is delayed until the wound can be cleaned properly.

In second intention healing, many of the same processes occur as in first intention healing. Plasma, proteins, and white blood cells accumulate in the wound; new capillaries begin to grow out of the wound edges; and epithelial cells begin to divide at the surface. However, because there is now a gap from one wound edge to the other, the dividing epithelial cells cannot cross the open space. Instead, they begin to migrate down the edges of the wound, and granulation tissue forms within the open wound area.

As soon as the cellular debris is cleaned and microorganisms (e.g., bacteria) are reduced in number, fibroblasts start to form collagen fibers. The speed of the process depends on the degree of contamination of the wound with microorganisms and cellular debris. The collagen fibers begin to accumulate with new capillaries to form granulation tissue. The wound edges grow toward each other until the defect is filled.

Frequently the surface of the wound is covered with dried plasma proteins, blood cells, and other debris to form a scab. The healing process continues under the scab. If no infection is present, these scabs are left in place.

Unless there has been extensive tissue loss, the surface of granulation tissue will eventually be covered with new epithelial cells. The extent to which epithelial cells can cover a wound is remarkable but is not without limits. Very large wounds may require special grafting techniques to be covered. The new skin does not grow hair follicles. Consequently, the resulting healed wound (scar) is hairless. When completely healed, the wound is somewhat contracted.

Some surgical textbooks discuss healing by third intention as a special case in which very large amounts of tissue have been lost. The principles of second intention healing still apply, except that more extensive granulation must take place before the wound heals. There are occasions when tissue loss is so extensive that the body cannot repair the wound, and if a limb is involved, amputation may be necessary to prevent the chronic suppuration of an irreparable wound.

Sutures and staples. Surgeons prefer to have most wounds heal by first intention. To keep the wound edges in side-to-side apposition, a mechanical force must hold the tissues together until initial healing allows the wound edges to remain in apposition. It is the purpose of sutures or staples to hold the wound edges together on a temporary basis, usually for the first 7 to 10 days of healing.

Suture Removal

In many hospitals, the technician is the individual responsible for removing sutures or staples from a healed incision. Knowing when an incision is properly healed is, in part, a matter of judgment that results from experience. Some general guidelines follow.

The attending veterinarian should always be consulted if any of the following conditions exist at the incision site at the time of suture removal: swelling, erythema (redness), a discharge of any sort, separation of the wound edges, or tissue protruding from the incision site. These conditions do not necessarily mean that a problem exists, but they are certainly signs that merit the attention of the attending veterinarian. After the incision is healed, the sutures are removed by gently applying traction to one of the free suture ends and cutting one side of the suture below the knot (Fig. 4-1). Use of a suture scissors is recommended to lessen the chance of cutting the skin by mistake. Gentle traction on the free end of the suture allows its removal from the skin. This process is repeated until all the sutures have been removed. Staples are removed with a special device that varies from one manufacturer to another. Instructions are provided with the staple removers. The date of suture or staple removal and the condition of the incision should always be noted on the patient's medical record.

Electrocautery

The conventional method for achieving hemostasis during a surgical procedure is to clamp the bleeding vessel with a hemostat and ligate the vessel with suture material. One alternative is to seal the vessel with a controlled electrical current that burns or cauterizes the bleeding end. This procedure is known as electrocautery; it achieves hemostasis by coagulating the ends of the bleeding vessels if the blood flow is not excessive. Electrocautery is particularly valuable in any surgery in which multiple small bleeders exist that would be difficult or time consuming to clamp and tie in the conventional manner.

Several manufacturers produce electrocautery units for surgical use. These range from simple battery-powered units to very powerful and sophisticated models. The technician must become familiar with the specifications for the particular type of equipment being used. Most types of equipment that are commonly used require that the patient be properly grounded. A ground is a wire that can transfer electrical

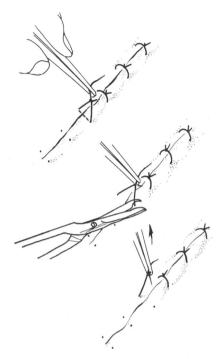

FIG. 4-1   One of free suture ends is gently elevated and the "hook" of suture scissors is placed inside the loop to cut the suture. After the loop has been cut, suture is removed by continuing to elevate the free end away from the skin.

current to a harmless place, usually to the ground. The ground can be a plate under the patient that is connected by wires to the electrocautery unit and to the ground wire present within the electrical outlet. An alternative to a plate under the patient is a metal rectal probe in the shape of a thermometer. The rectal probe is grounded in the same manner as the plate.

If the patient is not properly grounded (if the unit requires grounding), the electricity used for cauterization will travel along the path of least resistance, which may be the surgeon or the technician. Also, serious electrical burning of the animal can be caused by improper grounding.

Alcohol, ether, or other highly flammable materials should not be present when electrocautery is used. Portions of the electrocautery unit may be sterilized, usually the handles and wires, but not the cautery unit itself. The manufacturer's instructions must be carefully followed concerning sterilization techniques, maintenance, and the operation of the electrocautery unit.

The intensity of the current for electrocautery can be adjusted. The exact settings are determined by the veterinarian and depend, in part, on the type of tissue being cauterized.

The technician assisting in an operation that uses electrocautery must be very careful about sponging the blood. The field to be dried should be gently pressed with the gauze sponge to absorb the blood. Wiping a sponge across the field may disrupt clots that have already formed (either naturally or from electrocautery). Also, wiping with sponges too vigorously will usually increase the bleeding.

General Surgical Packs

In discussing individual operations, general surgical packs and special instruments are mentioned, and the special instruments are discussed as they apply to specific operations. However, instruments that are common to almost all operations are discussed in Chapter 3.

■ GENERAL RULES FOR THE TECHNICIAN IN SURGERY

The following checklists apply to all surgical procedures discussed in this text. The technician should make a habit of ensuring that every item on the checklist has been properly attended because inadequate or incorrect preoperative, operative, or postoperative care may cause complications. In addition to these general rules, each operation may require specific responsibilities for the technician. Such special procedures are included in the checklist for the specific operation.

Preoperative

1. Any consent or waiver forms used by the hospital should be signed by the owner before the patient is admitted. The owner should be given time to read and *understand* the forms being signed.
2. The technician should be sure that food and water have been withheld from the patient for the time period indicated by the attending veterinarian. Owners should be specifically asked if the pet has had *any* food or water. Some owners cannot resist giving at least a small amount of food or drink to their animals before coming to the veterinary facility.
3. The owner should be instructed when to call regarding progress reports on the patient. Specific times should be indicated rather than vague statements such as "sometime tomorrow."
4. Elective surgery patients should not be admitted unless they are relatively clean. A patient covered with mud, insects, or other debris may need bathing or grooming before surgery.
5. Any preoperative medications should be given in the correct dosages and at the correct times. With experience, the technician will be able to judge the flow of surgery so that if the surgical team is either ahead of or behind schedule, the times of medication can be adjusted accordingly. The ideal situation is one in which the next patient is completely prepared for surgery when the prior operation is being completed.
6. Any instruments or supplies necessary to perform the operation must be at hand, including scalpel blades, suture materials, needles, gowns, gloves, and drapes.
7. The appropriate area of the patient's body should be correctly prepared for surgery before the patient enters the operating room. This includes shaving, vacuuming loose hairs off the patient, and washing and disinfecting the appropriate area. Care should be taken to have the shaved area looking neat and symmetric.

Operative. When assisting during surgery, the technician should observe the following rules:

1. The technician should be familiar with the operation, especially as it pertains to the role of the assistant.
2. The technician should assist in a manner that will not block the surgeon's light or field of vision.
3. The technician should anticipate the instruments or supplies necessary for the particular operation and have them ready for the surgeon.
4. The technician should keep the surgical field dry by gently blotting with sponges. Excessive sponging may interfere with the surgical field.
5. The technician should keep the wound edges retracted so that the surgeon has maximum visibility. Excessive force that might injure the tissues should not be used.
6. When holding clamps on tissue or vessels that are to be ligated, the technician must hold the instruments in a manner that allows the surgeon easy access to placing the ligature material below the clamp. The clamp must then be repositioned to allow the surgeon maximum visibility to tie the ligature. (Refer to the discussion of operative technique under ovariohysterectomy for a discussion of double and triple clamping.)
7. When handling tissues, the technician must be as gentle as possible. Friable organs, such as the liver and spleen, are easily ruptured. Even moderate pressure on the pancreas may cause damage.
8. Appropriate scissors such as Mayo scissors are used to cut sutures or ligatures. The use of delicate dissecting scissors will needlessly dull them and alter the alignment of the scissor blades over time. The suture material should be cut with the tip of the scissors at the length indicated by the surgeon. The cut suture ends should not be allowed to remain in a body cavity or an incision.
9. If the surgeon is using a continuous suture pattern, the long loop of the suture material must be kept out of the surgeon's way. This usually requires the technician to have the free suture material on a side opposite the direction in which the surgeon is suturing. The technician may be required to rotate the long loop from side to side to keep it away from the surgeon's work area.
10. The technician should act as an extra pair of eyes and ears for the surgeon. Attention should not be solely focused on the surgical site so that the patient as a whole is neglected. The patient's breathing rate, blood color, and pulse should be monitored on a regular basis. The animal's condition throughout the operative procedure must be monitored.
11. If sponges were used inside the abdomen or chest cavities, the technician must ensure that they are all recovered. The best assurance is to know the number of sponges present at the start of surgery and account for the total amount of sponges before closure.

Postoperative. The technician should perform the following postsurgical responsibilities:

1. Patients should be carefully monitored for the recovery of swallowing reflexes so that the endotracheal tube can be removed.

2. Postoperative patients must remain warm. Heating pads, blankets, heating lamps, or other safe heating sources may be used. If blankets are used, they should be lifted occasionally to check the incisions and the general condition of the animal.

3. The cage should be changed as necessary to keep the patient clean and dry. A recovering animal must not be allowed to lie in feces or urine.

4. The patient's temperature and pulse as well as respiration must be systematically monitored. Major changes should be reported to the attending veterinarian. Memory must not be trusted. All preoperative, operative, and postoperative findings should be written on the patient's record and/or special anesthesia-recovery forms.

All patients should be carefully observed. Experience has shown that unusual cases are watched carefully but routine cases receive less attention. It is therefore true that routine cases may present the most surprises, many of which are unpleasant and can include cardiac and respiratory arrest.

The technician should watch specifically for the following signs in the postoperative period and should notify the attending veterinarian immediately if any occur:

1. Bleeding from the incision in larger amounts than the normal oozing that occurs during the first few minutes after surgery.

2. Loss of color or refill in the mucous membranes. If the patient's color is in doubt, the patient's hematocrit level should be checked as a baseline and rechecked in 15 to 20 minutes. A falling hematocrit level should be brought to the attention of the attending veterinarian.

3. Swelling of the operative site, including the abdominal or thoracic cavities or the incision itself.

4. Prolonged recovery from anesthesia or sedation (for the type of drug that was administered). Animals under anesthesia should be rotated from side to side (when this is possible) to avoid congestion of the lungs.

5. Separation of the incision edges.

6. Dehiscence (the opening of a surgical wound).

7. Dyspnea.

8. Vomiting. The patient should not be allowed to swallow vomitus because this may result in airway obstruction or aspiration pneumonitis.

9. Observing for chewing or licking at the incision site, in which case an E-collar should be placed over the animal's head to prevent the removal of sutures and opening of the surgical wound.

After the immediate postoperative period, the animal may be discharged to the owner's care at home or may remain hospitalized, depending on the nature of the surgery.

When the patient is discharged, the technician is responsible for the following procedures:

1. All medications prescribed by the veterinarian should be ready for the owner. The patient's name, the owner's name, the date, the veterinary hospital name and phone number, the name and strength of the medication, and clear directions for their use should be included on the label for the medication. Med-

---

Postsurgical Care

If your pet has had surgery, there are some simple rules to follow to avoid any damage to incisions and healing wounds.

1. Do not allow your pet to eat or drink immediately after arriving home because this may cause vomiting. After 1 hour you may allow small amounts of water until the animal is no longer thirsty.
2. Keep your pet as dry and as clean as possible.
3. Inspect the surgical site at least once each day.
4. Follow any special instructions about diet that you may have been given. Otherwise, resume your pet's normal diet.
5. Keep any bandages or dressings dry.
6. Be sure to observe any exercise restrictions the doctor has advised. Usually exercise should be limited to a leash only until the stitches are removed.

Be sure to notify the doctor if any of the following occurs:

1. Repeated vomiting
2. Extreme listlessness
3. Persistent bleeding
4. Excessive chewing at bandages or dressings
5. Stitches that are chewed or licked out
6. Loss of appetite that persists more than 24 hours

---

ication should *never* be dispensed in unmarked containers. Medications should only be dispensed in containers that comply with the pharmacy regulations for the state in which the veterinary hospital is located.

2. The owner should be reminded of any exercise restrictions after surgery.
3. The owner should be advised of any dietary restrictions.
4. The owner should be advised of the date and times for any return visits for dressing changes, suture removal, or other wound care procedures.
5. The owner should be advised to watch for danger signs.

Most owners are so happy and excited to see their pet (and vice versa) that they may not remember verbal instructions. It is highly recommended that a printed sheet of general instructions be given to the owner at the time of discharge (see the box above).

■ SURGICAL PROCEDURES
Reproductive Tract Surgery

Ovariohysterectomy (spay, neutering, OVH, OHE) (see Figs. 4-2 to 4-4)

Definition. An ovariohysterectomy is the removal of both ovaries and the uterus.

Indications. An ovariohysterectomy may be performed for the following reasons:

- Sterilization of the female dog or cat
- Elimination of estrous ("heat") cycles
- Some infections of the uterus, ovaries, or oviducts (also see Pyometra)
- Ovarian-induced hormone imbalances
- Some congenital abnormalities
- Neoplasms of the ovaries or uterus

Required instruments. In addition to the instruments in a general surgical pack, some veterinarians use a canelike or hooklike instrument to pull the uterine horn from the abdomen out of the incision. This comes in a variety of lengths and thicknesses and is referred to as a spay hook or a Snook hook.

Procedure. Most veterinary surgeons in North America use a ventral midline incision beginning just caudal to the umbilicus. (Some veterinarians, particularly those trained in Great Britain, use a flank incision for cats and small dogs.) The ventral midline incision is continued through the linea alba and peritoneum, which lines the abdominal cavity (Fig. 4-2). The left uterine horn and ovary are usually more caudal than the right and thus are easier to reach. When the surgeon isolates a uterine horn, it is first brought up and then out of the incision. Traction on the uterine horn exposes the ovary and ovarian pedicle (Fig. 4-3).

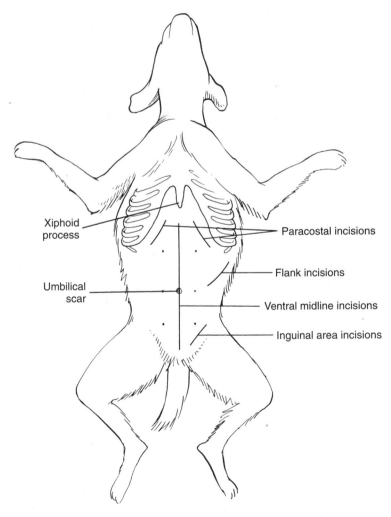

Xiphoid process

Umbilical scar

Paracostal incisions

Flank incisions

Ventral midline incisions

Inguinal area incisions

FIG. 4-2   Surgical incisions for abdominal procedures.

The exact method of traction and transection of the pedicle is a matter of individual preference for each veterinary surgeon. Triple clamping, double clamping, and clips are commonly used, depending on the surgeon's preference, as well as the size and condition of the patient.

Triple clamping involves placing three hemostatic forceps, such as Kelly or Crile forceps, across the uterine pedicle proximal to the ovary. The transection is made so that one forceps remains with the ovary and two are left proximal to the ovary. In the double-clamp method, only two clamps are used on the ovarian pedicle instead of three. This method may be used when the pedicle is small, such as in a cat or a small dog.

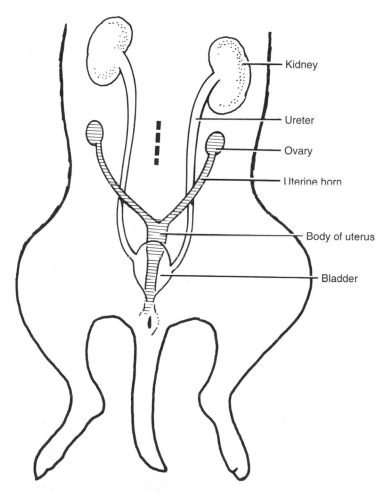

FIG. 4-3 Ovariohysterectomy. Ventral view showing relative position of ovaries, uterine horns, kidneys, and ureters. Dotted line indicates approximate location of incision preferred by many veterinarians.

The surgeon then ties suture material into the groove created by the forceps most distant from the ovary. If double or triple clamps are used, the surgical technician usually releases the clamp while the surgeon ties the ligature material. Practice by the two individuals working as a team will help the team develop efficiency of time and patient safety. The technician should not exert undue traction on the pedicle because this may result in a rupture of the pedicle and hemorrhage. The hemostatic clamp or clamps should be carefully rotated to allow the surgeon the best exposure for tying the knots.

If metal clips are used, the surgical technician usually loads the clip-applying forceps. This is of particular importance because the clip edges will not come together properly if they are not loaded correctly in the forceps. This can result in a slippage of the clips and postoperative hemorrhage.

The opposite ovary is removed in the same manner as the first. The uterine horns are then pulled cranially into the incision to expose the body of the uterus and the uterine blood vessels. The uterine body is fixed with either clips or clamps and transected cranial to the cervix. Care is taken to have adequate hemostasis and a smooth uterine "stump" to minimize the development of adhesions between the transected edge of the uterus and the urinary bladder. The uterine blood vessels are usually ligated separately from the uterus itself.

Closure of the abdomen is a matter of the surgeon's preference. Most surgeons prefer a three-layer closure: first layer, external rectus fascia; second layer, subcutaneous tissues; and third layer, skin. The three-layer closure minimizes the chances of wound dehiscence. The steps in preparing to perform a dog spay operation are presented in Fig. 4-4.

Role of the technician. Clients ask more questions about ovariohysterectomies than any other surgical procedure performed in the small animal hospital. The technician should be familiar with common attitudes and misconceptions about this surgical procedure to answer clients' questions about this operation.

Many individuals consider themselves knowledgeable about spaying dogs and cats, which probably accounts for the overwhelming amount of public misinformation regarding ovariohysterectomy. Even the name of the procedure causes confusion. Owners want their pets "spaded," "spade," "changed," or "altered." The most common term used when speaking to the public is *spay.* The past tense of *spay* is *spayed* not *spaded.* Even more confusion is caused by owners obtaining information concerning the spaying procedure from a misinformed individual. Most owners seem surprised when told that an ovariohysterectomy is a *major* surgical procedure that involves the removal of both ovaries and the entire uterus.

Some common misconceptions about the ovariohysterectomy are (1) it is beneficial for the pet to have at least one litter before surgery; (2) all spayed dogs and cats get fat; and (3) all dogs or cats over 3 years of age are too old to be spayed. All three of these statements are incorrect. Let us examine each claim so that the reader will be able to discuss ovariohysterectomy intelligently with an owner.

An argument against the first theory is that there are hundreds of thousands of pups and kittens destroyed each year because of a lack of homes. Every litter adds to this unresolved problem. Another argument is that it is generally easier to perform an ovariohysterectomy on a dog or cat before it has come into heat for the first time

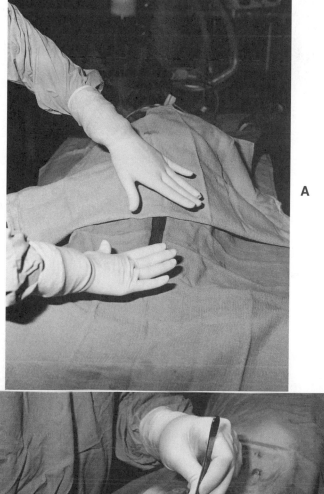

FIG. 4-4   Steps in preparing to perform a dog spay operation. **A,** The incision site is draped with four sterile towels. **B,** A ventral midline incision is made into the abdominal cavity.

Continued

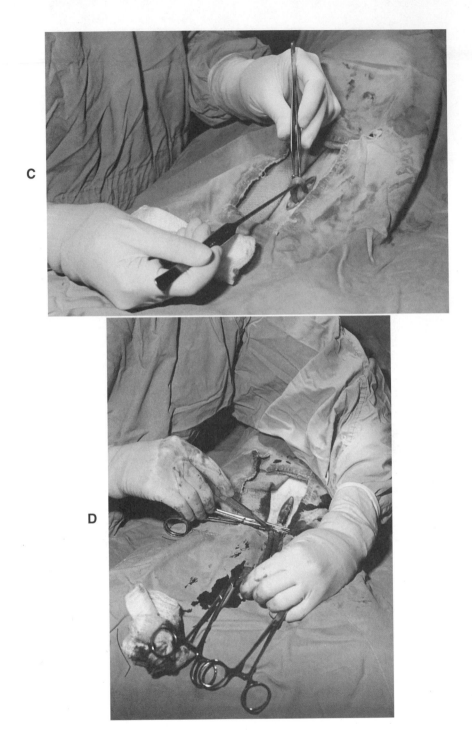

FIG. 4-4, cont'd   C, The horns of the uterus are pulled from the abdominal cavity. **D,** Each horn and ovary are detached from the body wall, clamped, and ligated.

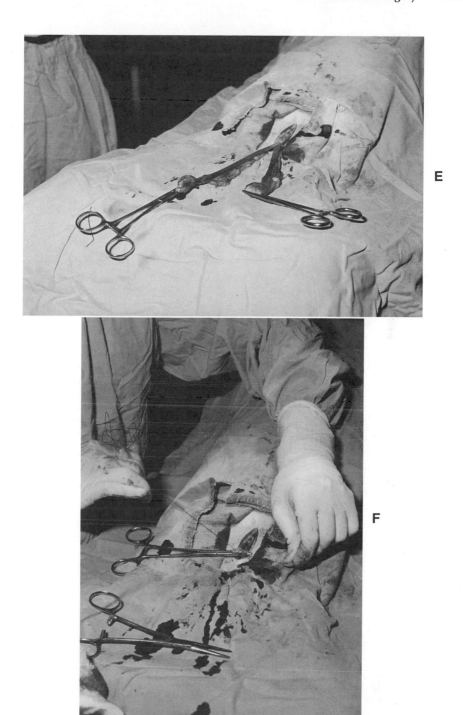

FIG. 4-4, cont'd   **E,** Both uterine horns and the ovaries are taken from the abdominal cavity.
F, The uterine stump is clamped, ligated, and excised.   *Continued*

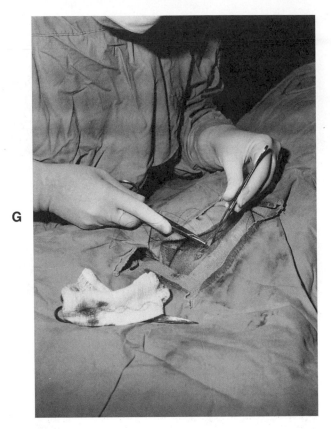

FIG. 4-4, cont'd   G, The incision is closed in layers. (Courtesy Angell Memorial Animal Hospital.)

because many structures of the reproductive tract enlarge after the first heat cycle. It is certainly easier to perform an ovariohysterectomy before the bitch or queen has had a litter. Pregnancy causes enlargement not only of the uterus but also of the associated blood vessels. The vascular and organ enlargement necessitates a larger abdominal incision, a longer surgical procedure, and a somewhat greater risk.

An additional advantage to performing an ovariohysterectomy before the first "heat" in dogs and cats is that when the ovaries are removed, the animal is not exposed to estrogens from the first estrous cycle. As a result, there is a marked decrease in the incidence of mammary tumors in female animals who have not had long-term exposure to estrogen hormones.

The second statement that bitches or queens get fat after an ovariohysterectomy is a commonly heard remark. It is true that some dogs gain weight after being neutered. This is most often caused by the owner who continues to feed the same intake of calories to a dog or cat who is becoming less active. Owners must be instructed to match the food intake with the activity level of their pet.

Finally there is the third theory. The reader should remember the following dictum of the profession: chronologic age is not as important as physical condition. A

2-year-old obese dog may be a greater surgical risk than a 10-year-old dog in excellent physical condition. One very important risk factor to consider is the animal's estrous cycle status. Most veterinary surgeons prefer not to perform surgery on a patient "in heat." Not only are the reproductive organs likely to be enlarged but also there is an increased tendency for the animal to bleed because increased estrogen levels have an adverse effect on blood clotting.

There are a number of potential disadvantages associated with an ovariohysterectomy:

- The animal's inability to reproduce if the owner should desire pups or kittens.
- The animal no longer has a source of estrogens. On occasion this may result in skin disorders.
- Urinary incontinence. Some older spayed bitches may involuntarily pass urine in their beds or around the house and not even be aware they are doing so. In this case some drugs may be prescribed by the veterinarian. Phenylpropanolamine is generally tried first. Some veterinarians believe that the urinary problem in some cases may be related to the development of a postoperative adhesion between the urinary bladder and the uterine stump.

When the animal has been presented for ovariohysterectomy, the technician should perform the following procedures.

Preoperative
1. General rules apply (see p. 264).
2. The technician should ascertain that the animal is a female and has had no previous ovariohysterectomy. To be certain no previous OHE has been performed, you may shave the midline to find a scar, or palpate the area to find a "suture line." This does *not* ensure that the surgery was a spay, however.

Operative
1. General rules apply (see p. 265).
2. The technician holds and then releases the clamping instruments when the surgeon ties the suture material into the grooves left by the clamps. It is important to hold the clamps in a position that allows the surgeon maximum visibility of the tissue being ligated.

Postoperative
1. General rules apply (see p. 265).
2. Some veterinarians prefer to use an abdominal bandage to cover the ventral incision. These dressings are sometimes referred to as belly bands. If the animal is sent home while wearing an abdominal bandage, the owner should be instructed to watch for a shift in the position of the bandage or any irritation caused by the bandage.

Pyometra (pyometritis)

Definition. Pyometra is an accumulation of pus within the uterus. Causative organisms, such as bacteria, may be present, or the pus may be sterile. Closed pyometras are those in which the cervix is closed and all the pus is retained within the uterus. Open pyometras are those in which the cervix is open so that some of the pus can drain out.

Indications. Pyometras are serious cases that challenge both medical and surgical skills. Endotoxins from bacteria can enter the bloodstream and damage many organs. If the toxins remain in the body for any length of time, permanent damage to vital organs, such as the kidneys, will result, and death can follow. Surgical removal of the infected uterus is indicated as soon as the patient is sufficiently stable to undergo surgery.

Required instruments. All instruments necessary to perform this operation are found in the general surgery pack. Some surgeons may request two larger Carmalts (see Fig. 3-43).

Procedure. From a technical point of view, a pyometra operation is an ovariohysterectomy. However, instead of normally strong and hollow uterine tubes, there are often massive, friable, fluid-filled uterine horns to be removed. The surgical technician must be particularly careful to handle tissues gently when assisting because the uterine wall is easily ruptured. Should this occur, it would cause serious abdominal contamination and potential fatal peritonitis postoperatively.

The abdominal incision is considerably longer than that used for an ovariohysterectomy to accommodate the removal of the greatly distended uterus. The uterus is gently lifted from the abdomen. The ovarian pedicle is isolated, fixed, and transected in much the same manner as for an ovariohysterectomy. The vascular supply to the uterus is usually greatly enlarged. The body of the uterus may be much smaller than the horns. If this is the case, the fixation of the uterine body above the cervix is the same procedure as for an ovariohysterectomy.

The uterus and ovaries should then be removed to a surgical bucket with the clamps left in place. The bucket should be taken out of the operating room before the clamps are removed. Any variance from this procedure could cause contamination of the operating room with pathogenic organisms or an undesirable, putrid odor. The technician must be certain that the clamps are recovered after completion of the operation.

Role of the technician

Preoperative

1. General rules apply (see p. 264).
2. Because of the very serious nature of the disease process, all questions by the owner regarding medical or surgical treatment and prognosis should be answered by the attending veterinarian.

Operative. Many surgeons have a surgical technician assist during the pyometra operation.

1. General rules apply (see p. 265).
2. The technician should be extremely careful when handling the uterus because it is quite friable and may rupture.

Postoperative

1. General rules apply (see p. 265).
2. Because pyometra patients are often high-risk patients, they require careful monitoring of all vital signs, including urinary output.
3. Large volumes of fluids are generally used before and during surgery, which should result in high urinary output. (The attending veterinarian should be notified if urinary output is less than expected.) As soon as the patient is ambulatory, she should be allowed frequent opportunities to urinate.

4. The common postoperative signs of problems listed on p. 266 should also be monitored. All medications indicated by the attending veterinarian should be given as scheduled.

Ceasarean section (C-section, section, hysterotomy) (Fig. 4-5)

Definition. Cesarean section is the removal of the fetus (fetuses) through an incision in the uterus and the abdomen, as opposed to the normal vaginal route of delivery. The operation derived its name from Julius Caesar, who supposedly was the first human to be so delivered. Many authors dispute the authenticity of the legend, but still it persists.

Indications. Cesarean sections are generally performed when birth through the vaginal canal is either difficult or impossible. Difficulties with the birth process are called *dystocias*. Such situations occur more frequently in the undersized, short-muzzled (brachycephalic) breeds in which the head of the fetus is quite large in relation to the rest of the body.

Bitches or queens who have had prior cesarean sections or pelvic injuries are also potential candidates for cesarean section, in which case the owner should be discouraged from breeding this animal again because of future complications.

Uterine inertia is another reason to perform a cesarean section. This is most easily described as the absence or weakness of the uterine contractions at the time of parturition. This most often occurs in small breeds with large litters, obese animals, or older animals over 5 years of age. Uterine inertia is very rarely seen in queens and mainly occurs in bitches.

The most common problems leading to dystocias are those relating to the malposition of the fetus. Pups or kittens may be presented in any conceivable position within the birth canal. In some positions, the pup or kitten will simply not fit through the birth canal. On occasion these problems can be corrected by external manipulation of the fetus into a correct position.

There are other less frequently encountered indications for cesarean section, such as neoplasms, infections, adhesions of the uterus, toxemias, and trauma, any of which may affect the uterus or birth canal and prevent a normal vaginal birth.

Required instruments. All instruments for a cesarean section are to be found in the general surgical pack.

Procedure. The entire surgical area must be well draped. The midline ventral abdomen is opened sufficiently to pull out the uterine horns without rupturing the gravid uterus. The surgeon will sometimes instruct a technician to help elevate the linea alba during its incision to prevent damage to the uterus, which usually lies directly beneath the incision.

The uterine horns are brought out of the abdomen and pulled in a caudal direction to expose the dorsal aspect of the uterine body. This is why the entire animal must be well draped. After incising the uterus on its dorsal surface, the surgeon removes the fetuses. Usually all those from one uterine horn are delivered before proceeding to the second horn.

A word of warning is imperative at this point. There is almost always some excitement in the operating room as the pups and kittens draw their first breath. It is

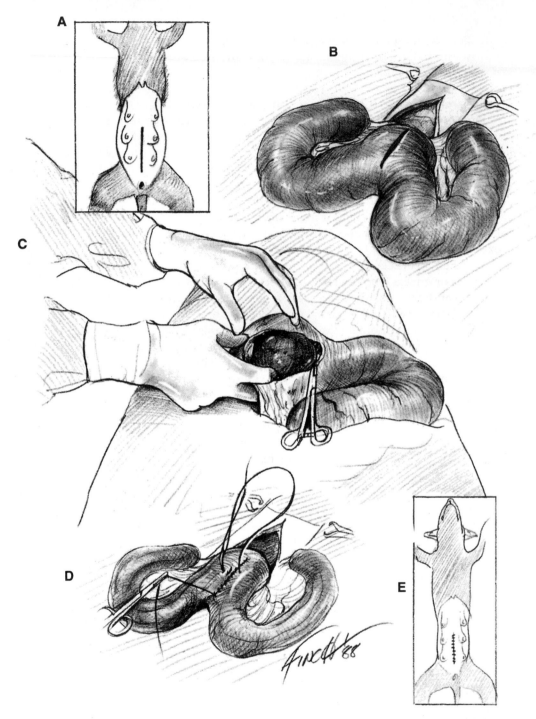

FIG. 4-5 Cesarean section. **A,** The animal is placed in standard dorsal recumbency, and a ventral midline abdominal incision is made. **B,** The uterus is extracted from the abdomen, and a hysterotomy incision is made on the uterine body. **C,** A fetus in the uterine body should be removed first. **D** and **E,** After the puppies have been removed, the uterine incision is closed. (From Caywood DD, Lipowitz AJ: *Atlas of small animal surgery,* St Louis, 1989, Mosby.)

very easy to focus attention on the newborn instead of on the bitch or queen. This is a potentially dangerous situation because the period immediately following the removal of the pups or kittens is one in which the circulation within the mother's body is undergoing a drastic change. The uterus, which occupied a large volume in the abdomen, is now greatly reduced in size; thus the venous circulation changes rapidly, predisposing the animal to shock. Accordingly the focus of attention still belongs on the bitch or queen.

The fluid rate should be monitored closely. For dogs the fluid protocol perioperatively is 20 ml/kg for the first hour and 10 ml/kg for each additional hour. For cats a constant 10 ml/kg/hr is maintained. Vital signs such as heart rate, color, pupil size, and blood pressure should be monitored carefully and the fluid rate adjusted accordingly.

The uterine incision is closed in whatever patterns the surgeon prefers.

Role of the technician

Preoperative

1. General rules apply (see p. 264).
2. Specific client questions regarding the prognosis should be answered by the attending veterinarian.
3. Some bitches or queens are presented after the delivery of part of the litter. The technician should place the newborn pups or kittens in a warm (91.4° F [33° C]), humid location to await their littermates who will be delivered by cesarean section. A human infant incubator is well suited for this purpose.

Operative. Many surgeons have a surgical technician assist during a cesarean section.

1. General rules apply (see p. 265).
2. The technician must be careful to support the gravid uterus when it is removed from the abdomen because its weight could cause a rupture of the ovarian pedicle if the uterus slides too far from the abdominal area.
3. The technician should assist the surgeon in removing the fetuses from the uterus. This often involves one person pushing as the other pulls. Care must be taken not to injure the neonates with excessive squeezing or pulling. Each fetus removed should be transferred to other attendants, being careful not to drop the newborn or to break sterility.

Postoperative

1. General rules apply (see p. 265).
2. One common problem in the immediate postoperative period is that the mother is placed with the newborn before she has recovered adequately from anesthesia. While in a semiconscious state, the bitch or queen may accidentally injure her young. The technician should wait until the mother's senses are completely restored to return the fetuses to their mother.

The membranous sac covering the body of the puppy or kitten must be ruptured to expose the head and nose. This should be done immediately on removal of the fetus from the uterus. The pups or kittens will still have placental tissues attached to the umbilical cord. The technician should be careful not to let the weight of the placental tissues hang from the pups or kittens without support because such tension on the umbilical cord can cause abdominal herniation at the umbilicus. The umbilical cords are usually tied with a nonabsorbable suture at least 1 cm away from the neonate's body.

The mouth, pharynx, and nares should be cleared of all fluids. The pup or kitten should be thoroughly dried by rubbing briskly but gently between the hands, using soft toweling. This rubbing activity simulates the mother's actions if she were awake. When the pups or kittens are dry and breathing well, they should be placed in a warm but humid atmosphere until they can be placed safely with their mother. An infant incubator is ideal if one is available. Occasionally some bitches (or queens) will be quite awake but will turn and attack a neonate and on some occasions devour it. This behavior seems to diminish a few days after a normal or cesarean birth. Careful monitoring of the mother is the best protection.

In most veterinary hospitals, the bars of the cage door are far enough apart to permit a pup or kitten to fall out onto the floor. Precautions must be taken to prevent this, especially in cages that are not at floor level.

Occasionally a pup or kitten will suckle on the suture ends instead of a nipple, which can open the incisional wound. For this reason internal absorbable sutures are often placed instead of external sutures. The incision should still be monitored closely for any disruption.

Bloody vaginal discharge is to be expected, but the volume of blood should not be copious. Heavy, unclotted bleeding or foul-smelling discharges should be reported to the attending veterinarian.

Many bitches and queens are possessive about their young and will not allow anyone to touch them. The mother should be approached slowly and with caution to avoid injury. The mother should be well aware of a human's presence before anyone enters her cage.

Hopefully the pups or kittens will nurse. If, for some reason, the pups or kittens cannot nurse, the pet's owner should be instructed how to hand-feed the young.

Many veterinarians prescribe dietary supplements for the nursing mother. Instructions for the administration of supplements or any other medications should be carefully explained to the owner.

No strenuous exercise is allowed until after the sutures are removed and the incisions are completely healed, no less than 3 weeks.

Canine castration (orchiectomy, altering, neutering)

Definition. Castration is a surgical procedure for the removal of the testes.

Indications. Dogs are castrated for the following reasons:

- Reduction of aggressive tendencies and/or the tendency to wander from home
- Sexual sterilization
- Reduction of the male trait of "marking" territory with urine
- Neoplasms of the testes or scrotum
- Traumatic wounds of the testes or scrotum that are too extensive to repair successfully
- Certain infections of the testes or scrotum
- Treatment of some conditions of the prostate gland that are caused by male hormone production

Required instruments. All the instruments necessary for castration of the dog are contained in the general surgical pack.

Patient preparation. General rules apply with one exception. When shaving an area for the castration of dogs it is recommended not to shave the scrotum to reduce skin irritation. The scrotum should be draped off from the surgical site, and the testes are manipulated through the drape.

Procedure. A midline incision is made on the cranioventral aspect of the scrotum. One testicle is pushed into the incision, and the fascia over the testicle is incised. Traction on the testicle accompanied by blunt dissection will expose the testicle, the spermatic cord, the tunics, and the vessels (Fig. 4-6).

At this stage of the operation there are two methods available to the surgeon, the "closed" and "open" techniques.

In the closed technique, the tunics are left in place and the entire spermatic cord is ligated with a double- or triple-clamping technique or wound clips. If the surgical assistant is holding the hemostatic clamps on the structure to be ligated, care must be taken not to exert too much traction because this may result in the rupture of the blood vessels inside of the tunics, causing retraction of the bleeding vessels into the abdomen.

In the open method the outer tunic is incised, exposing the spermatic vessels and spermatic cord. These structures are then ligated as described above. The cut tunic is then either crushed or ligated separately from the spermatic vessels and spermatic cord.

Some veterinarians tie the spermatic vessels and cord into a knot on themselves, thus negating any need for ligatures.

Regardless of which method is used, no tunic tissue can be allowed to protrude from the scrotal incision after surgery. Gentle outward traction of the scrotum will allow the tunics to retract toward the abdomen. If the tunics are allowed to form an adhesion with the scrotal skin, the wound will not heal properly.

Careful attention to hemostasis during surgery will help to prevent postoperative hemorrhage and swelling, which is common to this operation.

On occasion the entire scrotum is removed (scrotal ablation). This procedure is usually indicated in the presence of scrotal damage from trauma, infections, or neoplasms. If the scrotum is not removed, the skin tissue from this area will usually atrophy following surgery.

Subcutaneous and skin tissues are closed according to the surgeon's preference.

Role of the technician

Preoperative. Just as the technician should understand the common questions owners ask about ovariohysterectomy, the technician should also be able to answer questions about the castration of the dog and cat.

Most veterinarians prefer to castrate dogs and cats at a slightly older age than they neuter females. The most significant reason for this delay is that the testes produce the male hormone testosterone, which contributes to the growth process. Castration before 6 months of age may result in a stunting of the overall growth of the animal.

Owners should also be aware that if their purpose in castration is to reduce the aggressive behavior of a male animal, the effects are not immediate. If castration is

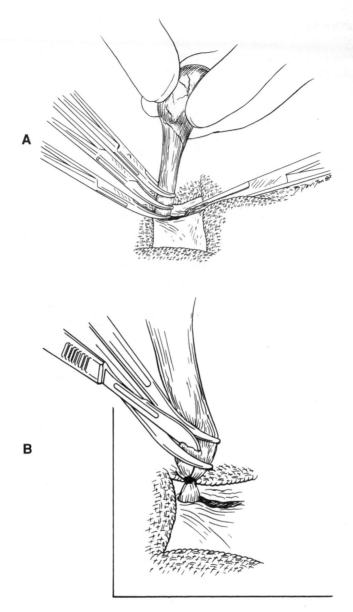

FIG. 4-6   Canine castration. **A,** Three clamps are placed on the spermatic cord. **B,** The cord is transfixed and ligated in the crushed area of the most proximal clamp. The cord is transected between the most distal clamps. (From Crane SW: Canine castration. In Bojrab MJ, editor: *Current techniques in small animal surgery,* ed 3, Philadelphia, 1990, Lea & Febiger.)

performed before 10 to 12 months of age, the operation often achieves the desired effect within a few months, but castration is no guarantee of good behavior. It is also true that the older the dog is before castration, the longer it will take to achieve a calming effect. If an older dog (above 4 to 6 years of age) is castrated, he may never cease being aggressive.

Males are capable of inseminating a female anytime after the onset of spermatogenesis, which might be as early as 4 to 5 months of age.

When the dog is presented for castration, the technician should perform the following procedures:

1. General rules apply (see p. 264).
2. The technician should verify that the animal is a male.
3. The technician should verify that both testicles are in the scrotum. (If both testes are not present, the procedure will differ from that described.)

Operative. Most veterinarians do not use an assistant in the canine castration operation.

1. General rules apply (see p. 265).

Postoperative

1. General rules apply (see p. 265).
2. Careful attention to hemostasis during surgery helps to control postoperative swelling; however, because of the vascular nature of the scrotal tissues, some swelling is common. It is sometimes helpful to apply a cold pack to the incision during the immediate postoperative period because the cold temperature will cause some local vasoconstriction and help prevent incision bruising.
3. Another possible problem is the dog's inclination to lick at the sutures after regaining consciousness. Soothing lotions or powders applied to the incision area may reduce the discomfort that causes the licking. Some dogs require an E-collar to prevent damage to the incision.
4. Owners should be advised to restrict the exercise of the castrated dog until the sutures are removed. Owners should also understand how and when to administer any prescribed medications.

Feline castration (Fig. 4-7)

Definition. The definition for canine castration applies to feline castration.

Indications. The first six indications listed under canine castration also apply to feline castrations. An additional reason is the elimination of the odor of tomcat urine.

Required instruments. All necessary instruments to perform a feline castration are to be found in the general instrument pack.

Procedure. All the surgical procedures discussed to this point are performed in an operating room under sterile conditions. Feline castrations should also be performed in a sterile manner; however, most veterinarians do not use the full cap-mask-gown technique for this operation. This is not an excuse for sloppy patient preparation or poor surgical technique.

Some technicians prefer to pluck the fur from the scrotal wall of the anesthetized cat, and others prefer to clip the fur. Either method is acceptable.

The only variation from the technique for canine castration is that the incisions for feline castration are made on the caudoventral aspect of each testicle. When clos-

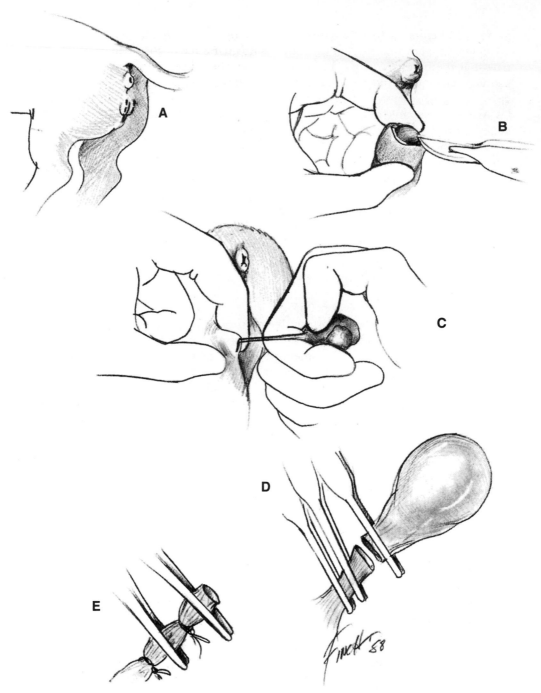

FIG. 4-7 Feline castration. **A,** The animal is placed in lateral recumbency and prepared. **B,** A skin incision is made in the scrotum directly over the testicle and extruded from the scrotum. **C,** The incision is carried through the spermatic fascia and the testicle. **D,** Three hemostatic forceps are placed on the tunic-covered spermatic cord, and it is transected. **E,** A ligature is securely placed around the cord beneath the forceps. (From Caywood DD, Lipowitz AJ: *Atlas of small animal surgery,* St. Louis, 1989, Mosby.)

ing, some veterinarians tie the spermatic vessels and cord into a knot on themselves, thus negating any need for ligatures.

The castration may be performed in either an open or closed manner. The only other variation is that no sutures are used to close the scrotal wound. The incision is left open to drain should fluid accumulate; however, it usually is closed by a scab within 1 or 2 days.

Role of the technician. The same responsibilities listed under canine castration apply to feline castration.

Other reproductive tract operations. Less commonly performed reproductive tract operations include episioplasty, episiotomy, removal of prostatic abscess or cyst, prostatectomy, and repair of vaginal prolapse.

Gastrointestinal Tract Surgery

There are many operations involving the gastrointestinal tract. Many of the operations are technically similar but vary as to location, such as the gastrotomy, duodenotomy, and jejunotomy (operations to make temporary openings in the stomach, duodenum, and jejunum, respectively).

Other operations are more specific to a particular site, such as a pyloromyotomy (an operation used to relieve constriction of the valve leading out of the stomach).

The scope of gastrointestinal surgery is too vast to discuss individual operations in any detail in this text; however, guidelines for the technician that are common to many gastrointestinal tract operations are discussed. In addition, two specific operations are described: the placement of a pharyngostomy tube and intestinal resection with anastomosis.

The gastrointestinal tract begins at the mouth and extends to the anus. At no point is the gastrointestinal tract consistently sterile. In other words, there are living organisms, such as bacteria, viruses, yeast, fungi, and parasites, present in the entire length of the gastrointestinal system. The variety and number of organisms found depend on the exact anatomic location.

Occasionally a veterinarian has the advantage of performing gastrointestinal surgery on an elective basis. This allows the withholding of food or other solids so that the gastrointestinal tract is emptied as much as possible. It also allows specific antimicrobial medications to be given to lower the population of organisms within the lumen of the gastrointestinal tract.

However, usually surgery of the stomach or intestines is an emergency, and therefore the tract contains varying amounts of food, fluids, stool, or foreign materials in addition to billions of microorganisms.

These comments emphasize the necessity of packing off as much as possible the portion of the gastrointestinal tract that requires surgery. This must be done to reduce contamination of the abdomen or thorax if the esophagus is the portion of the tract requiring surgery. If the surgeon or technician is careless and excessive contamination occurs, the risk of serious complications such as peritonitis or adhesions is greatly increased. The ability of the body to overcome infection is related in part to the number of contaminating organisms. The smallest possible amount of contamination will lessen the risk; however, the complete absence of contamination is the goal.

Antibiotics and abdominal drains are of great importance in treating and preventing infections related to gastrointestinal surgery. Irrigating the abdominal cavity after gastrointestinal surgery with a prewarmed antimicrobial solution helps to reduce the number of pathogenic organisms that remain on the peritoneum following the procedure.

The technician assisting during gastrointestinal surgery should pay close attention to the surgeon and the course of the operation. The surgical assistant must act as a sentinel for preventing contamination by alerting the surgeon to any possible contaminant in the sterile field.

Tissues often must be rotated or moved during the course of the surgical procedure. If the tissues are not held in the correct position, complications may develop, such as the uneven placement of sutures. Uneven sutures predispose the incision to leakage, which leads to infection.

The technician must be careful about which tissues are handled. Even slight pressure on the pancreas can cause the death of many cells and lead to serious complications. The liver and spleen are easily fractured or punctured. Tissue *must* be handled gently.

Assisting a surgical procedure involves more than just passing instruments. The technician also assists in monitoring the whole patient. During surgery of the stomach or intestines, the patient is often in an unbalanced metabolic state and therefore at greater risk. Vital signs, such as heart rate, tissue color, and bleeding tendencies, must be watched by the surgeon as well as the assisting technicians.

Pharyngostomy tube placement

Definition. Pharyngostomy tube placement is an operation in which an opening is made between the pharynx and the body wall in the upper neck. Through the opening a flexible tube is placed from the opening in the neck down the esophagus and into the stomach.

Indications. Any animal unable or unwilling to eat is a candidate for a pharyngostomy tube. The most common cause of being unable to eat would be trauma to the mouth area such as maxillary or mandibular fractures. Esophageal or oral surgery may also require the placement of a pharyngostomy tube during the initial healing phase.

A pharyngostomy tube is used to instill fluids or semisolids for nutritional purposes. Animals generally do not mind being fed via a pharyngostomy tube but might object vigorously to forced oral feeding.

Required instruments. Tubing of a size appropriate to the animal's esophagus is required. The gastric end should have side openings as large as possible without sacrificing tube strength. A cap should be available for the part of the tube left outside the body. Special pharyngostomy tubes are commercially available from several sources. All other instruments for this procedure are found in the general surgical pack.

Procedure. An oral speculum is used to hold the mouth open, and the animal is placed in right lateral recumbency. The surgeon locates the retropharyngeal pouch with the left hand. With the right hand, the surgeon uses a scalpel to make a small stab incision. The incision is made in the skin directly over the pouch, which is being marked by a finger from the left hand. The left hand is then withdrawn, and a curved forceps is brought to the retropharyngeal pouch. The tip of the forceps is forced through the lateral wall of the pharynx directly under the stab incision, then out through the skin. The tip end of the pharyngostomy tube is then grasped by the forceps tip and brought into the mouth. The surgeon removes the forceps and directs the tube down the esophagus to the stomach.

The tube may be sutured into place at the external opening. For additional support, the tube is taped to a bandage that has been loosely applied to the neck. The entire procedure usually takes less than 5 minutes. General anesthesia is usually necessary.

Role of the technician. Any syringe or fluid-holding device compatible in size to the tube may be used to administer liquids through the tube. The veterinarian calculates the volume of fluid and calories to maintain the patient and then divides this amount into multiple feedings. An excellent feature of the tube is that oral medications, such as vitamins and antibiotics, can often be mixed directly with food and fluids. This simplifies their administration for both the patient and the technician, particularly if jaw fractures are involved. The technician should always consult the veterinarian before mixing medications because some drugs may be inactivated by stomach acids and cannot be given with food.

The temperature of the food or fluids usually is not important; however, a hypothermic patient should not be given cold fluids. The fluids should not be given rapidly because this may cause a vomiting reaction, as will trapped air bubbles if the fluid being given is frothy. Foods must be small enough to pass through the tube. A blender usually suffices to mince most types of canned food if the food is mixed with an equal amount of water or saline.

After feeding, the technician should flush the tube with water and ensure that the cap is securely in place.

Stomach tubes may be left in place 1 or 2 days or as long as a few weeks, depending on the need for continued nutritional or fluid support.

The tube is removed by first removing the neck bandages and the suture or sutures holding the tube in place. The tube is then withdrawn, and the small opening into the pharynx is allowed to heal by second intention healing.

Intestinal resection and anastomosis (Fig. 4-8)

Definition. In intestinal resection and anastomosis a portion of the intestine is removed and the two remaining portions are joined together so that a continuous gastrointestinal tract is reestablished.

Indications. Whenever a section of intestine has been damaged so that it can no longer function properly, a resection and anastomosis are indicated.

Frequently the damage is a result of circulatory deficiencies. This may be indirectly caused by any condition that continuously expands the intestinal wall and stretches the blood vessels, thereby preventing a normal flow of blood to that area of the bowel. Foreign bodies are the most common cause of such stretching of the intestinal wall.

The circulatory damage may also be caused by the direct obstruction or rupturing of intestinal blood vessels, such as by an embolus or trauma. Regardless of whether the damage is direct or indirect, if a portion of the intestine remains without a blood

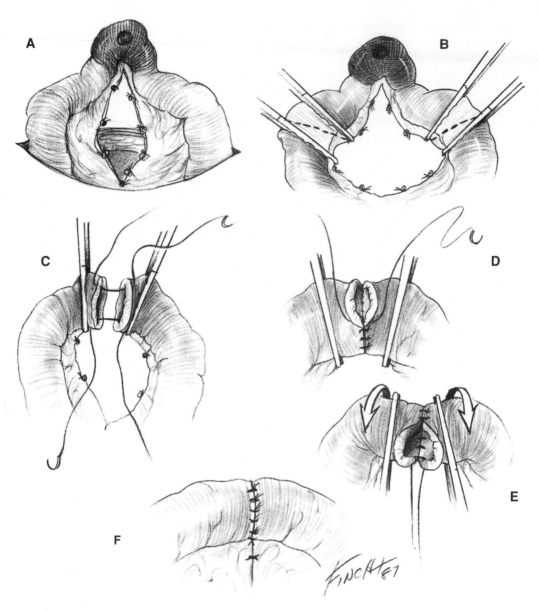

FIG. 4-8   Resection and anastomosis technique. **A,** The segment of intestine to be operated is elevated to a ventral midline abdominal incision. **B,** Forceps are placed on the bowel, which is then transected and removed. **C,** The inverting mucosa is trimmed. The bowel ends are brought close together, and sutures are placed at the mesenteric border and one at the antimesenteric border. **D,** The bowels are aligned and sutured. **E,** The bowel is turned to complete the circumferential placement of sutures. **F,** The forceps are removed after all sutures have been tied. (From Caywood DD, Lipowitz AJ: *Atlas of small animal surgery,* St. Louis, 1989, Mosby.)

supply for a critical period (usually measured in hours), death of the intestinal tissue will result. If it is not repaired, the animal will die from this type of injury.

Other indications for the removal of a section of intestine include irreparable traumatic lesions and neoplasms involving the wall of the intestine.

Required instruments. Many instruments have been developed to hold various parts of the intestinal tract. Among these is a body wall retractor to provide a constant opening to the gastrointestinal tract with a clear view of the surgical site. Another common instrument used in this surgery is the Doyen intestinal forceps. These have oblique serrations along the entire length of the forcep jaw used to occlude bowel to prevent spillage of its contents and reduce excess contamination. Despite the referral to several of these instruments as atraumatic, the technician should remember that all grasping instruments are traumatic to one degree or another. This is particularly true if the instrument is applied with more force than is indicated. For example, plain thumb forceps may kill many cells if used to grip the intestinal wall too tightly. Plain thumb forceps are relatively atraumatic when compared with rat-tooth thumb forceps. In many cases, human hands are the best "instruments" for holding gastrointestinal tract tissues.

The technician should become familiar with the name and care of the specific gastrointestinal tract instruments available at the facility.

Procedure. A long ventral midline incision is made to expose the abdominal cavity. The abdomen is explored in its entirety so that all lesions may be considered. The technician usually is directed to hold some tissues or organ in a particular position to allow a better view of the area being examined. Care must be taken to handle tissues gently and to avoid excessive traction on the abdominal viscera.

When the damaged intestine is localized, it is usually brought out of the abdominal incision to decrease the amount of intestinal leakage that may potentially contaminate the abdominal linings. The exteriorized bowel is then packed off with sponges or towels moistened with saline. The portion of intestine to be removed may be clamped with a crushing forceps. The portion to be saved is first "milked" to remove as much intestinal content as possible and then clamped with as little trauma as possible. Doyen clamps or the assistant's fingers are sometimes used for this purpose.

The blood supply from the mesentry is then isolated, clamped, and ligated. The surgeon will ensure that an adequate blood supply remains for the portion of intestine that is intact.

The intestine is then transected at an angle of approximately 30 degrees. This angle allows a larger lumen to be preserved at the anastomosis site and thus prevents a possible narrowing of the intestine at the surgical site. It also ensures an adequate blood supply to the border opposite the mesentery where the blood supply is usually less than at the mesenteric surface. The resected tissues and clamps are then placed in a container, which is removed from the operating room. The technician must ensure that the clamps are recovered after surgery.

The severed ends of the intestine are then placed near each other. Both the surgeon and the technician must ensure that the intestine is correctly aligned; that is, there is no twisting of the bowel or mesentery. The surgeon uses one of several suture techniques available to rejoin the intestine. After the completion of this phase, the surgeon may inject the segment (occluded at both ends) with sterile saline to check for leaks.

At this stage the surgeon will remove the contaminated packing and flush the abdomen with warm sterile saline. The surgeon will then replace all gloves and may request a replacement for all or some instruments and drapes with fresh, sterile equipment before completing the operation to decrease the chance of abdominal contamination. The mesentery is then rejoined with fine absorbable sutures. The surgeon will next flush the entire abdomen with warm sterile saline.

Before abdominal closure, the technician should be certain that all packing (sponges or towels) has been accounted for and removed from the abdomen. The abdomen is then closed in a routine fashion, except that many surgeons prefer to use nonabsorbable sutures in the fascial layer.

Role of the technician
Preoperative
1. General rules apply (see p. 264).
2. Because infection is of such great concern in this operation, the technician must ensure that the prescribed antibiotic therapy is administered *before* surgery. Often an intravenous antibiotic is given mixed with intravenous fluids. If intravenous antibiotics are prescribed, the technician must ensure that the correct form of the drug is administered. Many drugs come in both intramuscular and intravenous forms and should *not* be interchanged.
3. Extra sterile instruments, drapes, and gloves should be available if the surgeon desires a complete change after the anastomosis.

Operative
1. General rules apply (see p. 265).
2. The technician should constantly observe the surgical site to ensure that the packing is in place. In addition, the technician should observe for any leakage from the intestine itself, which the surgeon may not have seen, especially on the side opposite the surgeon's view.
3. When holding the intestines, only as much force as necessary should be used.
4. When holding the intestines in apposition for the anastomosis, close attention must be paid to the surgeon to continue rotating the intestine so that the sutures can be placed correctly.
5. Before closing the abdomen, the surgical team should check and recheck for foreign material in the abdomen (sponges, towels, instruments, suture strands, or needles).
6. The use of cold irrigation fluids should be avoided; prewarming fluids to 37° C is recommended.

Postoperative
1. General rules apply (see p. 265).
2. Any dietary restrictions should be followed carefully. This may include withholding food and water (NPO) for a short period following surgery.
3. The instructions regarding the route of administration for medications ordered by the veterinarian should be followed carefully.
4. The nature and frequency of bowel movements should be noted. If bowel movements are present, the technician should check for blood, formed stools,

and/or mucus. The presence of any of these factors should be recorded on the patient's record.

Other gastrointestinal tract operations. Gastrointestinal tract operations less commonly performed include cleft palate repair, colopexy, enterotomy, esophagotomy, esophagostomy, surgery for gastric torsion, pyloromyotomy, repair of rectal prolapse, and salivary mucocele.

Cutaneous and Subcutaneous System Surgery

Abscess

Definition. An abscess is a common septic lesion caused by bacteria and consists of a mass of pus surrounded by a fibrous tissue wall. Pus is the fluid that is formed from dead and disintegrating bacteria, white blood cells, enzymes, and products of chemical disintegration of body tissues, such as cells. Pus may also be mixed with serum, blood, or mucus.

A common cause of abscess formation in animals is a bite wound from another animal. However, a pathogen may settle in any part of the body as a direct result of a wound or indirectly through the circulatory system, termed a hematogenous spread. If the pathogen grows in body tissue and pus accumulates, an abscess may be formed.

Indications. The surgical indication for treating an abscess is to drain the purulent material from the body. This is significant because the purulent material may contain one or more toxins (produced by the infecting organisms and tissue breakdown) that can travel to other parts of the body via the circulatory system and cause a variety of clinical signs such as lethargy, fever, inappetence, localized redness, swelling, heat, and pain. If the original pathogens are still present in the abscess, these may also be spread by the circulatory system. When pathogens enter the bloodstream and spread to other tissue, the condition is known as *septicemia*. The lymph ducts are part of the circulatory system and may also spread toxins or pathogens.

Removing the pus from the body has the additional benefit of relieving the pain associated with the swelling that is caused by the size of the abscess. This is particularly important when the infection is near a movable joint or sensitive organ, such as the eye. Abscesses may interfere with the function of the affected part. As examples, an abscess of the prostate gland may cause difficulty in passing urine, or an abscess in a joint may render the patient unable to use that limb. Thus another indication for treating abscesses is to restore normal function to the affected part.

Required instruments. All general surgical packs contain the instruments used to open an abscess. Some veterinarians prefer the use of scalpels to make the opening; others prefer a special instrument that bores a round hole through the skin and subcutaneous tissues. This type of instrument is called a trephine. The most common one used is a Keys cutaneous punch, which is available in a variety of diameters from a few millimeters to 1 cm.

To keep the abscess drainage hole open after the surgical procedure, it may be necessary to use some sort of drainage system. The Penrose drain is the most common type of drain used; it is constructed of a thin, pliable latex. These drains allow fluid to seep along the latex by both gravity and capillary action. Other drains available are tube drains, which are more rigid than flat latex drains, providing a consistent lumen. These can be constructed of rubber, silicone rubber, polyvinylchromide, polyethylene, or other plastics. Sump pump drains are another type of tube drain but are double-lumen tube drains. Open suction drains are used for removing large quantities of fluids and are constructed by applying a vacuum to the drainage lumen of a sump drain. The closed drains are used where dependent drainage is difficult to establish or where a patient's posture frequently alters the point of dependency. These drains are constructed by applying negative pressure to a tube drain that does not have an air vent.

Procedure. The technique used to drain an abscess depends on its location, but the one constant principle is that ventral drainage must be established. Drainage is more effective if the abscess is allowed to drain with gravity, not against it.

The technician should clip and prep the area as in any other operation before any incisions are made. A sharp object such as a scalpel or trephine is used to make an opening in the skin. The wound is then extended by blunt dissection until the abscess itself is entered. Often a second, smaller hole is made on the dorsal aspect of the abscess to provide an exit for a drain.

Fluids, such as saline or a dilute chlorhexidene solution, are often used to flush purulent material and debris from the wound. It is important to avoid contaminating the flushing solution by allowing any contact between the fluid in the abscess and the fluid in the storage container. The technician should use only the fluid that is needed the first time or use fresh, clean transfer containers (e.g., syringes) if additional fluid is needed.

Role of the technician

Preoperative

1. General rules apply (see p. 264).
2. All preparations for surgery should be done with equipment and supplies that will not contaminate the sterile operating room. For example, clippers used to shave an abscessed wound site should never be used to clip the surgical site for an ovariohysterectomy.
3. The technician should be protected from direct contact with purulent exudate if the abscess is already draining. Disposable plastic or rubber gloves work well for this purpose.

Operative

1. General rules apply (see p. 265).
2. The surgeon often directs the technician to flush sterile saline or a dilute chlorhexidene solution into the abscess cavity to remove pus and debris.

Postoperative

1. General rules apply (see p. 265).
2. The drainage hole must be kept clean and open. A dilute chlorhexidene solution or plain warm water can be used for this purpose.
3. Any discharges that have dried onto the skin or fur below the drainage hole should be cleaned. This material is often uncomfortable, and the animal may react by chewing at the area or removing the drain if one is present. An E-collar should be placed routinely after any drain is placed as long as the drain is not in direct contact with the sharp edges of the collar.

4. The owner should be shown how to keep the area clean before taking the animal home.
5. The owner should be instructed to report any alterations in the drain if the animal is sent home with a drain in place. In general, drains are left in place until all drainage has stopped. This may vary in time from a single day to over a week.

Lacerations

Definitions. Lacerations may be defined as linear tears in any tissue (as opposed to punctures, which are usually round and small). Lacerations vary in length from a few millimeters to several centimeters. They most often involve skin, subcutaneous, and/or muscle tissue; however, corneal, lingual, gingival, and other types of lacerations are frequently encountered in veterinary practice.

Lacerations may be smooth or jagged. The resulting wound or wounds may be clean or contaminated and may be fresh or of long duration. All these factors must be considered in the treatment and nursing care of a lacerated wound.

Indications. The purpose of treating lacerations is to restore torn tissues to their original function. Open skin provides a portal of entry for pathogens. Tongue lacerations may prevent the animal from eating. Splenic lacerations can cause a fatal hemorrhage. All these examples are certainly indications for surgery; however, the technician should be aware that not all lacerations require surgical treatment. The size, the location, and the sterility of the laceration are all factors considered by the attending veterinarian. (See the section on wound healing, p. 4-2.)

Required instruments. All instruments required for routine laceration repair are found in the general surgical pack. Specialized instruments may be required to repair lacerations of tissues such as blood vessels, ligaments, eyes, and nerves, but these procedures are not discussed in this text.

Many veterinary hospitals keep separate emergency or laceration packs available that contain instruments specifically designed for treating skin lacerations. Generally the laceration pack is similar to the general surgical pack except that it contains fewer of each instrument. Surgical technicians should become familiar with the instrument and suture preference of the veterinarian or veterinarians with whom they work.

The surgical technician employed in a practice that uses surgical skin staples must become familiar with the care of the staples and the applying "gun." Care includes loading the gun, sterilizing the gun and the staples, and removing the staples when the wound has healed. Some smaller lacerations (less than 5 cm) that are fresh and clean can be stapled after preparing the wound without the use of anesthesia because the staples cause no more pain than the subcutaneous hypodermic injection of a local anesthetic drug. The increased patient safety and decreased treatment time should offset the increased cost of staples over conventional sutures, which usually require the use of a general anesthetic.

Procedure. The type, position, and age of the wound vary so widely from case to case that it is impractical to describe a specific procedure to treat lacerations; however, some general principles apply in each case.

Hemostasis. The technician may be the first hospital staff member to see an animal with a laceration. If hemorrhage is present, direct pressure is usually applied to promote hemostasis. This is a priority procedure. Clean or sterile gauze pads are ideal for this purpose. Studies of wound treatment in both human and veterinary hospitals have shown that open wounds are as likely to be contaminated in the hospital as at the time of the injury.

Cleansing. If wounds are to heal by primary intention, the wound must be clean, that is, free of dead tissues, foreign matter, and significantly high numbers of pathogens. Wounds must be properly prepared before surgery. The surgical technician should never debride the wound because this should be done by the attending veterinarian. The technician can, however, gently remove foreign material. A combination of plain thumb forceps and sterile irrigation usually suffices. The type of irrigating fluid used should be determined by the attending veterinarian. In general the fluids (often saline) should not contain sugars because they may provide nourishment for some bacteria present in the wound and allow them to overgrow the wound. Copious amounts of plain water should also be avoided because water is hypotonic and may damage adjacent cells that were previously uninjured.

It is very important to protect the open wound when the fur in the area is being clipped because hair is often a major source of wound contamination. The use of a vacuum while clipping is advised, as well as packing moistened gauze or sterile lubricating jelly in the wound to protect hair from falling into the open wound.

Drainage. If the wound accumulates fluid (serum or pus), drainage must be provided. The indications for drainage of lacerations are similar to those for abscessed wounds. Penrose drains are frequently used for this purpose. Many fresh, small lacerations will heal without drainage, but if fluid accumulation is anticipated, drainage is indicated. If the technician is careless about wound preparation for laceration repair, the result may well be an abscess, which would require additional surgery and cause greater risk for the animal.

When the wound has been properly prepared, the surgeon may then close the wound with either sutures or staples. Sterile drapes should be used to lessen the chance for wound contamination during wound closure.

Role of the technician

Preoperative

1. General rules apply (see p. 264).
2. Care must be taken during preparation of the patient to avoid contaminating the wound with hair or other debris.
3. Foreign debris should be removed from the wound with a plain thumb forceps or a similar instrument.
4. The attending surgeon may direct the technician to flush the wound with saline or other fluid before surgery.

Operative

1. General rules apply (see p. 265).
2. The technician should provide the surgeon with the desired suture material or materials and instruments.

Postoperative

1. General rules apply (see p. 265).
2. The technician may be directed by the attending surgeon to bandage or splint the closed wound to prohibit the animal from chewing at the sutures or sta-

ples. An E-collar may also be necessary. Dressings also support the sutured skin edges to keep them from separating.

3. The owner should be informed of any instructions regarding the care of dressings applied to the wounds.

Declaw (feline) (onychectomy)

Definition. Declawing is the surgical removal of the entire nail and third phalanx of the paws. In most circumstances, only the front paws are declawed.

Indications. Cats have a natural tendency to sharpen their claws and will sometimes use furniture legs or other furnishings for this purpose. Cats who destroy furniture or wall coverings may be candidates for declawing if they cannot be trained to use a scratching post. In most instances, removal of the front claws is sufficient to prevent damage to drapes, table legs, and other furnishings.

Required instruments. Some veterinarians prefer to use a small (no. 15) scalpel blade for the removal of the nail and third phalanx (Fig. 4-9). Others prefer a sterilized nail trimmer such as a White nail trimmer or a Resco nail trimmer.

Procedure. The paws must be thoroughly washed and prepared before surgery. For most short-haired cats, the hair on the feet is not clipped, but for long-haired cats it may be required. The technician should examine the cat for polydactyly (extra toes), and the surgeon should be informed if extra digits are present. Usually extra toes will appear on the medial aspect of the paw.

After the paw is washed, a tourniquet is applied firmly to the leg distal to the elbow to prevent radial nerve paresis and to control bleeding. If a nail clipper is used, the instrument is applied exactly at the joint, and the nail is amputated. A small scalpel blade may then be used to remove the remaining portion of the third phalanx, which the clipper is unable to reach. The procedure may be performed in much the same

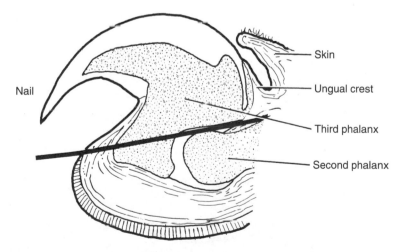

FIG. 4-9   Solid line shows correct line of incision with nail trimmer for removing entire nail and ungual crest. Note that a small portion of the third phalanx will be left. This small portion of bone is easily removed with scalpel. (Modified from Bojrab MJ, editor: *Current techniques in small animal surgery,* Philadelphia, 1975, Lea & Febiger.)

manner except that the scalpel blade alone is used throughout instead of the nail clipper. If a significant portion of the third phalanx is allowed to remain (Fig. 4-10), the cat may experience pain and the claw can grow back. It is important to be certain the entire third phalanx has been removed from *all* digits before bandaging the feet. A toe count should be done before bandaging to ensure that all five (or more) digits have been properly amputated.

Some surgeons prefer to close each toe with a fine absorbable suture such as 4-0 PDS or a surgical cyanoacrylate adhesive; others leave the incision open.

Some surgeons will bandage the foot after the declaw is finished. A recommended bandaging method is to apply a layer of gauze around the paw to a level above the carpus. Cotton is sometimes wrapped over the gauze, and an additional layer of gauze is applied over the cotton. Finally, tape or a finger of a surgical or exam glove (secured at the top of the bandage with tape) is applied over the cotton and the gauze to prevent the bandage from slipping off.

Role of the technician

Preoperative

1. General rules apply (see p. 264).
2. Before surgery, the owner should be informed that only the front feet of the cat will be declawed (unless hospital policy differs from this rule) and that the cat must not be left alone outdoors because cats are usually unable to climb trees and escape ground level danger or defend themselves against other cats or dogs.

Operative

1. General rules apply (see p. 265).
2. All materials should be readily available for bandaging the paws so that the first paw may be dressed before the second paw is begun. The technician will usually apply the bandages while the surgeon waits to declaw the other paw.

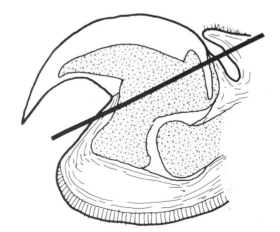

FIG. 4-10   Solid line shows an incorrect incision line. Note that some of the ungual crest will remain, as well as a significant portion of the third phalanx. If this incision line is not corrected, nail may well grow back. (Modified from Bojrab MJ, editor: *Current techniques in small animal surgery,* Philadelphia, 1975, Lea & Febiger.)

The tourniquet is left in place until the foot bandage is completed. Wasted time in bandaging prolongs the anesthetic period for the patient and increases tourniquet time.

Postoperative

1. General rules apply (see p. 265).
2. The technician should ensure that the dressings remain in place. When a cat recovers from anesthesia following a declaw, its first efforts may be to shake off the dressings. If the cat is successful, the paws may hemorrhage and require redressing. Foot bandages should be applied securely the first time because redressing a half-conscious cat can be a traumatic experience for the cat and the technician.
3. Some veterinarians prefer to remove the dressings the day after surgery; others leave the bandages on a day or two longer. When removing a declaw bandage, the technician should use bandage scissors, begin cutting from the top, and stop cutting before the toes are reached. If bleeding occurs, the attending veterinarian may request that a new dressing be applied.
4. The technician should advise the owner to substitute shredded paper for kitty litter until the incisions heal because the litter particles may adhere to the incision and cause irritation.

Orthopedics

Definition. Orthopedics is the surgical art that deals with injuries or diseases of the skeletal system.

Definition of terms

dislocation   A change in the normal anatomic relationships of the bones that form a joint (Fig. 4-11, *A*).

luxation   Synonymous with dislocation.

subluxation   A partial (incomplete) dislocation (Fig. 4-11, *B*).

fracture   A break in cortical bone or cartilage.

  articular fracture   A fracture involving a joint surface (Fig. 4-11, *C*).

  comminuted fracture   A fracture in which the bone is fractured into a number of fragments (Fig. 4-11, *D*).

  open fracture   A fracture in which one or more bone fragments from the fracture area have penetrated into the soft tissues (Fig. 4-11, *E*). The term is usually assumed to mean that the skin over the fracture is open. The fractured bone end may or may not protrude through the skin. Contamination of the bone is a potential complication.

  physeal fracture   A fracture at the physis (growth plate). This fracture is seen only in growing animals (Fig. 4-11, *F*).

  greenstick fracture   An incomplete fracture, not penetrating both cortices (Fig. 4-11, *G*). When bending of the bone occurs, the fracture occurs on the convex side of the bone. The term is sometimes used instead of "incomplete fracture," which is similar except that the bone is not bent.

  linear fracture   A fracture in which the fracture line runs parallel with the long axis of the bone.

  oblique fracture   A fracture whose angle is between horizontal and vertical (Fig. 4-11, *H*).

  spiral fracture   An oblique fracture that curves or winds around the bone (Fig. 4-11, *I*).

  transverse fracture   A fracture horizontal to the long axis of the bone; that is, the fracture is at right angle to the long axis of the bone (Fig. 4-11, *J*).

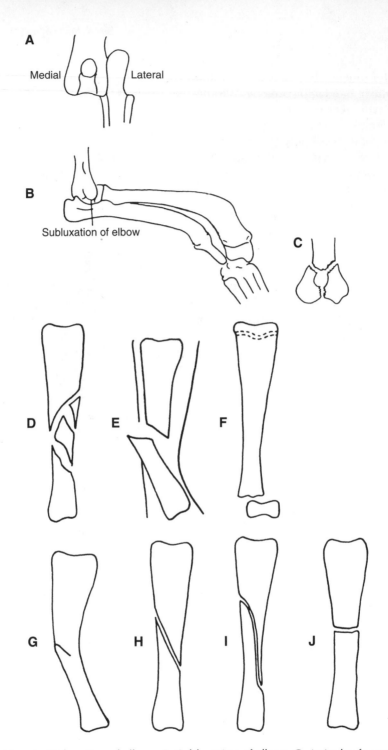

FIG. 4-11 **A,** Dislocation of elbow. **B,** Subluxation of elbow. **C,** Articular fracture (Y fracture). **D,** Comminuted fracture with multiple fragments. **E,** Open fracture; bone fragment has broken through skin. **F,** Physeal fracture occurs at or through epiphyseal plate. **G,** Greenstick fracture, an incomplete fracture in which partial continuity is maintained. **H,** Oblique fracture occurs at angle to long axis of bone. **I,** Spiral fracture curves around bone. **J,** Transverse fracture occurs at right angle to long axis of bone. (From Denny HR: *A guide to canine orthopaedic surgery,* London, 1980, Blackwell Scientific Publications.)

Required instruments. The specialized instruments for orthopedic surgery literally fill entire catalogs and are far too numerous to mention here. The technician must become familiar with the names and shapes of the instruments used in the specific practice, as well as the care and sterilization techniques specified by the manufacturer.

In general, orthopedic instruments resemble carpenter's tools. There are hammers (mallets), drills, chisels, saws, and fastening devices, such as nails, wires, screws, pins, and plates. Most instruments and fastening devices are made of stainless steel. Great care must be taken in their use because scratches, dents, or other imperfections may result in the mechanical failure of an orthopedic device.

Initial presentation of the patient. Fractures, unless they involve the skull bones, are rarely life-threatening emergencies. The technician is often the first hospital staff member to see an injured animal and must check for critical injuries. The technician should ensure that the animal can breathe in an unobstructed manner, that vital signs are stable, and that major hemorrhage is controlled. Under no circumstances should the technician administer any drugs without the direct approval of the attending veterinarian.

The animal should not be moved unless it is necessary and then only with proper support. Some nerve and blood vessel injuries occur not from the original trauma but from the improper handling of the animal after the injury. Bone fragments are often very sharp, and moving a fractured limb can be similar to cutting the leg with a scalpel.

Procedure. The repair of specific fractures is a subject that fills many veterinary textbooks and is certainly beyond the scope of this text. As with other portions of this chapter, the purpose is not to teach the technician how to perform surgery, but rather to acquaint the technician with a general knowledge of procedures. (See the selected readings at the end of the chapter for further information.)

External fixation (closed fracture reduction). In closed fracture reduction, the bones are manipulated into proper alignment and held in that alignment by the use of a solid external device (cast or external fixation device) attached to the fractured appendage. Anesthesia is required for proper closed reduction.

A wide variety of materials have been used for the external fixation of fractures. Because of the extreme variety in the size and shape of animals, veterinarians have been particularly inventive about developing external fixation devices to fit their patients.

Internal fracture reduction (open fracture reduction). The technician should remember that bone is a living tissue and must be handled accordingly. Unnecessary force can injure the living bone and cause complications. Bone is usually the deepest tissue within a limb and therefore is afforded poor drainage in the event of infection. Bone infections (osteomyelitis) are serious and difficult to treat. Proper patient preparation, surgical draping, and strict sterile operating technique are essential to prevent bone contamination during internal fracture repair. In addition, unnecessarily long surgical time can increase the possibility of postoperative bone and/or wound infection.

After the patient has been prepared for surgery, the soft tissues are dissected to expose the fractured portion of the skeleton. The technician must be very careful not to manipulate any bone fragments because nerve, muscle, or blood vessel damage may result. The surgeon directs the technician when and how to move the bone fragments.

The surgeon manipulates the bones into correct alignment; some sort of bone clamp often is used to hold the alignment while the fixation device, such as a pin, wire, or screws, and plate are implanted (Fig. 4-12).

After the bone is repaired, any damage to surrounding soft tissue is corrected and the wound is closed. Careful attention must be paid to hemostasis.

It is not unusual to use an external fixation device on a fracture after internal fixation has been completed. The external fixation device provides additional support, which may be necessary, particularly in the early phases of healing.

Closed reduction of luxations. The hip (coxofemoral joint) is the joint most commonly dislocated in dogs and cats; however, almost any joint may luxate.

If the veterinarian diagnoses a luxated joint, if the injury is fresh (treated within 24 hours), and if no other injuries are present, the luxation may sometimes be reduced with the patient under general anesthesia without the need for surgical intervention. Not all luxations are reduced successfully in a closed manner.

The successful reduction of a luxation entails adequate patient muscle relaxation (hence the anesthesia), a knowledge of the anatomy of the joint and surrounding tissues, and often a great deal of strength from the veterinarian and the technician. The technician must follow the veterinarian's instructions exactly to avoid injuring the patient more seriously.

Successful reduction of a luxated joint is often accompanied by a "crack" or "pop" sound as the bones slip back together. Postreduction radiographs are usually taken to ensure that the bones are in the correct position. Splints, dressings, or casts may also be used postoperatively to prevent the reluxation of the joint. These generally remain for 7 to 10 days.

Role of the technician

Preoperative
1. General rules apply (see p. 264).
2. To move a patient with an orthopedic injury, the technician must properly support the affected part or parts to prevent further injury to soft tissues.
3. The significance of proper patient preparation for surgery cannot be stressed too strongly. This includes clipping the fur, washing and disinfecting the surgical site or sites, and vacuuming stray hairs. Every effort must be made to avoid infections in orthopedic procedures.

Operative
1. General rules apply (see p. 265).
2. A technician who is assisting in an open surgical repair should be mentally and physically prepared. Orthopedic surgery requires careful attention to detail.

Postoperative
1. General rules apply (see p. 265).
2. If the technician is responsible for applying dressings or bandages, care must be exercised to apply pressure evenly and not too tightly. Particular attention should be paid to the limb and foot distal to the orthopedic injury. Mild swelling

Text continued on p. 307

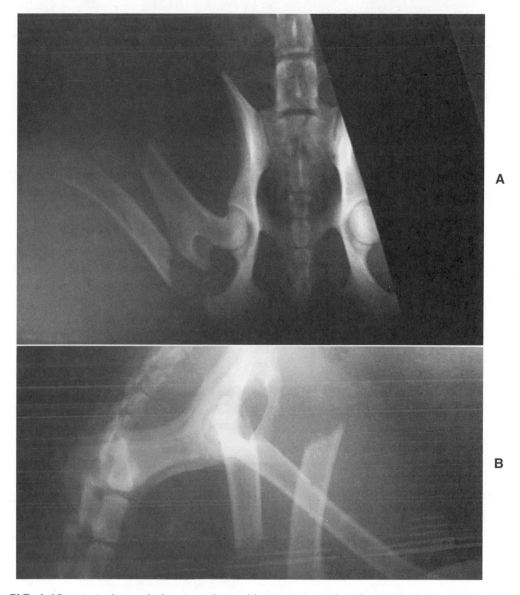

FIG. 4-12   **A,** Radiograph showing a femoral fracture. Ventrodorsal view of pelvis. **B,** Lateral radiograph showing femoral fracture.   *Continued*

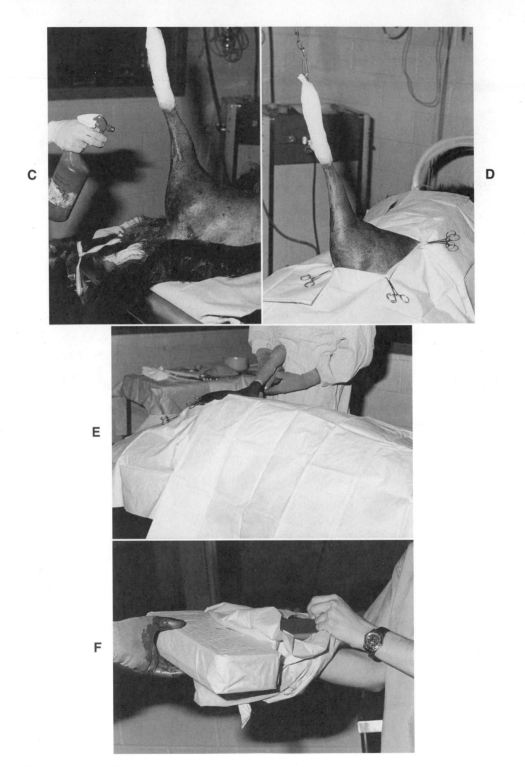

FIG. 4-12, cont'd **C,** Sterile preparation of surgical site before internal reduction. **D,** Surgical site is draped, and limb is extended to induce relaxation of muscles. **E,** The foot is wrapped to prevent contamination of the surgeon and the surgical site. **F,** Instruments are double wrapped and handed to the surgeon in a sterile manner.

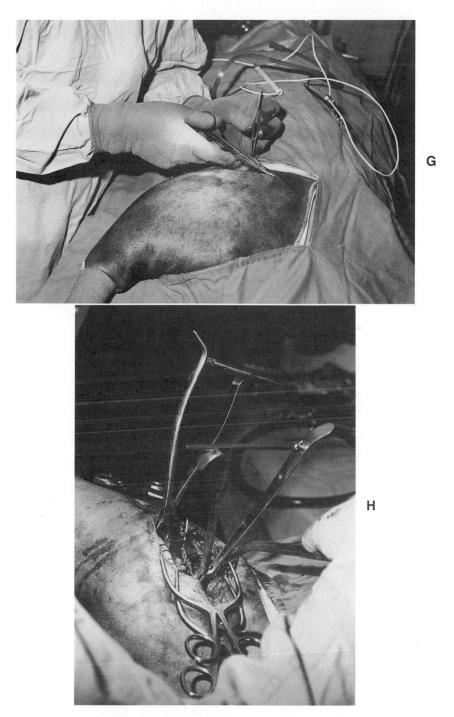

FIG. 4-12, cont'd   G, The surgeon makes the initial approach. **H,** Reducing the fracture using bone holding instruments.   *Continued*

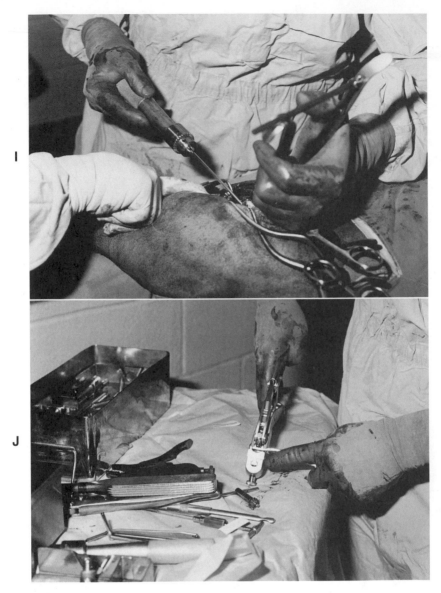

FIG. 4-12, cont'd   I, Intramedullary pins are used to align the fracture. The surgeon is driving the pin. **J,** Bone plates are bent to conform to the size and shape of the bone.

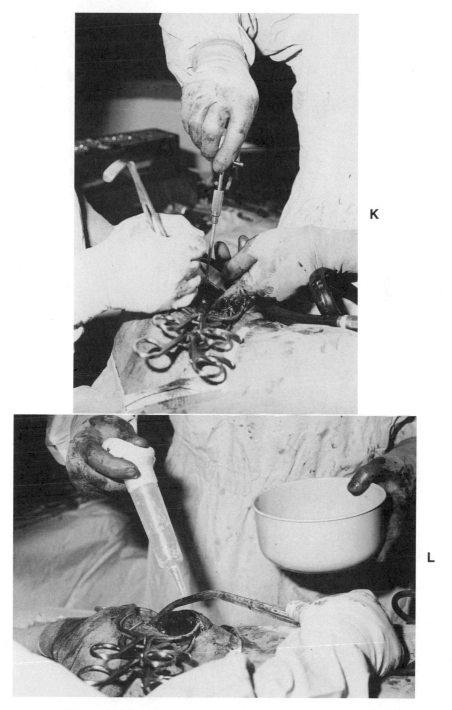

FIG. 4-12, cont'd **K,** Bone screws are used to hold the metal bone plates in place. **L,** Flushing with normal saline keeps the tissue moist.

Continued

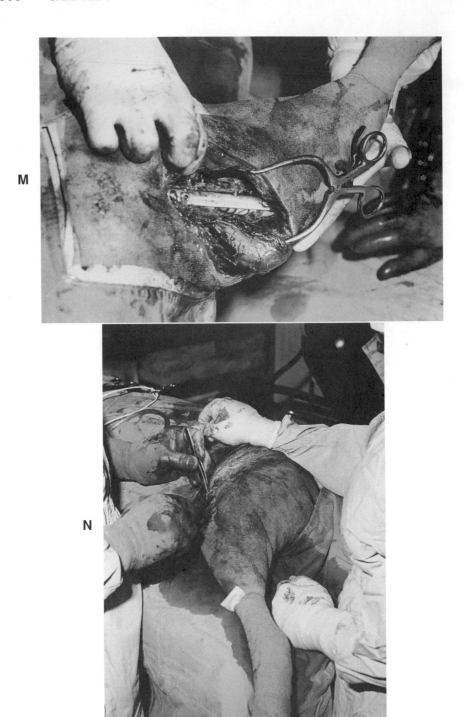

FIG. 4-12, cont'd **M,** Intramedullary pin and bone plates in place. **N,** The closure of the incision is done in several layers, usually ending with staples on the skin layer. (Courtesy Angell Memorial Animal Hospital.)

distal to the injury is to be expected. Persistent or excessive swelling may indicate that the dressing or splint has been applied too tightly. Excessively tight splints or bandages can cause necrosis or require the amputation of the toes and/or skin of the affected limb.

3. Casts and splints should not become wet. Cages should be kept clean to prevent urine, feces, or saliva from soiling the external fixation.
4. Patients must be prevented from thrashing during the immediate postoperative period because such activity may dislodge or damage the external fixation.
5. The list of possible problems caused by external fixation materials when the animal leaves the hospital is almost endless. The use of a splint or cast instruction sheet is highly recommended. The technician should be certain that the owner understands all instructions before discharging the patient (see box below).

Auditory System Surgery

Lateral ear wall resection (Zepp modified LaCroix operation) (Fig. 4-13)

Definition. A lateral ear wall resection is an operation to remove or transplant the lateral cartilaginous wall of the vertical ear canal to expose the horizontal canal and provide drainage for the ear.

Indications. Chronic infections in an ear usually cause a gradual thickening of the skin that lines the ear canal. This thickening reduces the circulation of air inside the ear, which ordinarily helps to dry the ear. In addition, ceruminous (waxy) materials or any type of pus cannot drain from a narrow ear canal as easily as from one with a wide diameter. The lack of air circulation and reduced drainage usually cause further infection, as well as self-mutilation by the animal, who will frequently scratch a

---

Care of Splints and Casts

If your pet has had a fracture or tendon injury, a splint or cast may be applied to the affected leg. Proper care of splints and casts is essential if the injury is to heal correctly. Movement at a fracture site can result in delayed healing or permanent deformity to the bone or nearby joints.
1. Do not allow your pet to eat or drink immediately after arriving home because this may cause vomiting. After 1 hour, you may allow small amounts of water at a time until the animal is no longer thirsty.
2. Inspect the splint or cast when you first arrive home with your pet so that you can detect any changes that may occur later.
3. Splints and casts *must* be kept clean and dry.
4. Feed your pet the normal diet unless a specific change has been advised.
5. Only allow as much exercise as the doctor has advised. Too much activity is the most common cause of postoperative complications.

Contact the hospital if any of the following occurs:
1. Your pet excessively chews its cast or splint.
2. The cast or splint on the leg changes position.
3. Bleeding or sore areas develop at the top or bottom of the splint or cast.
4. The leg swells above or below the cast or splint.
5. The splint or cast gets wet.

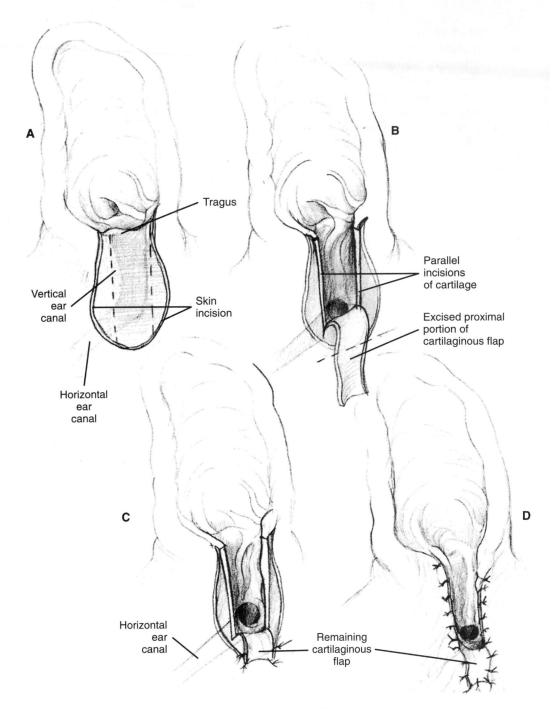

FIG. 4-13 Zepp lateral ear canal wall resection. **A,** Skin incisions. **B,** Incisions extend down the ventrical ear canal. **C,** The proximal portion of the flap is excised. **D,** Skin is sutured to cartilage margins. (From Caywood DD, Lipowitz AJ: *Atlas of small animal surgery,* St Louis, 1989, Mosby.)

sore ear. When this cycle cannot be broken by medical therapy, the animal may be a candidate for resection of the lateral ear wall.

Occasionally the operation is performed to relieve polyps or neoplasms from deep within the ear canal.

Required instruments. In addition to the instruments included in a general surgical pack, there are two instruments that are not essential for the operation but alleviate the surgical difficulty. The first is a cartilage scissors. These make clean cuts through the cartilage of the ear that needs to be excised. The other valuable surgical tool is an electrocautery system. The use of electrocautery is common in many operations; however, it is particularly valuable in any surgery where there are multiple bleeders that might be difficult or time consuming to clamp and tie in the conventional manner.

Procedure. Incisions are made in the skin parallel to and directly over the cranial and caudal walls of the vertical ear canal. The skin incisions are extended beyond the point at which the ear canal becomes horizontal. The skin and soft tissues between the incisions are resected, exposing the lateral aspect of the vertical ear canal. Parallel incisions are then made on the cranial and caudal aspects of the vertical ear canal to the level of the horizontal ear canal.

The resected cartilage is then pulled ventrally so that the *inner* surface of the vertical ear canal becomes the *outer* ventral wall below the horizontal canal. This cartilage flap is trimmed to fit the initial skin incisions made during the operation. The flap is sometimes referred to as a drainboard. Bleeders are often small and difficult to clamp and ligate. Electrocautery is used to provide hemostasis. The remaining cartilage is sutured to the skin edges.

Role of the technician
Preoperative
1. General rules apply (see p. 264).
2. The ear should be cleaned of debris before the surgical procedure. This includes the elimination of waxy discharges as well as purulent material. The technician should be careful not to traumatize the ear. Irrigation of the ear canal with a mild detergent solution may be necessary to loosen and remove accumulated wax, pus, and other debris.

Operative
1. General rules apply (see p. 265).
2. If electrocautery is used, the patient must be properly grounded. The technician should refer to the manufacturer's instructions.

Postoperative
1. General rules apply (see p. 265).
2. After surgery the incisions will probably be very tender to the patient. The technician should be gentle when cleaning the wounds.
3. Some veterinarians prefer to bandage the ear flaps (pinnae) over the head for a few days postoperatively to allow more air circulation around the incisions. When such dressings are removed, the technician must be careful not to cut into the ear flap itself.
4. The owners should be shown the proper procedure for caring for the ear at home. In particular, they should be warned not to put any solid objects such

as cotton swabs into the shortened ear canal. This caution is to prevent any damage to the tympanic membrane.

Other auditory system operations. Some other auditory system operations that are performed include ablation of the ear canal, removal of an aural hematoma, otoplasty (ear trimming), and bulla osteotomy.

Ophthalmic Surgery

Nictitating membrane flap placement (temporary tarsorrhaphy)

Definition. A nictitating membrane flap placement involves covering all or part of the cornea with the nictitating membrane, which is temporarily sutured into the desired position.

Indications. Nictitating membrane flaps are used whenever the cornea needs temporary protection. The most common indication is in the healing of deep corneal ulcers; however, they are also used in the repair of traumatic corneal injuries and following some intraocular surgical procedures. Flaps allow medications to be in direct contact with the cornea and also keep the cornea moist. These factors are useful in the medical treatment of some corneal diseases.

In effect, the nictitating membrane flap is a temporary bandage for the eye composed of a nonirritating, nonforeign tissue that the body will not reject. Flaps are often left in place for a few days to 2 weeks.

Required instruments. All instruments required for the placement of a nictitating membrane flap may be found in the general surgical pack. In addition, sterilized buttons, tubing, or other tension-absorbing materials should be available according to the surgeon's preference.

Procedure. Before any shaving or washing of the upper eyelid is begun, the eye must be protected. Most veterinarians prefer to apply an ophthalmic ointment to the eye, but the medication depends on the condition being treated. During surgical preparation of the upper eyelid, care must be taken not to allow hair or caustic material to contact the eye. Soaps and alcohols are examples of chemicals that should never contact the cornea.

Mattress sutures are placed starting from outside the upper eyelid, through the lid, into the nictitans, and out through the upper lid. The sutures are then tied with some means of support to avoid skin necrosis. Sterilized buttons or pieces of intravenous or latex tubing are often used for this purpose.

Role of the technician

Preoperative
1. General rules apply (see p. 264).
2. Any special sutures and/or tension-absorbing material should be readily available.
3. Hair or caustic chemicals should not be allowed to contact the cornea during the surgical preparation of the patient.

Operative
1. General rules apply (see p. 264).

Postoperative

1. General rules apply (see p. 265).
2. The technician should remember that the patient is temporarily blinded on the operated side and should therefore be approached slowly and with ample auditory warning. Some dogs may snap at people if startled.
3. The owner should be forewarned of the appearance of the operated eye. Because the globe of the eye is covered, some owners think that the eye has been removed.
4. The technician should carefully demonstrate to the owner the proper procedure for applying any medication to the eye.

Other ophthalmic system operations. Ophthalmic system operations that are less commonly performed include cataract removal, enucleation, iridencleisis, keratectomy, parotid duct transplant, and repair of distichiasis, ectropion, entropion, and prolapse of the harderian gland of the third eyelid ("cherry eye").

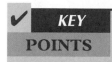

KEY POINTS

1. First intention wound healing is the healing of a wound without infection or excessive granulation tissue. It is sometimes referred to as side-to-side healing.
2. Second intention wound healing is the open healing of a wound by granulation. There may be some degree of suppuration (pus formation), which is the result of inflammation.
3. To keep the wound edges in side-to-side apposition, a mechanical force must hold the tissues together until initial healing allows the wound edges to remain in apposition. The purpose of sutures or staples is to hold the wound edges together on a temporary basis.
4. In many hospitals the technician is responsible for removing sutures or staples from a healed incision.
5. Electrocautery is the process of sealing a vessel, to achieve hemostasis, by burning or cauterizing the bleeding end with a controlled electrical current. This method is particularly valuable when multiple small bleeders would make clamping and tying vessels in the traditional manner difficult and time consuming.
6. General rules for the technician in the preoperative setting include the following: obtaining signatures on any consent or waiver form used by the hospital, making sure that food and water have been withheld from the patient for the time period required, instructing the owner when to call regarding progress reports, ensuring that elective surgery patients are relatively clean before they are admitted, ensuring that preoperative medications are given in the correct dosages and at the correct times, gathering any instruments or supplies needed for the operation, and preparing the patient's body for surgery.

Continued

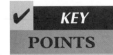
KEY POINTS

7. Preparing a patient's body for surgery before the patient enters the operating room includes shaving, washing, and disinfecting the appropriate area, as well as vacuuming loose hairs off the patient.

8. When assisting during surgery, the technician should be familiar with the operation and the technician's role; assist in a way that does not block the surgeon's light or field of vision; anticipate and provide the instruments or supplies necessary for the particular operation; keep the surgical field dry by blotting with sponges; keep the wound edges retracted, hold instruments in a manner that allows the surgeon easy access; handle tissues as gently as possible; use appropriate scissors; keep any long loops of suture material out of the surgeon's way; act as an extra pair of eyes and ears for the surgeon; and ensure that all sponges are recovered.

9. The technician's postoperative duties include monitoring patients for recovery of swallowing reflexes; keeping postoperative patients warm and checking incisions and general condition of the patient; changing cages as necessary to keep the patient clean and dry; and systematically monitoring the patient's temperature, pulse, and respiration.

10. Specific signs the technician should watch for and notify the physician of in the postoperative period include bleeding from the incision in larger amounts than normal; loss of color or refill in the mucous membranes; swelling of the operative site; prolonged recovery from anesthesia or sedation; separation of the incision edges; dehiscence; dyspnea; vomiting; and sutures or staples missing from the incision.

11. On patient discharge, the technician is responsible for the following procedures: ensuring that prescribed medications are ready for the owner and are thoroughly labeled; reminding the owner of any exercise restrictions; and advising the owner of any dietary restrictions, date and times for return visits, and danger signs to watch for at home.

12. Ovariohysterectomy is the removal of both ovaries and uterus for any of the following reasons: sterilization, elimination of estrous cycles, infection, ovarian-induced hormone imbalances, extensive traumatic injuries, some congenital abnormalities, and neoplasms of the ovaries or uterus.

13. Pyometra is an accumulation of pus within the uterus. Surgical removal of the infected uterus is indicated as soon as the patient is sufficiently stable to undergo surgery.

14. Cesarean section is the removal of the fetus through an incision in the uterus and abdomen instead of the normal vaginal route. Cesareans are performed when birth through the vaginal canal is either difficult or impossible.

15. Canine castration is a surgical procedure for the removal of a dog's testes. Dogs are castrated for the following reasons: to reduce aggression or wandering, sexual sterilization, reduction of territory "marking," neoplasms of the testes or scrotum, severe, traumatic wounds of the testes or scrotum, certain infections, and some conditions of the prostate gland.

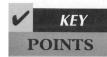

16. Feline castration has the same indications as canine castration, with the addition of elimination of the odor of tomcat urine.

17. In gastrointestinal surgery, as much of the gastrointestinal tract as possible must be packed off to reduce contamination of the body cavity. In addition, the technician must act as a sentinel for preventing contamination.

18. In pharyngostomy tube placement, an opening is made between the pharynx and body wall in the upper neck and a flexible tube is run down the esophagus and into the stomach to feed an animal unable or unwilling to eat (usually as a result of trauma to the mouth area).

19. In intestinal resection and anastomosis, a portion of the intestine is removed and the two remaining portions are joined together in a reestablished, continuous gastrointestinal tract. It is used whenever a section of intestine has been damaged and made dysfunctional.

20. An abscess is a circumscribed collection of pus, usually resulting from the introduction of pathogenic organisms under the skin (i.e., a bite wound) that requires draining.

21. Lacerations are linear tears in any tissue; treatment is done to restore torn tissues to their original function.

22. Declawing is the surgical removal of the entire nail and third phalanx of the paws. In most circumstances, only the front paws are declawed.

23. Orthopedics deals with injuries or diseases of the skeletal system.

24. The following terms are important in orthopedics: dislocation, luxation, subluxation, fracture, articular fracture, comminuted fracture, open fracture, physeal fracture, greenstick fracture, linear fracture, oblique fracture, spiral fracture, and transverse fracture.

25. The technician must become familiar with the names and shapes of the orthopedic instruments used in the specific practice.

26. The main orthopedic surgical procedures are closed fracture reduction and open fracture reduction.

27. A lateral ear wall resection involves the removal or transplant of the lateral cartilaginous wall of the vertical ear canal to expose the horizontal canal and provide drainage for the ear. It is indicated for chronic ear infections that have caused a thickening of the skin that lines the ear canal.

28. Nictitating membrane flap placement involves covering all or part of the cornea by suturing the nictitating membrane into place as needed. This is done whenever the cornea needs temporary protection.

▼ REVIEW QUESTIONS

1. What is first intention wound healing?

2. What is second intention wound healing?

3. What is the purpose of sutures or staples?

4. Why does a technician have to know about removing sutures or staples?

5. Describe the general guidelines for removing sutures.

6. What is electrocautery?

7. Describe the general rules for the technician in the preoperative setting.

8. What is involved in preparing a patient's body for surgery before the patient enters the operating room?

9. What general responsibilities does the technician have when assisting during surgery?

10. What are the technician's postoperative duties?

11. What specific signs should the technician watch for and notify the physician of in the postoperative period?

12. What are the technician's responsibilities during patient discharge?

13. Provide the definition, indications, and instruments needed for an ovariohysterectomy.

14. What common misconceptions may clients have about the ovariohysterectomy?

15. Describe the technician's responsibilities in ovariohysterectomy.

16. Provide the definition, indications, and instruments needed for a pyometra.

17. Describe the technician's responsibilities in pyometra.

18. Provide the definition, indications, and instruments needed for a cesarean section.

19. Describe the technician's responsibilities in cesarean section.

20. Provide the definition, indications, and instruments needed for canine castration.

21. Describe the technician's responsibilities in canine castration.

Continued

22. Provide the definition, indications, and instruments needed for feline castration.

23. Describe the technician's responsibilities in feline castration.

24. What special precautions must be taken in gastrointestinal surgery?

25. Give the definition, indications, and instruments needed in pharyngostomy tube placement.

26. Describe the technician's role in feeding a patient through a pharyngostomy tube.

27. Define and identify indications and special instruments used in intestinal resection and anastomosis.

28. What are the technician's responsibilities in intestinal resection and anastomosis?

29. What is an abscess? What special instruments might be needed for its treatment?

30. What are the technician's responsibilities in abscess drainings?

31. Give the definition, indications, and instruments needed in treating lacerations.

32. What is the technician's role in treating lacerations?

33. Give the definition, indications, and instruments needed in declawing.

34. What is the technician's role in declawing procedures?

35. What is orthopedics?

36. Define the following orthopedic terms: dislocation, luxation, subluxation, fracture, articular fracture, comminuted fracture, open fracture, physeal fracture, greenstick fracture, linear fracture, oblique fracture, spiral fracture, and transverse fracture.

37. Identify the main orthopedic surgical procedures.

38. In general, what is the role of the technician in orthopedic surgery?

39. Give the definition, indications, and special instruments needed for a lateral ear wall resection.

40. What are the technician's responsibilities in lateral ear wall resection?

41. Give the definition, indication, and special equipment needed for nictitating membrane flap placement.

42. What are the responsibilities of the technician in nictitating membrane flap placement?

ANSWERS FOR CHAPTER 4

1. First intention wound healing is the healing of a wound without infection or excessive granulation tissue. It is sometimes referred to as side-to-side healing.

2. Second intention wound healing is the open healing of a wound by granulation. There may be some degree of suppuration (pus formation), which is the result of inflammation.

3. To keep the wound edges in side-to-side apposition, a mechanical force must hold the tissues together until initial healing allows the wound edges to remain in apposition. Sutures or staples hold the wound edges together on a temporary basis, usually for the first 7 to 10 days of healing.

4. In many hospitals, the technician is the individual responsible for removing sutures or staples from a healed incision.

5. General guidelines for removing sutures include the following: The attending veterinarian should always be consulted if any of the following conditions exists at the incision site: swelling, erythema, discharge, separation of wound edges, or tissue protruding from the incision. Sutures are removed by gently applying traction to one of the free suture ends and cutting one side of the suture below the knot. Use of a suture scissors is recommended to lessen the chance of cutting the skin. Repeat until all sutures are removed.

6. Electrocautery is the process of sealing a vessel, to achieve hemostasis, by burning or cauterizing the bleeding end with a controlled electrical current. This method is particularly valuable when multiple small bleeders would make clamping and tying vessels in the traditional manner difficult and time consuming. Most types require that the patient be properly grounded.

7. General rules for the technician in the preoperative setting include obtaining signatures on any consent or waiver form used by the hospital; making sure that food and water have been withheld from the patient for the time period required; instructing the owner when to call regarding progress reports; ensuring that elective surgery patients are relatively clean before they are admitted; ensuring that preoperative medications are given in the correct dosages and at the correct times; gathering any instruments or supplies needed for the operation; and preparing the patient's body for surgery.

8. Preparing a patient's body for surgery before the patient enters the operating room includes shaving, washing, and disinfecting the appropriate area, as well as vacuuming loose hairs off the patient.

9. When assisting during surgery, the technician should be familiar with the operation and the technician's role; assist in a way that does not block the surgeon's light or field of vision; anticipate and provide the instruments or supplies necessary for the particular operation; keep the surgical field dry by blotting with sponges; keep the wound edges retracted, hold instruments in a manner that allows the surgeon easy access; handle tissues as gently as possible; use appropriate scissors; keep any long loops of suture material out of the surgeon's way; act as an extra pair of eyes and ears for the surgeon; and ensure that all sponges are recovered.

10. The technician's postoperative duties include monitoring patients for recovery of swallowing reflexes; keeping postoperative patients warm and checking incisions and general condition of the patient; changing the cage as necessary to keep the patient clean and dry; and systematically monitoring the patient's temperature, pulse, and respiration.

11. Specific signs the technician should watch for and notify the surgeon of in the postoperative period include bleeding from the incision in larger amounts than normal; loss of color or refill in the mucous membranes; swelling of the operative site; prolonged recovery from anesthesia or sedation; separation of the incision edges; dehiscence; dyspnea; vomiting; and sutures or staples missing from the incision.

12. On patient discharge, the technician is responsible for the following procedures: ensuring that prescribed medications are ready for the owner and are thoroughly labeled; and reminding the owner of any exercise or dietary restrictions, date and times for return visits, and danger signs to watch for at home.

13. Ovariohysterectomy is the removal of both ovaries and uterus for any of the following reasons: sterilization; elimination of estrous cycles; infection; ovarian-induced hormone imbalances; extensive traumatic injuries; some congenital abnormalities; and neoplasms of the ovaries or uterus. In addition to the general surgical pack, a canelike or hooklike instrument called a spay hook or a Snook hook is sometimes required for ovariohysterectomy.

14. Some common misconceptions clients have about the ovariohysterectomy are (1) it is beneficial for the pet to have at least one litter before surgery; (2) all spayed dogs and cats get fat; and (3) all dogs or cats over 3 years of age are too old to be spayed.

15. In addition to the general rules, the technician should perform the following procedures for an ovariohysterectomy:

    Preoperative. The technician should ascertain that the animal is a female and has had no previous ovariohysterectomy.

    Operative. The technician holds the instruments in a position that allows the surgeon maximum visibility of the tissue being ligated and then releases the clamping instruments when the surgeon ties the suture material.

    Postoperative. If the animal is sent home wearing an abdominal bandage, the owner should be instructed to watch for a shift in its position or any irritation caused by the bandage.

16. Pyometra is an accumulation of pus within the uterus. Surgical removal of the infected uterus is indicated as soon as the patient is sufficiently stable to undergo surgery. In addition to the general surgical pack, Rochester-Carmalt forceps may be necessary.

17. In addition to the general rules, the technician should perform the following procedures for pyometra:

    Preoperative. The technician should ensure that all the clients' questions about treatment and prognosis are answered by the attending veterinarian.

    Operative. The technician must be extremely careful when handling the uterus to avoid rupture.

    Postoperative. The technician must carefully monitor all vital signs, including urinary output. Because of the large volumes of fluids used, as soon as the patient is ambulatory, the technician should ensure that the animal is allowed frequent opportunities to pass urine. Monitor carefully for common postoperative signs of problems.

18. Cesarean section is the removal of the fetus through an incision in the uterus and abdomen, instead of through the vaginal route. Cesareans are performed when birth through the vaginal canal is either difficult or impossible. The general surgical pack provides everything needed, but a warm place for the pups or kittens and clean, dry toweling should be provided.

19. The technician should perform the following procedures during a cesarean section:

    Preoperative. The technician should ensure that all the clients' questions about treatment and prognosis are answered by the attending veterinarian; if the patient is presented after delivery of part of the litter, the technician should place the newborn pups or kittens in a warm, humid location.

    Operative. The technician must be careful to support the gravid uterus to avoid rupture; also, the technician should assist in removing fetuses from the uterus.

    Postoperative. The technician ensures that the mother's senses are completely restored before returning the pups to their mother.

20. Canine castration is a surgical procedure for the removal of a dog's testes. Dogs are castrated for the following reasons: to reduce aggression or wandering; sexual sterilization; reduction of territory "marking"; neoplasms of the testes or scrotum; severe, traumatic wounds of the testes or scrotum; certain infections; and some conditions of the prostate gland. All instruments needed are provided in the general surgical pack.

21. In addition to the general rules, the technician should perform the following procedures for canine castration:

    Preoperative. The technician should answer client questions, particularly about appropriate ages for castration and expected results; the technician should also verify that the animal is a male and that both testicles are in the scrotum.

    Postoperative. The technician must pay careful attention to postoperative swelling, with the use of cold packs if needed; the technician should also ensure that the dog does not lick the sutures; finally, the technician must advise owners on exercise restrictions and medication requirements.

22. Feline castration has the same indications as canine castration, with the addition of elimination of the odor of tomcat urine. All instruments needed are in the general instrument pack.

23. In addition to the general rules, the technician's further responsibilities in feline castration are the same as those for the canine castration.

24. In gastrointestinal surgery, as much of the gastrointestinal tract as possible must be packed off to reduce contamination of the body cavity. In addition, the technician must act as a sentinel for preventing contamination.

25. In pharyngostomy tube placement, an opening is made between the pharynx and body wall in the upper neck and a flexible tube is run down the esophagus and into the stomach to feed an animal unable or unwilling to eat (usually as a result of trauma to the mouth area). In addition to the general surgical pack, the pharyngostomy requires a flexible tubing with a cap.
26. In feeding a patient through a pharyngostomy tube, the technician should (1) consult the veterinarian before mixing medications with food; (2) blend food with water for administration; (3) administer food slowly; and (4) flush tube with water after each feeding and ensure that the cap is in place.
27. In intestinal resection and anastomosis, a portion of the intestine is removed and the two remaining portions are joined together in a reestablished continuous gastrointestinal tract. It is used whenever a section of intestine has been damaged and made dysfunctional. Special instruments are used to hold various parts of the intestinal tract.
28. In intestinal resection and anastomosis, the technician's responsibilities are threefold:

    Preoperative. The technician must ensure that the prescribed antibiotic therapy is administered before surgery. Extra sterile instruments, drapes, and gloves should be available if the surgeon desires a complete change after the anastomosis.

    Operative. The technician should ensure that the packing stays in place, that no leakage has occurred, and that intestines are held gently and in rotation, as needed, during anastomosis so that sutures can be placed correctly. The technician must also ensure that no foreign materials are left in the abdomen (sponges, towels, etc.).

    Postoperative. The technician should monitor and report any change in drainage or bowel movements. The technician should ensure that correct dietary restrictions and medication instructions are followed.
29. An abscess is a circumscribed collection of pus, usually resulting from a puncture wound, that requires draining. Although general surgical packs contain everything needed for drainage, a trephine and drainage system may also be required.
30. In abscess drainings, the technician's responsibilities are threefold:

    Preoperative. The technician must be protected from direct contact with purulent exudate and must ensure that equipment and supplies used do not contaminate the sterile operating room.

    Operative. The technician may be required to flush sterile saline or other solution into the abscess cavity to remove pus and debris.

    Postoperative. The technician should ensure that the drainage hole is kept clean and open, that dried discharges on nearby fur or skin are cleaned off, and that the owner is instructed in proper care and monitoring of the site after discharge.
31. Lacerations are linear tears in any tissue; treatment is done to restore torn tissues to their original function. No special instruments in addition to the general surgical pack are required.
32. In treating lacerations, the technician's role includes the following:

    Preoperative. The technician ensures that the wound is not contaminated with debris; foreign debris should be removed from the wound with a plain thumb forceps or similar instrument. The technician may be required to flush the wound before surgery.

    Operative. The technician provides the surgeon with the desired materials and instruments.

    Postoperative. The technician may be required to bandage the wound or place an E-collar to prohibit the animal from chewing sutures; the technician must also instruct the owner on how to care for the dressings.
33. Declawing is the surgical removal of the entire nail and third phalanx of the paws. In most circumstances, only the front paws are declawed. In addition to the general surgical pack instruments, some veterinarians prefer to use a small scalpel blade (no. 15) or sterilized nail trimmer.
34. In declawing procedures, the technician's role includes the following:

    Preoperative. The technician must inform the owner that only the front paws will be declawed and that after surgery cats must not be left alone outdoors because they will be unable to defend themselves from other animals.

    Operative. The technician will usually apply the bandages while the surgeon waits to declaw the other paw. The tourniquet is left in place until bandaging is complete.

    Postoperative. The technician must ensure that dressings remain in place until the veterinarian indicates their removal. Then the technician is usually the one to remove them. Finally, the technician should advise the owner to substitute shredded paper for kitty litter until incisions heal.

35. Orthopedics deals with injuries or diseases of the skeletal system.
36. The following terms are important in orthopedics:
    dislocation   A change in the normal anatomic relationships of the bones that form a joint
    luxation   Synonymous with dislocation
    subluxation   A partial dislocation
    fracture   A break in cortical bone or cartilage
    articular fracture   Fracture of a joint surface
    comminuted fracture   Bone fracture in fragments
    open fracture   Fracture with bone fragments penetrating soft tissue
    physeal fracture   Fracture at the epiphysis (growth plate)
    greenstick fracture   Incomplete fracture, not penetrating both cortices
    linear fracture   Fracture parallel with long axis of the bone
    oblique fracture   Fracture whose angle is between horizontal and vertical
    spiral fracture   Oblique fracture that curves or winds around the bone
    transverse fracture   Fracture horizontal to the long axis of the bone
37. The main orthopedic surgical procedures include closed fracture reduction, open fracture reduction, and closed reduction of luxations (dislocations).
38. In general, the role of the technician in orthopedic surgery is as follows:
    Preoperative. The technician must properly support affected parts to prevent further injury and must ensure proper patient preparation for surgery.
    Operative. The technician must be prepared for the tedium of this type of surgery.
    Postoperative. The technician must use extreme caution in applying bandages and splints and must protect casts and splints from moisture and be sure the owner is well educated in their care. Patients must be prevented from thrashing during the immediate postoperative period.
39. A lateral ear wall resection involves the removal or transplantation of the lateral cartilaginous wall of the vertical ear canal to expose the horizontal canal and provide drainage for the ear. It is indicated for chronic ear infections that have caused a thickening of the skin that lines the ear canal. In addition to the general surgical pack a cartilage scissors and electrocautery system are used.
40. The technician's responsibilities in lateral ear wall resection include the following:
    Preoperative. The technician should prepare the ear without traumatizing it.
    Operative. The technician must ensure that the patient is grounded if electrocautery is used.
    Postoperative. The technician must be gentle when cleaning wounds and removing dressings and must show owners how to care for the ear at home. In particular, owners should be warned not to put any solid objects such as cotton swabs into the shortened ear canal.
41. Nictitating membrane flap placement involves covering all or part of the cornea by suturing the nictitating membrane into place as needed. This is done whenever the cornea needs temporary protection. In addition to the general surgical pack, sterilized buttons, tubing, or other tension-absorbing materials should be available.
42. The responsibilities of the technician in nictitating membrane flap placement are as follows:
    Preoperative. The technician should ensure that special sutures and/or tension-absorbing materials are available and that hair or caustic chemicals do not touch the cornea during surgery.
    Operative. Duties are the same as those for general surgery.
    Postoperative. Because the patient is temporarily blinded on the affected side, the technician should approach slowly and with ample auditory warning. The owner should be forewarned of the appearance of the operated eye and should be taught the proper procedure for applying medication to the eye.

SELECTED READINGS

Bojrab MJ et al: *Current techniques in small animal surgery,* vol 2, Philadelphia, 1997, Lea & Febiger.
Bongura: *Kirk's current veterinary therapy. XII. Small animal practice,* Philadelphia, 1995, WB Saunders.
Fuller RJ: *Surgical technology: principles and practice,* ed 3, Philadelphia, 1994, WB Saunders.
Harvey CE et al: *Small animal surgery,* Philadelphia, 1990, JB Lippincott.

Piermattei DI: *Handbook of small animal orthopedics and fracture repair,* Philadelphia, 1997, WB Saunders.

Slatter DH, editor: *Textbook of small animal surgery,* ed 2, Philadelphia, 1993, WB Saunders.

Stone EA, Barsanti JA: *Small animal urologic surgery,* Philadelphia, 1986, Lea & Febiger.

Swain SF, Henderson RA: *Small animal wound management,* Baltimore, 1990, Lea & Febiger.

Whittick WG: *Canine orthopedics,* ed 2, Philadelphia, 1990, Lea & Febiger.

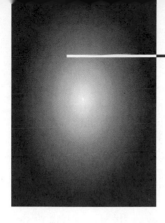

CHAPTER **5**

Surgical Emergencies

PERFORMANCE OBJECTIVES

After completion of this chapter the student will:

Restate the clinical signs, classifications, and treatment of shock.

Demonstrate an understanding of the proper restraint of trauma patients.

Explain the primary objectives and sequence of events in cardiopulmonary resuscitation.

Recognize and describe the various causes and presenting signs of respiratory emergencies.

Demonstrate the application of knowledge of the four spinal functions to evaluate the spinal trauma patient.

Identify the causes and treatment of anesthetic emergencies from among the major categories.

Define the principles of evaluating ophthalmic emergencies.

Describe the postoperative nursing care of gastrointestinal patients.

List the major urinary emergencies.

Tell the signs of impending dystocia.

Surgical emergencies occur frequently and unexpectedly in veterinary medicine and demand rapid recognition and therapy. A well-educated technician can be an invaluable asset to any veterinarian who must work promptly and effectively to correct a surgical emergency. The primary objectives in this chapter are twofold. The first is to familiarize the technician with the common emergencies of each of the six body systems so that the technician can easily recognize these crises. The second objective is to explain the basic therapy involved in the reversal of these emergencies so that the technician can anticipate the instruments and medicines needed for each situation. The technician can act as a sentinel for the veterinarian and maximize the efficiency of the veterinarian by being prepared. Reading this chapter will help the technician to understand the basic sequence of events that can be expected and the rationale behind the treatment of each emergency.

■ SHOCK

Shock is a descriptive term used to denote any condition in which there is inadequate tissue perfusion leading to cellular hypoxia, metabolic acidosis, and ultimately cell death. It could be argued that shock is a medical emergency, but because it can occur and seriously complicate any surgical emergency, it has been included in this chapter. It is imperative to realize that in any crisis accompanied by shock, shock must be successfully reversed or the treatment of the emergency will fail. Shock has been divided into four basic classes:

1. *Hypovolemic shock* is caused by loss of blood, plasma, or fluids leading to decreased circulating blood volume. Hypovolemic shock is the most common type of shock seen in dogs and cats. Perhaps the most common form of hypovolemic shock is hemorrhagic shock, which results from acute blood loss, such as in lacerations, surgery, or ruptured abdominal organs. Other causes of hypovolemic shock include fluid losses from vomiting and diarrhea, excessive diuresis, plasma losses caused by burns, and fluid sequestration, which can occur when large areas of tissues are bruised or crushed.

2. *Distributive (vasculogenic) shock* refers to a state in which the intravascular fluid remains the same but the vascular space is increased. Examples of distributive shock include asepsis and anesthetic overdose. Unlike other forms of shock, this type may respond to drugs that constrict blood vessels (alpha-stimulators) or mixtures of constrictors and dilators of blood vessels (alpha- and beta-stimulators).

3. *Cardiogenic shock* occurs when the heart loses its ability to pump blood and cardiac output fails. In this case myocardial failure may be caused by dysrhythmias, valvular insufficiency, or congenital defects.

4. *Obstructive shock* is caused by a restriction in the flow of blood. Examples include gastric dilation/volvulus (GDV), cardiac tamponade, pneumothorax, and cecal syndrome of heartworm disease.

It is important to note that although the causes of shock may vary, the basic sequence of events in shock is essentially the same. If the technician can achieve a thorough understanding of these events, the clinical signs will become obvious. No single clinical sign is adequate to identify shock.

Clinical Signs of Shock

- Tachycardia
- Hypotension: prolonged capillary refill time and weak pulse
- Rapid respiration
- Hypothermia
- Weakness, restlessness, and depression
- Reduced urine output
- Coma and dilation of pupils

Pathophysiology of Shock

Shock is precipitated by any event that decreases cardiac output and blood pressure. The body responds by stimulating the sympathetic nervous system and the adrenal gland to cause arterial vasoconstriction and contraction of the spleen. This shunts blood away from the skin and intestinal viscera and maintains the volume of blood circulating to the vital organs. The heart rate increases, further increasing cardiac output. The kidney attempts to maintain the circulating blood volume by retaining sodium and water. This is mediated by two hormones, renin and antidiuretic hormone (ADH), and causes decreased urine output. If decreased tissue perfusion persists, the classic signs of hypothermia (weakness, mental confusion, weak pulse) will develop.

An inadequate delivery of oxygen to the tissues results in cell anoxia and the accumulation of lactic acid, which causes metabolic acidosis. Blood becomes trapped in the capillaries because the small arterioles lose tone and the veins remain constricted. At this point the shock is rapidly becoming irreversible. The terminal event in all forms of shock is cardiopulmonary arrest (Fig. 5-1).

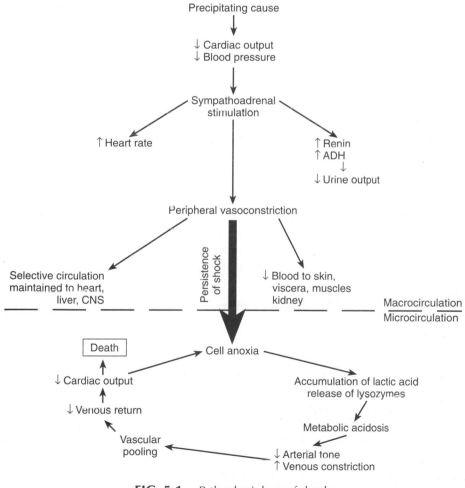

FIG. 5-1   Pathophysiology of shock.

Target organs. In the past it has been common to speak of target organs with regard to shock. These organs were thought to be the most susceptible to the effect of shock and differed in each of the domestic animals. The intestinal tract was listed as the target organ for the dog and horse, and the lungs were cited for the cat and cow. As more has been learned about shock, the realization has developed that it is in fact a multisystem disorder and that no part of the body remains unharmed. However, it is still helpful to understand how shock affects each of the major organs both as a prognostic tool and as a guide to the potential complications of shock.

Blood flow to the heart itself is decreased only if more than 20% of the total blood volume is lost. If blood pressure is maintained above 70 mm Hg, the coronary blood flow remains adequate. (The pulse is palpable at 70 mm Hg or greater.) As blood flow to the heart is decreased, cardiac function and compliance decline, end-diastolic pressure rises, and blood flow to the heart is further compromised. The heart rapidly loses its ability to compensate for the already lowered cardiac output.

Reduced blood flow to the brain results in a reduced capacity to function not only because of lowered oxygen tension but also because of a depletion of the brain's supply of glucose, which is its greatest source of energy. Cerebral blood flow remains adequate until mean systemic arterial pressure falls below 60 mm Hg. Clinical signs of hypoxic encephalopathy include transient ataxia, confusion, and stupor.

Reduced blood flow to the kidney must be prolonged to cause renal failure. Clinical signs that reflect kidney damage include oliguria, glucosuria, and specific gravities that decrease with each sequential sample.

The lungs often are the most damaged by shock. The common causes of shock (trauma of the upper abdomen and thorax) cause direct physical damage to the lungs. Damaged tissues often release various vasoactive chemicals that have an adverse effect on the alveolar capillaries, and these capillaries are also the site at which platelet aggregates and microclots in transfused blood are filtered out of the circulation. The actual act of resuscitation can also be harmful to the lung. Care must be taken in all shock patients to minimize these secondary pulmonary changes. Respiratory failure is also a well-recognized problem in humans 24 to 72 hours after shock has been treated (shock lung or acute respiratory distress syndrome [ARDS]). Dogs appear to be less susceptible to ARDS than cats or humans.

The most common complication of shock in the intestinal tract is hemorrhagic enteritis that causes a loss of plasma into the lumen of the gut. The mediators of this complication are endotoxins in septic shock, ischemia in hemorrhagic shock, and vascular stasis in other forms of shock.

■ MANAGEMENT OF THE TRAUMA VICTIM

Initial contact of the trauma patient with the veterinary hospital may be through the technician. A quick assessment of the victim's vital signs will allow the technician to determine the severity of the injury, not only so that first aid can be given but also so that the veterinarian can be informed. The animal's level of consciousness, its breathing, heart rate, and femoral pulse should be quickly assessed. Any arterial bleeding should be controlled. The color of the mucous membranes and the capillary refill time should be checked. The animal's ability to walk on its own, deformity of any limbs, the presence of pain, and the temperature should be noted. The strength of the pulse is a crude measurement of the animal's blood pressure. Any differences between the heart rate (the rate auscultated at the chest) and the pulse is called a pulse deficit and denotes an inefficient contraction of the heart. The technician should work with speed and above all should remain calm. Both the owner and the patient will be frightened and unpredictable. The technician should be systematic in the precursory examination. It should be remembered that many of the ugliest injuries are not life threatening, and an apparently insidious problem can in fact kill the animal. The ultimate responsibility of determining the prognosis and correct therapy belongs to the veterinarian. The key role of the technician is in assessment of the patient and anticipation of the therapy.

Restraint and transportation of an injured animal often present a challenge to the technician (Figs. 5-2 and 5-3). *Any* animal in pain may bite, so the technician must be prepared to muzzle the patient (Fig. 5-4, p. 330). Care should be taken to balance the importance of maintaining the animal's ability to breath with human safety. Human safety always comes first. Most animals will assume the least painful position to guard broken bones or to allow maximum excursion of the chest, and

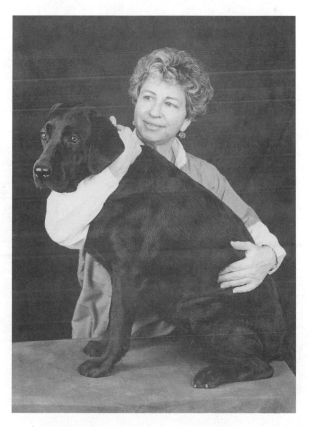

FIG. 5-2 Manual restraint of dog.

the animal should be allowed to remain in that preferred position. Any animal that cannot walk or is suspected of having a spinal injury should be transported with a stretcher. A stretcher can be made from a board, any stiff object, or a blanket held at the corners. The technician should slide or lift the patient onto the stretcher, keeping the spine level and straight (Fig. 5-5, p. 331). If the animal needs to be restrained on the stretcher, it should not be strapped so tightly that breathing is hampered. The technician must move slowly and with caution. Rough handling and excitement may worsen any existing pain and shock (Figs. 5-6 and 5-7). Temporary splints are often unnecessary at the hospital, but if needed in the field, they can be

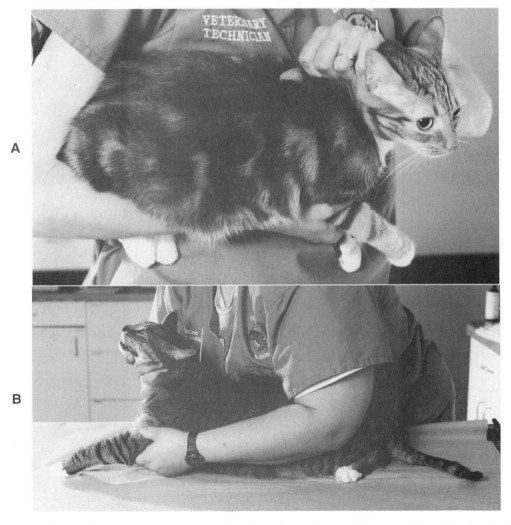

FIG. 5-3   **A** and **B,** Demonstration of effective form of manual restraint of cat. One hand of holder grasps cat's forelegs and supports body while other hand restrains head and neck.

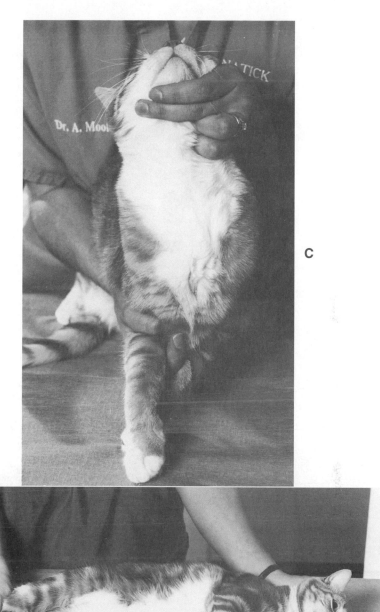

C

D

FIG. 5-3, cont'd   **C,** Alternative method of restraint is to hold all four feet with one hand while grasping fur at nape of neck with other hand. **D,** The correct way to employ the lateral cat stretch.

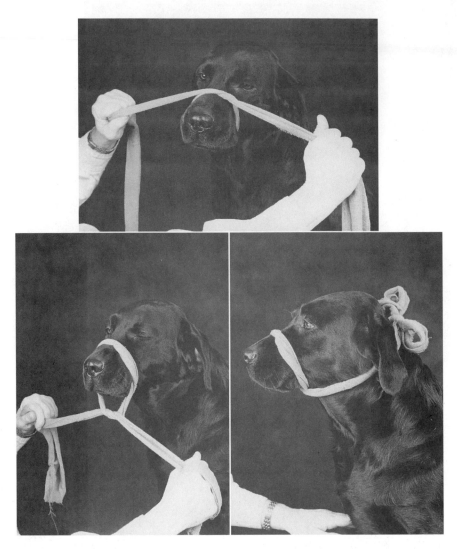

FIG. 5-4   To muzzle dog, use strip of gauze 2 to 3 feet in length. Make overhand loop, place loop over dog's muzzle, and pull tight. Secure knot under jaw, bring two free ends to back of head, and tie bow behind ears.

fashioned from any rigid object that will successfully support the size and contour of the fractured limb. In most cases tranquilizers are unnecessary and contraindicated. Their pharmacologic properties usually lower blood pressure and alter the animal's level of consciousness in a manner that interferes with any neurologic evaluations for the presence of head injuries. Analgesics are often indicated but should only be administered after evaluation by and under the direct supervision of the attending veterinarian.

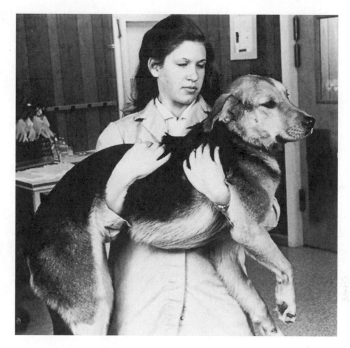

FIG. 5-5   Correct method for lifting trauma victim.

■ CARDIOPULMONARY EMERGENCIES
Respiratory and Cardiac Arrest

Respiratory and/or cardiac arrest can develop during any surgical procedures. Their incidence increases in emergency surgery because the patient may already be severely compromised. In any emergency, the probability of poor oxygen delivery to the heart increases and anoxia is the greatest inciting cause of arrest. Cardiac arrest can also be precipitated by overdoses of any anesthetic and is an inherent risk of all surgical procedures that must be minimized.

Respirations must be monitored closely in the surgical patient, and the technician must realize that respiratory arrest frequently is the antecedent to cardiac arrest. Cardiac arrest is the absence or cessation of any effective contraction of the heart. The electrical activity of the heart may vary from asystole (no P waves, no electrical activity) to ventricular fibrillation. In addition to anesthetic overdose and shock, cardiac arrest may be caused by anoxia of the heart muscle, coronary artery disease (uncommon in animals), myocardial disease, electrical shock, primary lung or airway disease, head trauma, or toxemia. Vagal stimulation can also precipitate cardiac arrest. This should be remembered during intubation, cervical spinal procedures, and neck and chest surgery so that manipulation of the vagus nerve can be avoided.

The classic signs of cardiac arrest are the absence of pulse, heartbeat, and respiration. Crisis signs that may precede cardiac arrest include cyanosis, dysrhythmias with pulse irregularities, a decrease in blood pressure, and a prolonged capillary refill time. Respirations may become more shallow and rapid, bleeding from wounds

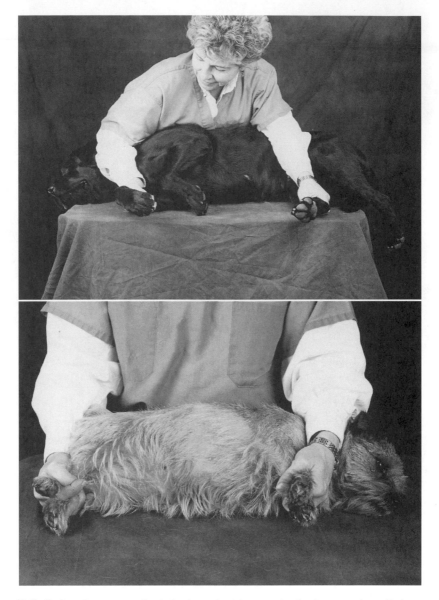

FIG. 5-6   Correct methods for lateral table restraint for large and small dogs.

or incisions may stop, the bladder and anus may relax, the skin may seem cool to the touch, and the pupils may begin to dilate.

The primary objectives in the treatment of cardiac arrest are to maintain the circulation that delivers oxygen to the tissues and to reestablish the normal electrical activity of the heart. It is almost impossible for one person to successfully resuscitate an animal. For this reason, the technician becomes an integral part of a team that must work in a coordinated and orderly fashion to accomplish these objectives.

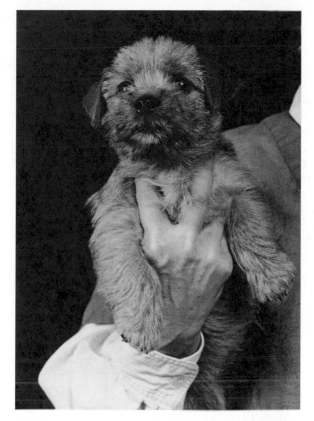

FIG. 5-7   Correct method for carrying an injured puppy.

An organized team allows simultaneous treatments and administration of fluids and drugs and can greatly increase the chance of a successful CPR. All available personnel should be trained to be functional members of the team. Equipment, drugs, and supplies should be located in one place at all times. A CPR flowsheet should be posted.

Cardiopulmonary resuscitation (CPR). After confirming a diagnosis of cardiac arrest, the technician and veterinarian must act quickly to try to reverse the arrest using CPR. The technician should remember the following:

A = Airway
B = Breathing
C = Circulation
D = Drugs
     Electrocardiographic monitoring
     Treatment of dysrhythmia
     Continued monitoring and support

Airway
1. Pull tongue forward.
2. Swab or suction the entire oral cavity.
3. If a foreign body is suspected, administer the Heimlich maneuver using sub-diaphragmatic thrusts with the fist of one hand or use a long forceps to extract the foreign body.
4. Intubate the trachea whenever possible; less desirable alternatives are to use a face mask, nose-to-mouth resuscitation, or an Ambu bag.

Breathing
1. Commence positive pressure ventilation using 100% oxygen. Ventilate at 30 to 35 breaths per minute.

Circulation

Closed chest massage. Standard cardiopulmonary resuscitation technique may prove ineffective in animals that weigh over 20 kg, are very obese, or have barrel-shaped chests.

TECHNIQUE
1. Place animal in right or left lateral recumbency.
2. Place the heel of the palm of the left hand over the precordium in small animals and more dorsally in larger patients.
3. Place the heel of the right hand over the left as shown in Fig. 5-8 and apply short, quick compressions of 120 per minute.
4. Apply simultaneous positive pressure ventilation (PPV) during the active phase of chest compression at the rate of one PPV per every four chest compressions.

Open chest CPR. This may be the best method for animals weighing over 20 kg. Thoracotomy is indicated when in the judgment of the team leader closed chest massage is unlikely to be successful. Thoracotomy is indicated only in a well-equipped central hospital.

TECHNIQUE
1. Animal is placed in right lateral recumbency, and an area over the fifth and sixth intercostal spaces is quickly clipped and painted.
2. A thoracotomy incision is made and incised down to the pleura.
3. Rib spreaders are used for retraction, and the heart is lifted from the opened pericardium.
4. Eighty to one hundred manual compressions per minute are applied.
5. After resuscitation, the thorax is lavaged with normal saline, a chest drain is put in place, and antibiotic therapy is instituted. The incidence of infection after emergency thoracotomy is reportedly low to nonexistent.

Drugs commonly used in CPR and shock treatment *(Table 5-1)*

Fluids. Ideally, all surgical patients should have an IV drip started before the procedure. Anesthetic induction results in a decrease in blood pressure, and the procedure itself represents an insult that can further compromise adequate tissue perfusion. When shock is treated, fluids should be administered rapidly, ideally through one or two large-bore catheters. (See Figs. 5-9 and 5-10.)

Intravenous administration of a crystalloid replacement fluid, such as Ringer's lactate solution, or any fluid that contains sodium, potassium, chloride, and bicarbonate should be dripped at a rate of 5 to 10 ml/kg/hr of anesthesia. Where clinical

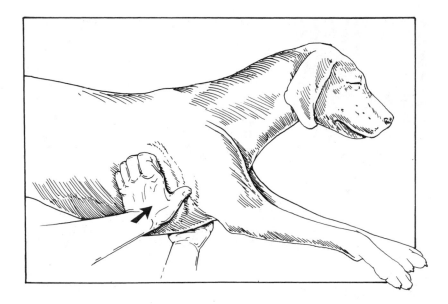

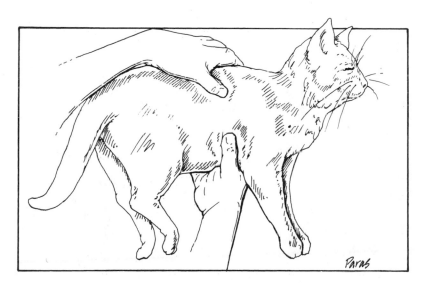

FIG. 5-8   External cardiac massage in the dog and cat. (From Muir WW et al: *Handbook of veterinary anesthesia,* 2nd ed, St Louis, 1995, Mosby.)

signs indicate hypovolemia, more aggressive blood volume restoration is required. In this instance, amounts of 40 to 90 ml/kg or more may be needed to stabilize the signs of hypovolemia.

Colloids are solutions that contain large–molecular weight particles that do not readily leave the intravascular space. Colloids may be used alone or in addition to crystalloids. Colloids include hetastarch, pentastarch, and dextran.

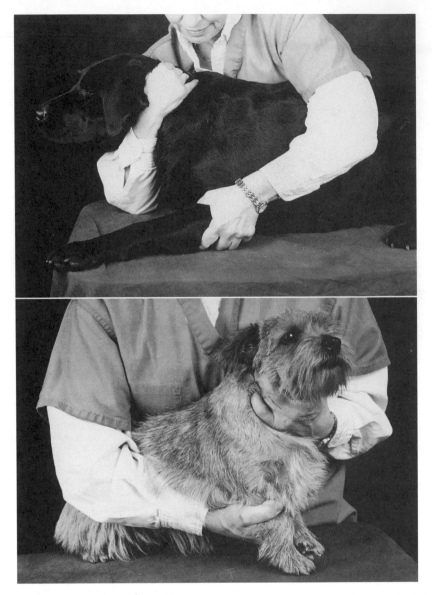

FIG. 5-9   Methods for holding off the cephalic vein for venipuncture in large and small dogs.

Where there has been hemorrhage or when the animal is anemic (packed cell volume below 20%), the crystalloids are fairly ineffective in restoring adequate volume. In these cases, whole blood should be administered at the rate of 5 to 10 ml/kg/hr. Transfusions should increase the recipient's packed cell volume (PCV) by 1% for each milliliter per kilogram administered. Administer until the PCV rises above 20% again. If fresh whole blood is not available, autotransfusion may be considered if the

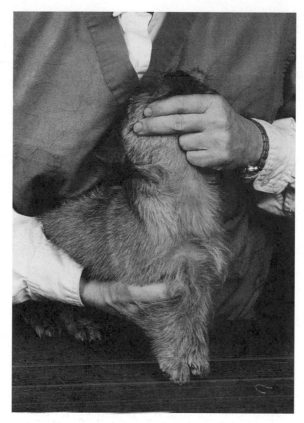

FIG. 5-10 Holding a puppy for venipuncture or drug administration via the jugular vein.

animal is hemorrhaging into the pleural or abdominal cavities. Blood is carefully aspirated out of the space, kept from coagulating, and administered via an intravenous infusion set equipped with a filter.

Sympathomimetics. These agents include dopamine, dobutamine, ephedrine, and mephentermine as first choice drugs. They are used to increase myocardial contractility and arterial blood pressure, thereby positively affecting tissue perfusion.

If these drugs fail to adequately increase blood pressure, more potent alpha agonists might be used with caution because they act primarily by constricting blood vessels. These drugs include morepinephrine, metaraminol, phenylephrine, and methoxamine.

Antidysrhythmics. Anticholinergics and sympathomimetics with beta-agonist action are used to treat cardiac dysrhythmias, such as bradycardia or premature ventricular contractions.

These drugs include lidocaine, propranolol, verapamil, and phenytoin.

Glucocorticosteroids. Steroids appear to have several beneficial effects in all forms of shock. These agents act to maintain cell membrane integrity and improve cellular

TABLE 5-1

Drug Dosages for CPR in Dogs and Cats

Drug	Dosage
Epinephrine	0.2 mg/kg IV; 0.4 mg/kg IT (diluted with equal volume of saline), every 3 to 5 min as needed; also can use IO (previously recommended: 0.1 to 0.5 mg/10 kg), 1:1000 = 1 mg/ml
Methoxamine	0.1 to 0.2 mg/kg IV; can use IT
Metaraminol	0.1 to 0.2 mg/kg IV
Mephentermine	0.1 to 0.5 mg/kg IV
Phenylephrine	0.01 to 0.1 mg/kg IV
Norepinephrine	0.01 to 0.1 mg for average dog
Dopamine	Dogs: 5 to 15 µg/kg/min; cats: 1 to 5 µg/kg/min CRI; can use IO
Sodium bicarbonate	0.5 to 1 mEq/kg initial dose; up to 8 mEq/kg if prolonged arrest and/or CPR
Do *not* give IT; can use IO
Calcium chloride (10%)	0.1 to 0.26 ml/kg IV (or 1.5 to 2 ml/dog)
Calcium gluconate (10%)	0.1 to 0.3 ml/kg IV; can use IO
Dexamethasone SP	4 mg/kg IV; can use IO
Atropine	0.01 to 0.02 mg/kg IV, IM, IT, IO
Lidocaine	Dogs: 2 mg/kg, up to 8 mg/kg IV; cats: 0.25 to 0.5 mg/kg slowly IV; can use IT or IO

From Nelson RW, Couto CG: *Small animal internal medicine,* 2nd ed, St Louis, 1998, Mosby. *IT,* Intratracheally; *IO,* intraosseously; *CRI,* constant-rate infusion.

metabolism. They increase capillary blood flow and help support effective heart muscle action. Their benefits in improving survival far outweigh the adverse effects of immune system depression and retarded wound healing. Examples of these drugs include prednisone, hydrocortisone, and dexamethasone.

Antibiotics. Antibiotic treatment is probably not indicated in mild hypovolemia or cardiogenic shock states. It is used prophylactically in septic shock.

Diuretics. Reduced visceral perfusion is reflected in reduced urinary output. Inadequate renal blood flow may proceed to renal shutdown without timely therapeutic intervention. Loop diuretics such as furosemide and osmotic diuretics such as mannitol are given until the oliguria or anuria is corrected and urine flows at a rate of about 0.5 to 1 ml/kg/hr.

Trauma

Respiratory tract trauma can cause lacerations and fractures of the larynx and trachea. The severity of the clinical signs is directly proportional to the amount of airway obstruction that develops after the injury. Lacerations of the airway produce subcutaneous emphysema. This leaking develops as air becomes trapped between the skin and subcutaneous tissues. Minor lacerations need not be repaired, and mild subcutaneous emphysema usually resolves with time. A major leakage of air or bleeding lacerations should be explored and repaired surgically by suturing the defect. Fractures of the upper airway are both difficult to diagnose and to treat. If severe occlusion of the airway occurs, the animal's breathing will become loud and sonorous. The presence of loud breathing, dyspnea, and cyanosis should alert the technician to an impending crisis in which a tracheotomy may be necessary. This will be discussed later in the section concerning airway obstruction.

Fractures of the ribs become surgical emergencies when they directly lacerate the underlying lung parenchyma or seriously diminish excursions of the chest. Interference with normal thoracic motion can occur when several ribs in a row are fractured, allowing the chest wall to give way or to flail with each change in thoracic pressure. Compressed pieces of rib must be elevated surgically and wired or pinned to the remaining fragments, and chest wall rigidity must be returned. A number of procedures using interlacing wires or Teflon splints sutured to the ribs have been used successfully.

Surgical emergencies of the heart are rare. Most patients with gunshot wounds or avulsion of major vessels do not survive the trip to the veterinary hospital. Other patients with blunt trauma to the heart may be completely asymptomatic or develop medical problems, such as dysrhythmias.

Pleural effusion in the trauma patient becomes an emergency when the lungs can no longer expand to provide adequate oxygenation of the blood. Pneumothorax is the presence of air in the pleural cavity and can result from penetrating wounds, esophageal foreign bodies, pneumonia, or other causes. Hemothorax is the presence of blood in the chest. These often occur together. Causes of pleural effusion that can develop slowly yet become an emergency when the animal begins to decompensate include chylothorax, pyothorax, and neoplasia. The result in each of these is atelectasis of lung tissue. The patient is dyspneic and often stands with the neck extended and the legs abducted to allow maximum excursion of the chest and intake of oxygen. Cyanosis is common. As more lung tissue is displaced by fluid or air, the severity of the clinical signs increases. Often the patient is frightened and the temperature is elevated. The diagnosis of pleural effusion depends on auscultation, percussion of the chest, radiography, and thoracentesis (aspiration of the chest). The primary aim in therapy is to remove as much air or fluid as possible so that the functioning lung capacity can return to normal. This can best be accomplished by thoracentesis or the insertion of a chest tube. The chest tube is usually inserted at the animal's seventh or eighth intercostal space with a local anesthetic (Fig. 5-11). If fluid is present, the tube is inserted in the ventral third of the rib space because gravity will cause fluid to lie ventrally in the chest. If air is present, the tube is usually inserted in the dorsal third of the rib space. The technician may often be required to suction the chest tube periodically after its insertion. Accumulation of pleural air may be so rapid that continuous suction is necessary. Failure to reduce the flow of air may be an indication for exploratory surgery.

Another condition that can decrease the size of the pleural cavity is a diaphragmatic hernia with prolapse of the abdominal viscera into the chest. Diaphragmatic hernias can be insidious and not discovered for weeks or months after an injury. They can, in fact, be congenital (pericardioperitoneal) and not diagnosed for years. They become surgical emergencies when the extra viscera in the chest cavity physically compresses lung tissue or causes secondary pleural effusion.

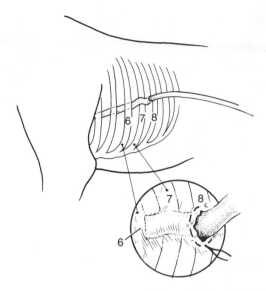

FIG. 5-11   Chest tube is inserted through small skin incision. Tube is passed through sub-cutaneous tissue and enters chest one or two rib spaces away. It is anchored in place with purse-string suture.

Diaphragmatic hernias are repaired through a ventral midline abdominal incision. The abdominal viscera are returned to the abdomen, and the torn diaphragmatic muscle is sutured. The technician may be called on to help the patient breath during this surgery because positive pressure ventilation must be maintained until the diaphragm is repaired and again becomes an airtight seal.

Airway Obstruction

The causes of airway obstruction are varied and almost innumerable. Trauma caused by fractures of the airway has already been discussed. Airway occlusion may be caused by epistaxis or the swelling of surrounding soft tissues after an injury. Foreign material, such as bones, food, vomitus, mucus, and chemicals, can obstruct the airway. Infections such as abscesses and necrotic laryngitis as well as tumors can also be a cause. Neuromuscular disorders, including esophageal paralysis and laryngeal spasm, may result in airway occlusion. Unfortunately, the brachycephalic breeds have an anatomic conformation that predisposes them to upper airway obstruction.

Airway obstructions are characterized by noisy, open-mouthed breathing. The noise is produced by the passage of air through a narrowed channel. It may be low-pitched and gurgling (sonorous) or harsh and high-pitched (stridor). The type and location of the noise can be an important aid in determining the cause of the obstruction. Often a history of decreased exercise tolerance, cyanosis, increased respiratory effort, choking, gagging, and collapse is reported. Heat prostration may be precipitated by this condition because of inadequate air exchange, increased muscle activity, and fright.

Therapy. The ultimate priority in the treatment of all airway obstructions is to relieve the obstruction and return oxygenation to normal. The technician should aid the veterinarian in examining the mouth and pharynx quickly. Any foreign material should be removed, and hemorrhage should be controlled. If the patient is unconscious, intubation should be attempted. If the obstruction cannot be relieved, it should be bypassed with a temporary tracheostomy. In most cases, a tracheostomy is performed with few minutes to spare. An experienced technician can assist the veterinarian and eliminate valuable minutes from the length of the procedure. A tracheostomy is performed with the animal in dorsal recumbency; the neck is supported by several towels or sandbags. The ventral aspect of the neck caudal to the larynx should be prepared for sterile surgery. A curved metal or plastic tracheostomy tube, approximately one third smaller than the lumen of the trachea, should be readied for insertion. The tracheostomy tube is inserted caudal to the second or third tracheal ring. Anesthesia and oxygen can be administered through the tracheostomy tube immediately after insertion. The tube is then sutured to the skin of the neck.

The anatomic obstructions usually require corrective surgery at some point in their course. When the crisis can be eliminated with oxygen and sedation, the surgery can be postponed and performed when the patient is more stable. Each of the corrective operations is designed to excise the obstructing tissue (Table 5-2). Many of these patients also have tracheostomy tubes postoperatively. The tracheostomy site must be kept clean and free of mucus. It is advisable to suction the inside of the tube frequently for the first 24 hours postoperatively to remove blood and debris. This must be done using sterile technique. The tracheostomy tube must remain patent to ensure the animal an adequate airway.

All airway obstructions are serious and often life threatening. If the patient is discovered by the technician, immediate veterinary help should be sought. The animal

TABLE 5-2

Anatomic Conformations That Predispose to Airway Obstruction

Conformation	Breeds affected	Surgical correction
Elongation of soft palate	Bulldog, pug, Pekingese, Boston terrier, beagle, cocker spaniel	Excision of excess tissue
Eversion of lateral ventricles of larynx, arytenoid cartilage collapse	All brachycephalic breeds	Excision of prolapsed tissue
Vocal cord paralysis	St. Bernard, husky, Bouvier des Flandres, other large breeds	Unilateral or bilateral laryngectomy with excision of vocal cord
Tracheal collapse	Chihuahua, Pomeranian, Yorkshire terrier, poodle, Maltese	Tracheal prostheses

should be handled with a minimal amount of excitement. The technician should be prepared to assist the veterinarian in removing foreign objects, administering anesthesia, and inserting a tracheostomy tube. The technician should also be aware of the nursing problems that can occur postoperatively in the obstructed patient.

■ ANESTHETIC EMERGENCIES

No matter how often we anesthetize animals or how familiar we are with anesthetics, from time to time anesthetic emergencies or complications arise. The best defense against such complications is to be adequately prepared by being familiar with the patient's health status, understanding the anesthetic equipment and drugs, and providing alert, active monitoring of the patient. The first rule when an anesthetic emergency arises is DO NOT PANIC.

The majority of anesthetic emergencies fall into the following four categories: (1) anesthetic equipment failure, (2) cardiovascular system, (3) respiratory system, and (4) neurologic and metabolic emergencies.*

I. Equipment failure
   A. Complication: failure to keep patient anesthetized
      1. Predisposing factors
         a. Endotracheal tube improperly placed, missized, kinked, or disconnected from machine; cuff not inflated
         b. Vaporizer disconnected, set incorrectly, or not calibrated
         c. Anesthetic machine leaks or has inadequate flow; CO_2 absorbent exhausted
         d. Patient in respiratory depression (hypoventilation)
         e. Often tank is turned off or empty
      2. Symptoms
         a. Patient awake or responding to pain
         b. Hypertension
         c. Tachycardia
      3. Treatment and resolution: systematically check patient, endotracheal tube, and anesthetic machine. Checking the anesthetic equipment before use will eliminate many potential problems. Before anesthesia is administered, assess the patient's status to determine if anything could predispose the patient to respiratory depression. If equipment failure is the problem, correct it or change equipment.
   B. Complication: animal in an excessively deep plane of anesthesia
      1. Predisposing factors
         a. Vaporizer: incorrect vaporizer setting, inaccurate vaporizer calibration, incorrect anesthetic in vaporizer
         b. Machine: vaporizer placed incorrectly in circuit
         c. Patient: low body temperature, preexisting disease, drug interactions and combinations

---

*By permission of Dr. A. Faggella.

2. Symptoms: pupils dilated, absence of reflexes, bradycardia, no muscle tone, hypotension, hypoventilation
3. Treatment and resolution: examining equipment before use will eliminate many potential problems. Decrease or turn off vaporizer setting. Empty reservoir bag and fill with pure O_2, ventilate patient. Antagonize any injectable drugs if possible.

II. Cardiovascular system
  A. Complication: bradycardia
    1. Predisposing factors
      a. Anesthetic drugs—anesthetic plane
      b. Increased vagal tone
      c. Surgical manipulation
      d. Hypothermia
      e. Late stages of hypoxia
      f. Metabolic problems
    2. Symptoms
      a. Heart rate
        (1) Less than 60 beats/min in dogs
        (2) Less than 100 beats/min in cats
    3. Treatment and resolution
      a. Determine cause
      b. Lighten anesthetic plane if possible
      c. Administer atropine or glycopyrrolate
      d. Keep patient warm
      e. Correct electrolyte abnormalities
      f. Support ventilation
  B. Complication: tachycardia
    1. Predisposing factors
      a. Anesthetic plane—too light
      b. Hypotension
      c. Hypovolemia
      d. Shock
      e. Inadequate ventilation
      f. Drug induced—e.g., ketamine, atropine, glycopyrrolate
      g. Hyperthermia
    2. Symptoms
      a. Heart rate
        (1) Greater than 120 beats/min in large dogs
        (2) Greater than 140 beats/min in medium dogs
        (3) Greater than 150 beats/min in small dogs
        (4) Greater than 200 beats/min in cats
    3. Treatment and resolution
      a. Assess anesthetic depth—adjust as needed
      b. Provide adequate fluid support
      c. Support ventilation

       d. Maintain normothermia
       e. See sections on hypotension, shock, and malignant hyperthermia

C. Complications: cardiac dysrhythmias
  1. Predisposing factors
    a. Anesthetic plane—too light or too deep
    b. Sensitization of heart to epinephrine
    c. Anesthetic drugs
    d. Electrolyte imbalance
    e. Hypoxemia, hypercarbia
    f. Acid-base imbalance
    g. Vagal or sympathetic reflexes
    h. Surgical stimulation or manipulation
  2. Symptoms
    a. Irregular pulse and pulse pressure
    b. Pulse deficits
    c. Irregular heart sounds
    d. Hypotension
    e. Pallor, cyanosis
    f. Poor capillary refill time
    g. Abnormal ECG tracing
  3. Classification of dysrhythmias
    a. By heart rate
      (1) Bradydysrhythmias—less than 60 beats/min
      (2) Tachydysrhythmias—greater than 170 beats/min
    b. By sight of origin in heart
      (1) Supraventricular
      (2) Ventricular
      (3) Junctional
  4. Prevention of anesthetic-related dysrhythmias
    a. Preoperative patient evaluation
    b. Correct electrolyte balance, hydration, and acid-base abnormalities before anesthesia
    c. Proper anesthetic drug selection and knowledge of drug actions
    d. Ventilatory support
    e. Cardiovascular support—fluids
    f. Proper anesthetic depth
  5. Treatment and resolution
    a. Correct underlying cause
      (1) Acid-base balance
      (2) Electrolytes
      (3) Ventilation
      (4) Fluid therapy
      (5) Assess anesthetic depth
    b. During anesthesia most dysrhythmias are caused by errors in technique or judgment, inappropriate drug selection, or problems related

to metabolic or ventilatory status and *not* by primary myocardial disease.

   c. Not all dysrhythmias require treatment. In general only those that interfere with efficient ventricular function or predispose to ventricular fibrillation or cardiac arrest are treated.

   d. Administer specific drug therapy

D. Complication: anemia

  1. Predisposing factors

    a. Hemorrhage

    b. Chronic disease

    c. Hemodilution—redistribution, fluid therapy

    d. Splenectomy, amputation

  2. Symptoms

    a. Hematocrit (Hct) level less than 21%; hemoglobin level less than 8 g/dl

    b. Pallor

  3. Treatment and resolution: whole blood transfusion

E. Complication: hypotension

  1. Predisposing factors

    a. Hypovolemia—hemorrhage, fluid deficits

    b. Decreased cardiac output; decreased venous return

    c. Peripheral vasodilation

    d. Anesthetic drugs

    e. Surgical manipulation

    f. Hypoxemia

    g. Cardiac dysrhythmias; bradycardia

    h. Improper use of ventilator

  2. Symptoms

    a. Poor peripheral pulses

    b. Prolonged capillary refill time

    c. Pallor

    d. Blood pressure measurement

      (1) Normal systolic: 100 to 160 mm Hg

      (2) Normal diastolic: 60 to 90 mm Hg

      (3) Normal mean: 80 to 120 mm Hg

    e. Oliguria, anuria

  3. Treatment and resolution

    a. Provide fluid support—crystalloids, colloids

    b. Adjust ventilator

    c. Decrease anesthetic depth

    d. Correct cardiac dysrhythmias

    e. Administer vasoactive drugs (under veterinarian's direction only)

      (1) Dopamine: 3 to 5 μg/kg/min

      (2) Dobutamine: 3 to 5 μg/kg/min

      (3) Ephedrine: 0.05 to 0.5 mg/kg

      (4) Calcium chloride: 0.05 to 0.1 ml/kg of 10% solution
      (5) Phenylephrine: 0.01 to 0.1 μg/kg
F. Complication: shock
  1. Predisposing factors
    a. Hypotension
    b. Cardiac dysrhythmias
    c. Hypovolemia
    d. Other cardiovascular disturbances
    e. Anesthetic drugs
    f. Metabolic problems
    g. Sepsis
  2. Symptoms
    a. Tachycardia
    b. Tachypnea
    c. Weak, thready pulse
    d. Prolonged capillary refill time
    e. Hypotension
    f. Pallor or injected mucous membranes
    g. Cool extremities
    h. Decreased urine output
    i. Hypothermia
    j. Early septic shock exhibits signs of a hyperdynamic circulatory system and may include bounding pulses, decreased capillary refill time, hypotension
  3. Treatment and resolution
    a. Fluids—crystalloids, colloids
    b. Oxygen
    c. Corticosteroids—controversial but proven effective in acute hemorrhagic (hypovolemic) shock and early septic shock
    d. Antimicrobials
    e. Sodium bicarbonate
    f. Vasoactive drugs
    g. Antiprostaglandins (e.g., Banamine)
    h. Naloxone
G. Complication: cardiac arrest
  1. Predisposing factors
    a. Inadequate ventilation—respiratory arrest
    b. Cardiovascular disturbances
    c. Anesthetic overdose
    d. Hypothermia
    e. Acidosis and other metabolic derangements
    f. Hemorrhage, anemia
  2. Symptoms
    a. Respiratory arrest
    b. No heart sounds
    c. Lack of pulses

       d. Dilated pupils
       e. Lack of bleeding from surgical sites
       f. ECG changes—ECG may be normal
    3. Treatment and resolution
       a. Intubate if not already done
       b. Ventilate—continuous ventilation
       c. Apply effective thoracic compression—large dogs may need open chest CPR
       d. Interpose abdominal compressions if possible
       e. Administer drug therapy as indicated by ECG
          (1) Epinephrine—intratracheal (IT), intravenous (IV), or intracardiac (IC)
          (2) Methoxamine—IT, IV
          (3) Atropine—IT, IV
          (4) Bicarbonate—IV
          (5) Fluids—IV
          (6) Steroids—IV
       f. Defibrillation—if ECG indicates ventricular fibrillation
       g. After resuscitation, may need inotropic support from dopamine or dobutamine
       h. Evaluate central nervous system (CNS) status and provide support and protection as needed
III. Respiratory system
  A. Complication: respiratory depression
    1. Predisposing factors
       a. Anesthetic drugs
       b. Anesthetic plane—too deep
       c. Surgical positioning
       d. CNS disease
       e. Hypocarbia
       f. Metabolic disease
    2. Symptoms
       a. Respiratory rate alone is not an indicator of adequate ventilation
       b. Decreased tidal volume or minute volume
       c. Breathing pattern may be regular or irregular
       d. Cyanosis not a reliable indicator—may or may not be present
    3. Treatment and resolution
       a. Support ventilation—manual and/or ventilator if available
       b. Lighten anesthetic plane
       c. Analyze blood gas if possible
       d. If possible correct underlying metabolic problem before anesthesia
       e. If possible correct surgical positioning
  B. Complication: abnormal breathing patterns
    1. Predisposing factors
       a. Anesthetic plane—too light or too deep
       b. Anesthetic drugs

      c. CNS disease or injury

      d. Surgical positioning or surgical manipulation

      e. Equipment malfunction or destruction

      f. Thoracic wall injury or impediment

      g. Hypercarbia; hypoxemia

  2. Symptoms

      a. Respiratory depression

      b. Abnormal breathing patterns

      c. Obstruction

        (1) Increased "work" or effort of breathing

        (2) Decreased excursion of chest or reservoir bag

        (3) Increased abdominal breathing and movement of diaphragm and accessory muscles of respiration

        (4) Cyanosis

        (5) Increased resistance, decreased compliance

        (6) If not intubated, upper airway obstruction may cause increased inspiratory stridor

        (7) In deep anesthetic planes, signs may be decreased or absent

      d. Parenchymal diseases (signs similar to obstruction with changes in lung sounds [rales, crackles, dullness])

      e. Pleural space disease (similar to obstruction)

      f. Thoracic wall abnormalities (flail chest; collapse of wall on inspiration)

      g. Neuromuscular disease

        (1) May see "jerky" respiration

        (2) Decreased excursion of thoracic wall musculature

        (3) Intercostal and diaphragmatic paralysis

      h. CNS disease

        (1) Respiratory depression

        (2) Abnormal breathing patterns

  3. Treatment and resolution

      a. Support ventilation/intubate

      b. Lighten anesthetic plane

      c. If respiratory obstruction—determine if upper or lower airway

      d. If pulmonary edema—administer diuretics

      e. If pleural space disease—consider using chest drainage system

      f. Check for equipment problems

      g. Guide all therapy by patient response to therapy and blood gas analysis, if available

C. Complication: endotracheal tube

  1. Predisposing factors

      a. Endotracheal (ET) tube wrong size

      b. Cuff improperly inflated

      c. ET tube obstructed or kinked

      d. ET tube in esophagus

      e. ET tube in bronchus

      f. ET tube disconnected from machine

2. Symptoms
   a. Inability to ventilate animal
   b. Patient awake or in light anesthetic plane
   c. Erratic respiration—increased ventilatory effort
   d. Cyanosis (may be intermittent)
3. Treatment and resolution
   a. Check for "breath sounds" in chest
      (1) If heard only on one side—endobronchial intubation—pull tube back or change to shorter tube
      (2) No sounds heard—esophageally intubated or tube obstruction—change and reintubate
      (3) Faint breath sounds but inability to adequately inflate chest—ET tube too small, cuff problem, or partial obstruction; change tubes
   b. Check all connections
      (1) NOTE: All cases of inadequate ventilation may cause the following:
         (a) Hypoxemia
         (b) Hypercarbia
         (c) Hypotension
         (d) Tachycardia
         (e) Decreased cardiac output
         (f) Shock
         (g) Cardiac arrest
      (2) DO NOT rely on the appearance of cyanosis as an indication of inadequate ventilation.
D. Complications: postoperative respiratory complications
   1. Respiratory depression
      a. Predisposing factors
         (1) Anesthetic drugs
         (2) Hypothermia
         (3) Surgical procedure
         (4) Pain
         (5) Obesity
         (6) CNS injury
         (7) Hypocarbia from overventilation
      b. Symptoms and problems
         (1) Hypoventilation—shallow and/or slow respirations
         (2) Prolonged recovery
         (3) Poor gas exchange—hypoxemia, hypercarbia
         (4) Pulmonary atelectasis—leads to further impairment of gas exchange
      c. Treatment and resolution
         (1) Support ventilation
         (2) Reverse anesthetic drugs when possible
         (3) Provide analgesia as needed
         (4) Provide heat

          (5) Determine CNS injury
          (6) Administer respiratory stimulants (Dopram)
   2. Postoperative dyspnea
     a. Predisposing factors
       (1) Upper airway obstruction
       (2) Pleural space disease or injury
       (3) Parenchymal disease or injury
       (4) Drug induced, i.e., neuromuscular blocking drugs
     b. Symptoms and problems
       (1) Increased stridor
       (2) Increased respiratory effort
       (3) Cyanosis
     c. Treatment and resolution
       (1) Determine if upper or lower airway obstruction
       (2) Provide ventilatory support
       (3) Apply the same therapy as that used for clearing airway during CPR

IV. Central nervous system disturbances
  A. Complication: cerebral edema
    1. Predisposing factors
     a. Hypoxemia
     b. Metabolic imbalance
    2. Symptoms
     a. Irregular respirations
     b. Coma
     c. Tachycardia
     d. Dilated pupils, blindness, nystagmus
     e. Sweating
     f. If conscious, decreased mentation
    3. Treatment and resolution
     a. Dexamethasone: 2 to 4 mg/kg IV
     b. Correct electrolyte and acid-base balance
     c. Mannitol: 2 g/kg IV
     d. Dimethyl sulfoxide (DMSO): 2 g/kg IV
     e. Oxygen
     f. Ventilatory assistance

V. Vomiting, aspiration, regurgitation
  A. Predisposing factors
    1. Feeding before anesthesia
    2. Drugs
    3. Light anesthesia
    4. Stress, excitement
    5. Surgical manipulation
  B. Symptoms of aspiration
    1. Coughing (if awake)
    2. Cyanosis
    3. Bronchospasm

4. Apnea or tachypnea
5. Airway obstruction
6. Pulmonary edema
7. Pneumonia
C. Prevention
  1. Withhold food 12 hours before anesthesia
  2. Avoid stress and excitement
  3. Use rapid induction technique for animals with history of vomiting
  4. Use cuffed endotracheal tube until reflexes are regained
D. Treatment and resolution
  1. If vomiting or regurgitation occurs
    a. Put animal in sternal recumbency
    b. Move head side to side to clean mouth
    c. Suction pharyngeal area
  2. If aspiration occurs
    a. Clean airway
    b. Provide oxygen
    c. If possible, lavage tracheobronchial tree with sterile saline
    d. Administer aminophylline and corticosteroids if bronchospasm present
    e. Administer antibiotics—broad spectrum
    f. Apply chest coupage
VI. Malignant hyperthermia
A. Definition: a pharmacogenetic, hypermetabolic state leading to uncontrolled increases in temperature and metabolic crisis. Usually diagnosed in retrospect.
B. Predisposing factors
  1. Inheritance
  2. Infection
  3. Anesthetic drugs
    a. Inhalational agents
    b. Succinylcholine (muscle blocking agent)
    c. Parasympatholytics
    d. Ketamine
  4. Environmental stress and excitement
C. Clinical signs—early
  1. Muscle rigidity
  2. Elevated body temperature
  3. Tachycardia and tachydysrhythmias
  4. Skin: warm, flushed, progressing to cyanosis
  5. Blood pressure: initial increase then profound decrease
  6. Marked tachypnea and hyperventilation; respiratory and metabolic acidosis
D. Late signs
  1. Muscle rigidity
  2. Increased core body temperature (108° to 110° F)

3. Electrolyte abnormalities
4. Metabolic acidosis (severe)
5. Hemolysis, coagulopathy
6. Acute renal failure
7. Hypoglycemia
8. Cerebral edema
E. Treatment and resolution
1. Remove triggering agents
2. If malignant hyperthermia is known, pretreat animal with dantrolene
3. Provide fluids
4. Administer dantrolene
5. Restore electrolyte balance
6. Decrease body temperature
7. Provide oxygen
8. Administer diuretics
9. Administer corticosteroids

■ NEUROLOGIC EMERGENCIES
Trauma

Brain injury may result from any of the following: direct trauma from compressed skull fractures, hemorrhage, rapid movement of the head causing the brain to deflect off the opposite side of the skull (contrecoup), edema of the brain tissue, exposure of the brain to the outside environment, embolization or infarction of cerebral arteries, hypoxia, anoxia, and lack of the vital nutrient glucose. The level of consciousness exhibited by the animal is perhaps the best indicator of the severity of the injury. The normal animal should be alert and oriented. As the animal deteriorates neurologically, it will become confused, dazed, semicomatose, and comatose.

For the most part, trauma to the brain is a medical emergency. There are only two surgical procedures to consider, and they are not commonly performed in veterinary medicine. The first procedure is the elevation or removal of depressed pieces of fractured skull. The second operation that can be performed is the craniotomy. This operation requires a skilled surgeon and an accurate diagnosis. It is reserved for the removal of intracranial hematomas, aneurysms, and masses and for the immediate relief of elevated intracranial pressure.

Spinal Cord Injury

Fractures and dislocations of the vertebral column are more often the cause of a surgical emergency than skull fractures. All injuries to the spine that result in serious neurologic deficits or an unstable vertebral column should be considered surgical emergencies. This is also true of patients that are affected by disk disease and are showing severe neurologic deficits or are continuing to deteriorate despite medical therapy.

Patient evaluation. The evaluation of the neurologic patient is based on the alterations of four spinal functions. Decreased conscious proprioception and ataxia are the first deficit to develop. Conscious proprioception is the ability of the animal to realize the position of its foot. This can be tested by knuckling the toes; the animal should return the foot to a normal weight-bearing posture. The second function to be affected is voluntary movement of the legs. Signs of the loss of this function can vary from weakness (paresis) to complete paralysis. The third function that is lost is superficial or skin pain. This is often difficult to assess. Deep pain is the last function to disappear. The ability to feel deep pain is tested by pinching the animal's toes with a hemostat. The animal must show some conscious recognition of pain. This might include whining or looking at the painful stimulus. Simple withdrawal of the leg can occur through a local spinal reflex, so it is not a sign of intact deep pain response.

The signs associated with spinal cord injury are caused by damage to the various nerve fibers in the spinal cord. When the spinal cord is damaged or compressed, one typically sees that larger nerve fibers (conscious proprioception) lose function before small (pain) fibers do. A foraminotomy refers to the removal of the root of the intervertebral foramen. A fenestration refers to the creation of a window in the anulus fibrosus to remove disk material from the intervertebral spaces. A ventral slot procedure refers to the creation of an opening in the ventral aspect of the intervertebral space. The veterinarian will choose among these surgical procedures based on the anatomy of the area affected and the problem that needs to be corrected.

Surgery is indicated after the vertebral column is unstable or to decompress the spinal cord. The need for surgery is up to the veterinarian. The decision will be based in part on the severity of neurologic signs, the stability of the vertebral column, time since the initial trauma, and progress of neurologic signs.

Therapy. Following the neurologic examination, the veterinarian localizes the site of the injury through the use of spinal reflex tests, plain radiography, and myelography. Vertebral fractures can be repaired by cross-pinning, by plating the vertebral bodies or spines, or by using bone cement. Body casts have been routinely unsuccessful because they are heavy and do not adequately stabilize the spine. The relief of spinal cord pressure from a protruding intervertebral disk is accomplished through any number of surgical procedures. The removal of the dorsal bony roof of the spinal canal is termed a dorsal laminectomy. A hemilaminectomy procedure removes one half of the roof. A foramenotomy refers to the removal of the roof of the intervertebral foramen. A fenestration refers to the creation of a window in the annulus fibrosus to remove material from the intervertebral space. A ventral slot procedure refers to the creation of an opening in the ventral aspect of the intervertebral space. The veterinarian will choose among these surgical procedures based on the anatomy of the area affected and the problem that needs to be corrected.

The technician plays a role in three different therapeutic phases of treating the neurologic patient. First, the technician is helpful in assessing the extent of the injury and detecting any deterioration of the patient's condition. Immediately notifying the veterinarian can save valuable time and could even change the overall prognosis. Second, the technician may be asked to assist in spinal surgery. The technician should become familiar with the specialized instruments used in spinal surgery. Last, the technician is responsible for postoperative nursing care. All neurologic patients should be placed on racks, grates, or waterbeds and closely confined. Urinations should be noted because some spinal patients lose bladder control. Each animal should be lifted and turned with a conscious effort to keep the spine straight and rigid. Daily checks should be made for the return or improvement of each of the four spinal functions. Care must be taken to prevent decubital sores in paralyzed patients. Frequent turning, adequate padding, and whirlpool treatments can minimize these. Initial rapid therapy followed by diligent nursing care can often return a spinal patient to a viable and manageable pet.

■ OPHTHALMIC EMERGENCIES
Trauma

The greatest barrier that must be overcome when dealing with ocular trauma is the fear of looking at an injured eye. Although the eye is indeed a fragile organ, it is also treatable, and the technician should not be overwhelmed by it. Two cardinal rules should be followed with respect to eye injuries: the eye must be kept moist, and immediate veterinary attention should be sought. To evaluate the injury, the technician should first obtain a history from the owner concerning the type of trauma, when it occurred, any exposure the animal had to chemicals, and any preexisting eye problems. The animal should be approached slowly and warned of any approach. Most eye injuries are quite painful, and if the animal was suddenly blinded, it will also be frightened. Any obvious loss of vision, any edema and hemorrhage around the eye, and the size and position of the globe within the orbit should be noted. The technician should be systematic and consistent in assessing the injury. The exterior structures of the eye are examined first (eyelids, third eyelid, conjunctiva, cornea); then the anterior chamber is examined. The technician should be prepared to institute first aid. Any hemorrhage should be controlled with pressure and cold packs. When dry or exposed, the eye can be irrigated with any commercial eye wash or saline. The amount of disfigurement present does not necessarily correspond to the severity of the problem, and the prognosis for all surgical problems is more optimistic if treatment is not delayed.

Proptosis of the Globe

Proptosis is a prolapse of the entire globe beyond the socket and eyelids. This can occur because the dog does not have a complete bony orbit and is especially a problem in the brachycephalic breeds in which the eyes normally protrude. The source of proptosis may be trauma, such as blows to the head, bite wounds, hemorrhage behind the eye, or retrobulbar masses. A proptosis can also be caused by overzealous restraint of the animal. During the initial examination the amount of dryness of the eye, the deviation of the globe, and the pupil size should be noted, and this information should be reported to the veterinarian. If the pupil is dilated, the prognosis for sight is guarded. After a quick examination, the technician should moisten the eye. The technician should continue to irrigate the eye and apply cold compresses to the lids until the patient is seen by the veterinarian. It will probably be necessary for the veterinarian to anesthetize the animal to reinsert the eye. This can be accomplished by using muscle hooks or by enlarging the palpebral fissure with a lateral canthotomy. After the globe is replaced, the eyelids are usually sutured closed (temporary tarsorrhaphy) for 2 weeks. The prognosis for the return of vision is proportional to the amount of damage done to the optic nerve by stretching and the duration of the proptosis.

Conjunctival and Eyelid Injuries

Conjunctival and eyelid injuries are usually lacerations, bite wounds, or hemorrhages. Chemosis or edema of the conjunctiva can also occur and may follow wounds, exposure to chemicals, or infections by upper respiratory viruses. Lacerations of the eyelids should be repaired as soon as possible and with minimal debridement. Lacerations of the conjunctiva rarely need to be sutured unless the lids are involved or the lacerations are quite large.

The conjunctiva and lids should first be examined carefully for foreign bodies and debris. Injury to the cornea should always be ruled out. Cold compresses can be used to minimize lid swelling, and large E-collars can be applied around the animal's neck to prevent self-trauma. When preparing the eyelids for surgery, hair clipping must be done very gently or immediate swelling of the lids will occur. The veterinarian may prefer gentle irrigation with eye solutions rather than the routine surgical soap preoperative scrub. Before soap is used around the eye, a protective ointment should be applied to the globe. Lid defects are usually sutured with small ophthalmic instruments and sutures. The conjunctival wound is sutured in one layer, followed by a skin closure. Postoperatively, cold packs will help decrease eyelid swelling and pain. The patient should be watched closely to prevent it from removing sutures and to keep the sutures from rubbing against the cornea.

Corneal Injuries

All corneal injuries are emergencies. They tend to be extremely painful, and they directly threaten the integrity of the globe. As the depth of the corneal injury increases, the problem becomes a surgical emergency. There are many types of corneal injuries. An abrasion is a superficial linear scratch in the corneal epithelium. An ulcer is a denuded, craterlike lesion that is superficial and may only affect the epithelium or can also involve the stroma, or central corneal layer. As more stroma is lost, the cornea may become dependent on one last fragile barrier called Descemet's membrane. An ulcer that destroys stroma to this membrane is called a descemetocele. If the membrane is ruptured, the anterior chamber has been penetrated, aqueous humor usually leaks from the eye, and the iris falls forward to plug the leak. This protruding mass is termed an iris prolapse. Ulcers are diagnosed with the use of fluorescein stain. When the epithelium is interrupted, the stroma retains stain and the ulcer turns a brilliant yellow-green. An exception to this is the descemetocele. In this lesion, the stroma is destroyed and Descemet's membrane that remains does not retain the fluorescein. On careful examination you will note a ring of stain that highlights the exposed stroma around the circumference of the ulcer.

If the corneal injury is superficial, medical therapy may suffice. If it is deep or has occurred in a breed of dog that is predisposed to corneal injuries (brachycephalic breeds), surgical intervention will be necessary. The cornea can be protected by performing a temporary tarsorrhaphy or a third-eyelid flap. A soft contact lens can also be inserted into the eye. If a descemetocele is threatening the eye, further support is given by making a conjunctival flap. A ruptured descemetocele always demands prompt surgical attention. As soon as possible the exposed iris should be excised, the anterior chamber re-formed, and the pupil dilated. If possible the corneal defect should be sutured, or conjunctival flap surgery may be performed. Sterility must be closely maintained during this procedure. Remember that ointments should never be used in the eye if the cornea is penetrated because the petrolatum base causes severe inflammation within the eye. Because they delay healing, steroids should never be used topically on an injured cornea. The postoperative care of corneal injuries is similar to that of eyelid emergencies.

Perforating Wounds

The most common perforating wounds of the cornea result from gunshot wounds or flying glass. It is important to determine the points of entry and exit and the trajectory the object has taken. If the foreign body remains within the globe, its exact location must be determined. If it is found in the cornea or anterior chamber, it can often be removed surgically, but if it remains in the posterior chamber or vitreous, surgical removal becomes extremely difficult. Blindness may result from retinal injuries, and enucleation may be necessary. It is also important to determine the chemical composition of the foreign body to determine future complications:

• Inert, mild damage	• Severe inflammation, probable loss of the eye
Gold	Copper
Silver	Bronze
Stone	Brass
Carbon	Iron
Glass	Steel
Plastic	Wood
Rubber	

Intraocular foreign bodies are very serious and usually require referral of the patient to a hospital capable of sophisticated intraocular surgery.

Lens Luxation

Another ocular emergency that often requires referral of the patient to a veterinary ophthalmologist is luxation of the lens. The lens is a clear, ovoid structure that normally rests behind the iris. It is held in place by microscopic fibers called zonules. In some animals, there may be a malformation of the zonules, which can cause a predisposition toward lens luxations, or the fibers may break from trauma, allowing for movement of the lens. If the lens falls into the anterior chamber, it is seen grossly as a milky, translucent disc behind the cornea. A posterior lens luxation is more difficult to diagnose. Lens luxations constitute surgical emergencies because secondary glaucoma or prolapse of the vitreous may result. Lens extraction is best completed by a veterinarian specially trained in this field.

Protocol for Technician in Treating Ophthalmic Emergencies

1. Obtain a quick, complete history from the owner.
2. Perform a systematic examination of the structure of the eye.
3. Lavage the eye vigorously, but gently.
4. Correct any obvious problems:
   a. Proptosis: moisten and apply cold compresses.
   b. Foreign body: flush loose matter out of the eye.
   c. Control hemorrhage.

   d. Control swelling of the lids with cold compresses.
   e. Calm the animal and the owner.
   f. Assess any other injuries.
5. Seek immediate veterinary attention.
6. Keep the eye moist.
7. Apply E-collar to prevent self-mutilation.

■ GASTROINTESTINAL EMERGENCIES
Oral and Esophageal Trauma

Oral trauma may be caused by blows or injuries to the head or by the lodging of foreign bodies within the mouth and pharynx. Fractures of the teeth and mandible are not usually surgical emergencies unless occlusion of the airway is threatened. Hemorrhage must be controlled, whether from fractured bones or lacerations of the tongue and gingiva. Often this requires examination with the patient under anesthesia and the ligation or cautery of arterial bleeders. If airway obstruction occurs, the insertion of a tracheostomy tube may be necessary.

Oral foreign bodies are a common problem in dogs because dogs are indiscriminate eaters and chewers. Common foreign materials include bones, sticks, fishhooks, needles, balls, and porcupine quills. Indications of such trauma include salivation, pawing at the mouth, rubbing the face, pain when opening the mouth, and hysteria. A thorough examination of the mouth may require deep sedation or anesthesia. Radiographs of the head can occasionally aid in localizing the foreign bodies. Caution must be taken when examining the oral cavity of animals who have a history of salivation and choking. The examiner should always wear gloves to provide protection from infectious diseases, such as rabies, which can portray the same clinical signs. Once the foreign body is found, it should be removed manually. In the case of a string foreign body the string should be secured and the veterinarian should decide if extraction is appropriate. The technician should remember that postoperatively these animals may have painful mouths. Soft, soothing, lukewarm foods and liquids should be offered.

Once they are swallowed, foreign bodies tend to lodge in one of the three areas at which the esophagus naturally narrows: the thoracic inlet, the base of the heart, and the hiatus of the diaphragm. If the foreign material does not completely obstruct the esophagus, the patient may actually show few clinical signs. The foreign body may be found incidentally or after the esophagus has ruptured, resulting in severe inflammation and infection of the mediastinum. Animals with occlusive foreign bodies show excessive salivation, lethargy, and anorexia. The animal may retain the ability to swallow liquids without difficulty, but solid foods will be regurgitated within minutes after the animal has eaten. Diagnosis of esophageal foreign bodies may depend on a plain radiograph, a barium swallow, or a direct endoscopic examination of the esophagus. The primary therapeutic objective is to remove the foreign material. It is preferable to retrieve the foreign body with an endoscope or to push the object into the stomach rather than to perform a thoracotomy. Surgery of the thoracic esophagus is difficult and often causes major complications, such as infection and stricture. Once the foreign material has been removed, food should be withheld for 24 to 48 hours and then liquids should be initiated. Salivation can be controlled with drugs such as atropine. Sedation is used if the animal exhibits pain. The technician should keep in mind the potential for stricture development in these patients.

Wounds of the esophagus are generally confined to the cervical esophagus because the thoracic portion is protected by the chest wall. Fight wounds, lacerations, and deep puncture wounds should be explored surgically to repair esophageal tears and to allow adequate drainage. A common sequela of esophageal wounds is stricture, and this may not develop until weeks after the original insult.

Blunt Abdominal Trauma

Because so many animals are hit by automobiles, trauma to the abdomen is frequently encountered in veterinary medicine. The cause of the injury can be penetrating or blunt and nonpenetrating. Lacerations of the abdominal organs may follow penetrating wounds. Penetrating wounds should always be surgically explored. Contusions, ruptures, hematomas, or avulsions of organ attachments may result from blunt trauma. It is often difficult to determine whether blunt abdominal trauma is actually a surgical emergency. The technician can provide important information about the vital signs and patient status that will aid the veterinarian in making this decision.

Hemorrhage from blunt trauma may be mild or may result in profound hypovolemic shock. As with other trauma victims, the first procedure must be to correct any life-threatening problems and to reverse shock. The persistence of shock despite massive fluid replacement or sequential decreases in the hematocrit may indicate continued bleeding that requires surgical intervention. The palpation of abdominal masses may indicate hematomas of the spleen or liver. Gradual enlargement of the abdomen signifies the presence of free fluid, such as blood, urine, intestinal contents, or peritonitis fluid. Abdominal pain is often present but is a nonspecific sign. Because a subjective history cannot be obtained, it is difficult to localize and quantitate the pain. The onset of vomiting, depression, and diarrhea within 24 hours of the injury warrants examination for damaged abdominal viscera. The absence of urination, the presence of gross hematuria, or the development of uremia may denote severe urinary tract trauma. Assessing abdominal injuries may be frustrating because many of these clinical signs are subtle and nonspecific. The veterinarian must often depend on ancillary diagnostic aids to reach a decision concerning the proper therapy for these patients.

Sequential measurements of the animal's vital signs often reveal subtle deteriorations in the patient's condition. The technician usually has the opportunity to detect such changes. Plain and contrast radiography, abdominal paracentesis, catheterization of the urinary tract, and laboratory tests can also help to determine a diagnosis. These trauma patients become surgical candidates if a definite intraabdominal injury has been determined or if an injury is suspected but cannot be ruled out by any other method. The surgical procedure of choice is exploratory laparotomy.

A complete and thorough examination of all abdominal organs can be done through a ventral midline incision. As each organ is examined, corrective surgical steps can be taken to repair the injury (Table 5-3). Strict measures must be taken to prevent infection and to allow the drainage of fluid from the abdomen. Postoperatively these patients may require diligent nursing care. The patient's temperature,

TABLE 5-3		
Blunt Abdominal Trauma and Surgical Therapy		
Organ	Type of injuries	Corrective procedures
Diaphragm	Tear, rupture	Suturing of defect
Liver	Fracture, laceration	Suturing of defect, closing of defect with omentum, and resection of isolated lesion or lobe
Gallbladder and bile ducts	Laceration, rupture, or avulsion	Ligation of injured ducts, suturing of defects, removal of gallbladder, and anastomosis of gallbladder to intestine
Spleen	Hematoma, laceration, or rupture	Partial or total splenectomy
Pancreas	Crushing injury or hematoma	Partial pancreatectomy
Gastrointestinal tract	Hematoma, laceration, rupture, avulsion of mesenteric attachment, infarction, or incarceration	Suturing of defects, segmental resection, and anastomosis
Urinary tract	Hematoma, contusion, rupture, avulsion of renal blood vessels, obstruction, pelvic fractures	Repair of blood vessels, suturing of ruptures, nephrectomy, anastomosis of the ureter, catheterization, urethrostomy

heart rate, pulse, and urine output should be monitored. Intravenous fluid therapy is often required. Any drainage of fluid from abdominal drains should be noted. The development of vomiting, increasing abdominal pain, or hemorrhage should be brought to the attention of the veterinarian. These patients are not out of danger until 72 hours have passed, during which time the animal has stable vital signs, a cessation of pain, and a return of appetite and normal activity.

Acute Abdomen

The term *acute abdomen* is used to describe any syndrome that causes severe abdominal pain. Signs that are referrable to abdominal organ disease, such as vomiting, anorexia, dehydration, diarrhea, and lethargy, may also accompany this pain. One of the most difficult diagnostic decisions a veterinarian must make is whether an acute abdomen is a medical or surgical problem. The differential diagnosis of acute abdominal disease is varied.

Differential diagnosis of acute abdomen syndrome

Surgical

Gastrointestinal obstruction, intussusception, linear foreign bodies, ulceration/rupture, incarceration, infarction, or volvulus

Splenic torsion

Testicular torsion

Uterine torsion

Pyometra

Ruptured bladder

Ureteral calculi

Prostatic abscess

Ruptured abdominal neoplasia

Medical

Pancreatitis

Bacterial, viral, or hemorrhagic gastroenteritis

Nephritis

Endometritis

Prostatitis

Adrenocortical insufficiency

It is beyond the scope of this chapter to describe the numerous methods and procedures to achieve an exact diagnosis in the acute abdomen patient; however, this chapter does describe the major gastrointestinal emergencies and their surgical correction.

Intestinal Surgical Emergencies

Intestinal obstructions are frequently caused by foreign bodies, strictures, adhesions, or tumors. The severity of the clinical signs determines the speed with which the obstruction must be relieved. Most foreign bodies lodge in the pylorus of the stomach, the duodenum, or the proximal jejunum. They can often be removed by simple gastrotomy or enterotomy techniques. The intestine is incised near, but not over, the obstruction. The offending material is removed and the intestine sutured. Any technician assisting the veterinarian during intestinal surgery must remember that this area is filled with bacteria. Strict attention must be paid to asepsis by isolating the portion of the gut being operated from the rest of the contents of the abdomen. Care must also be taken in handling intestinal tissue so that the blood supply is not compromised and the mucosa is not crushed. Linear foreign bodies such as strings do not usually cause an obstruction, but they can cause pleating and perforation of the intestines. It is sometimes necessary to perform multiple enterotomies to remove the entire length of string. If the obstruction results from a tumor of the intestine or if an obstruction has caused secondary necrosis, total resection of a portion of the gut may be necessary. Enough tissue is removed to totally excise the lesion and to allow healthy tissue to be anastomosed. The common technique used is an end-to-end anastomosis (see Fig. 4-8, p. 288), but variations, such as end-to-side or side-to-side procedures, can be used. All are designed to allow normal patency and function of the gut postoperatively.

An intussusception is the prolapse or telescoping of a segment of intestine into the lumen of the adjacent intestine. It is often associated with the hypermotility that accompanies diarrhea, intestinal parasites, tumors, or previous intestinal surgery. Intussusception is frequently a problem in younger animals, and the most common location is the ileocecal junction. An intussusception may cause an incomplete or complete obstruction. If the intussusception is actively sliding and unfolding, it may disappear and reappear during sequential examinations. During an exploratory laparotomy the lesion is usually reduced (manually pulled apart) or resected. If the intussusception can be reduced, the sliding segment can be sutured or anchored to nearby gut to prevent a recurrence. If the intussusception is resected, an end-to-end anastomosis is done. It is not uncommon for intussusception to recur postoperatively. Medical efforts must be instituted to relieve any contributing problem such as diarrhea or parasites.

Volvulus, or twisting of the intestine, is rare. When it occurs, the clinical signs are identical to those of acute intestinal obstruction. The treatment of volvulus consists of rerotating the gut into a normal position and resecting any areas that are not viable. A serious potential complication of volvulus is endotoxic shock. Large numbers of bacteria in the affected loop of intestine die during a volvulus. When the volvulus is corrected, a massive release of endotoxins can precipitate shock. The technician should be prepared to aid in the treatment of this serious complication.

Incarceration, or trapping of the intestines, is caused by mesenteric, umbilical or inguinal, and paracostal or diaphragmatic hernias. The mesenteric blood vessels are often twisted or constricted, producing rapid ischemia to the gut. The pathologic changes in the intestines in this emergency are similar to those in infarction of the gut. Infarction occurs any time the blood supply to the intestine is interrupted. Treatment of these disorders demands rapid surgical attention. The incarceration must be relieved and the hernia repaired. If the affected intestine is not viable, it should be resected. Infarctions are usually irreversible and necessitate resection of the affected area. Endotoxic shock is also a potential complication in these crises.

Ulceration of the gastrointestinal tract is rare in animals. It may result from bacterial infections, drug toxicities, or neoplasia, such as mast cell tumors. The diagnosis of intestinal ulceration is difficult. Therapy may involve medical correction or removal of the cause, treatment of shock, and resection of the affected segment of gut.

Postoperative care. Postoperative nursing care of all gastrointestinal patients is similar. If infection within the abdomen is anticipated, postoperative monitoring is essential. The patient should be given nothing by mouth for 24 to 48 hours. After this time, broth or baby foods can be started with a gradual conversion to solid foods within 3 days if vomiting does not occur. The critical period for leakage or dehiscence of the surgical site and development of peritonitis is usually 3 to 4 days. Body temperature, the presence of abdominal pain, and the activity of gut sounds should be monitored closely during this time. Ancillary medical therapy includes intravenous or subcutaneous fluids and antibiotics.

Gastric Dilation/Volvulus

Gastric dilation/volvulus (GDV) is commonly known as bloat. It tends to occur in large, deep-chested breeds of dogs such as Great Danes, St. Bernards, Irish setters, Doberman pinschers, and German shepherds. It has been seen in smaller dogs and other animals such as cats and rabbits. It can occur at any age and is an extremely complex medical and surgical emergency. GDV can occur with or without torsion of the stomach.

The exact etiology of GDV has not yet been determined. The heritability of the disorder is unknown. Typically GDV occurs after the recent ingestion of a large meal or large quantities of water followed by exercise. A mechanical obstruction to the outflow of the stomach, such as pyloric stenosis, a foreign body, or a tumor, could be involved but is uncommon. GDV develops as an accumulation of gas and fluid in the absence of vomiting or pyloric emptying. The major sources of gas are aerophagia, the fermentation of food, and the formation of carbon dioxide from stomach acid reacting with bicarbonate.

The clinical signs of GDV provide an easy diagnosis; they are severe abdominal distention, marked salivation, frequent unsuccessful attempts to vomit, abdominal pain, and dyspnea. Tympany of the abdomen may develop. The animal's behavior may range from nervousness to depression. As the stomach enlarges to fill the entire abdomen, pressure on the great veins decreases the venous return to the heart, and shock develops. The shock is further complicated by the release of bacterial endotoxins into the circulation through the devitalized gastric wall.

The term *gastric torsion* is actually a misnomer. A torsion is produced by a twisting along the object's long axis. The stomach, when it rotates, actually turns like a pear might turn on its stem. A more accurate description would be volvulus of the stomach. The stomach may twist 90 to 360 degrees. When this occurs, the esophagus and duodenum become occluded. The greater omentum and spleen usually follow the stomach as it twists, and a splenic torsion may result. The reason for the progression of a gastric dilation into a volvulus is unknown (Figs. 5-12 and 5-13). It is thought that the stomach may shift to the areas of least resistance as it enlarges within the abdomen or that the violent smooth muscle contraction and the efforts to vomit may cause the stomach to move.

Therapy. GDV is an urgent, complex, life-threatening emergency. It is not immediately necessary to differentiate a simple dilation from a volvulus. Three major objectives in the treatment of GDV must be accomplished: (1) the reversal of shock, (2) the immediate relief of gastric distention, and (3) the stabilization of the patient until surgery can be performed.

The technician should next obtain a stomach tube. The distance from the point of the dog's nose to the xyphoid of the sternum is the length of tube that is needed to reach the stomach. The technician should assist the veterinarian in trying to pass the tube. This should be attempted with the animal placed in a variety of positions or after mildly sedating the animal if the first attempt is unsuccessful. If all attempts to pass the stomach tube fail, the distended stomach may be trocarized with several 18-gauge needles.

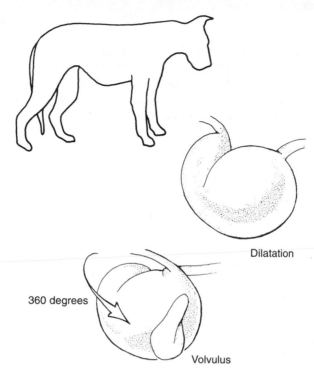

FIG. 5-12   Representation of acute gastric dilation with 360-degree volvulus. Arrow indicates direction of rotation. (From Van Kruiningen HJ, Gregoire K, Meuten DJ: *J Am Anim Hosp Assoc* 10:294, 1974.)

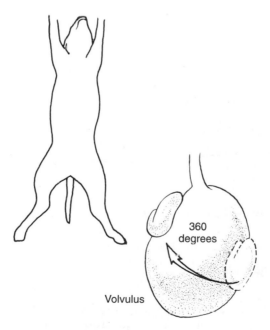

FIG. 5-13   Ventrodorsal view of 360-degree volvulus. Note clockwise rotation of stomach and spleen. (From Van Kruiningen HJ, Gregoire K, Meuten DJ: *J Am Anim Hosp Assoc* 10:294, 1974.)

Food should be withheld, and the technician should prepare for the probability of surgery. Surgery is recommended for those patients in whom the distention cannot be relieved by other means, to examine the health of the stomach, and to determine the presence of volvulus. Even if a patient has a simple dilation, some preventive surgical procedure is advisable because GDV can recur.

At the time of surgery, any rotation of the stomach is relieved, and nonviable areas are excised. A splenectomy may be necessary for splenic torsions. Preventive techniques are numerous, and the choice is based on the surgeon's preference. To date there is no single technique that is routinely successful in preventing GDV. Procedures that may be performed include several varieties of gastropexy (suturing the stomach to the abdominal wall). Numerous articles have been written about the various surgical techniques, and it is up to the veterinarian to choose the most appropriate surgery for each case.

Postoperative care. GDV patients require intensive nursing care postoperatively. Tachydysrhythmias are common, usually require medical treatment, and can be life threatening. Heart rate, pulse, and ECGs should be monitored for the first 48 hours. The detection of pulse deficits is particularly significant. Intravenous fluid therapy is always necessary. The patient should not be fed by mouth for 2 days. Water and gruel can be started on the third day. Stomach size must also be watched closely. Abdominal girth is measured just behind the ribs while the animal is standing. Care must always be taken to watch for recurrence of GDV.

The technician can also play an important role in educating clients in the early detection and prevention of GDV. Any owner of a large-breed dog should be prepared for the possibility of bloat.

Home advice: the treatment of GDV

Seek immediate veterinary attention. Because the exact etiology is unknown, there is no foolproof way to prevent GDV. Several steps have been shown to decrease the incidence of GDV, however, and the technician should be familiar with these steps.

Home advice: the prevention of GDV
- Food
  Avoid single large meals.
  Feed two or three small meals per day.
  Do not allow access to food storage areas.
  Soak all meals with warm water before feeding.
- Water
  Do not allow intake of large amounts of water at one time.
- Exercise
  Do not allow your pet to exercise for 1 hour after each meal.

■ URINARY EMERGENCIES
Blunt Trauma

Serious injury to the kidney is uncommon because it is not fixed in a rigid position within the abdomen. Blunt trauma, especially from automobile accidents, can cause subcapsular hematomas or contusions, a rupture of the kidney, or an avulsion of the renal blood vessels. Subcapsular hematomas rarely cause clinical signs. If the kidney is ruptured, urine-induced peritonitis or retroperitoneal hematomas may develop. An avulsion of the renal blood vessels precipitates acute hemorrhagic shock, and few of these patients survive long enough for surgery. Clinical signs for which the technician should be alert are shock, pain in the area of the kidneys, and an enlarging abdominal mass and hematuria. Diagnosis is difficult, and the veterinarian often depends on laboratory tests, radiography, and abdominal paracentesis to determine the existence of renal trauma. The ultimate objectives of therapy are to maintain adequate kidney function, control hemorrhage and shock, and repair the damage if possible. If the kidney can be saved by repairing blood vessels or suturing ruptures in the pelvis or renal parenchyma, these techniques should be tried initially. If these fail, or the extent of the injury is irreversible, a unilateral nephrectomy should be undertaken. Animals normally can survive with only one functioning kidney.

Trauma to the ureter occurs from injuries, calculi, or poor surgical technique. Clinical signs may not develop for several hours to several days later. The opposite kidney and ureter will compensate. Leakage of urine into the abdomen will produce peritonitis. Secondary obstruction of the ureter will result in hydronephrosis. If the injury is discovered early, anastomosis of the ureter should be attempted. If hydronephrosis has already destroyed a major portion of the renal parenchyma, a unilateral nephrectomy is the therapy of choice.

Most bladder ruptures develop from trauma to a full bladder or overzealous pressure on an obstructed bladder. Death secondary to bladder rupture may occur within 24 hours or several days later. The clinical signs associated with bladder rupture are shock, abdominal pain, hypothermia or hyperthermia, and hematuria or anuria. The technician should remember that the presence of urine on catheterization of the bladder does not preclude a rupture. A double-contrast cystography may be necessary to completely rule out bladder trauma. In the therapy of this emergency, not only must the bladder be surgically repaired, but also uremia and peritonitis must be combatted.

The causes of urethral trauma include pelvic fractures, bite wounds, catheterization, and calculi. The animal may be totally unable to pass urine or may do so only with great difficulty. Leakage of urine into the surrounding tissues will cause severe cellulitis. If possible, the urethra is catheterized and the catheter is left in place for 2 to 3 weeks while the urethra heals. In rare cases in which patency of the urethra cannot be reestablished, perineal or antepubic urethrostomies may be necessary to establish an exit route for urine.

Urethral Obstruction

Feline lower urinary tract disease (FLUTD) is the clinical condition that occurs as a result of cystitis and/or urethritis. It presents an array of symptoms including frequent voiding of often bloody urine, urinating in inappropriate areas, and partial or complete obstruction of the urinary tract. Many factors may induce these effects and cause FLUTD. These may include infectious organisms, neoplasms, trauma, toxins, and irritation of the mucosa from urinary crystals or calculi. The smaller urethra of the male cat makes the incidence of obstruction higher in this gender. Castration does not affect this statistic. The actual obstruction may be composed of mucin or crystalline plugs of struvite, calcium, or magnesium. The most common location for an obstruction is the proximal end of the penis. The cat may have an increased frequency of urination, hematuria, and stranguria before the obstruction. Once the urethra is completely occluded, the cat will frequently strain to urinate without result, creating the appearance that it is constipated. If uremia develops, the cat becomes anorexic and depressed and may vomit. Terminal hyperkalemia will produce bradycardia and coma. The bladder will occasionally rupture.

The first step in relieving the emergency is to establish the patency of the lower urinary tract by passing a urinary catheter. If this cannot be accomplished, the bladder should be emptied via cystocentesis, and an emergency perineal urethrostomy is performed (Figs. 5-14 and 5-15). When a urethral catheter is passed, it usually is sutured in place for 1 or 2 days. The technician may be required to supervise the maintenance of the catheter and to administer ancillary drugs such as IV fluids, antibiotics, urinary acidifiers, antispasmodics, and special foods. If sedation or anesthesia was necessary for catheterization of the urethra, these patients can be expected to have prolonged recovery periods from the present underlying uremia. Careful attention should be taken to prevent hypothermia.

Urethral obstruction in dogs, as in cats, is usually a disease of the male. Cystic calculi can often be passed successfully in the female but commonly lodge at the os penis of the male. Although rare in dogs, urethral obstruction may develop secondary to prostatic infection or tumor and tumors of the bladder. Cystic calculi in dogs are divided into two classes, primary and secondary. Primary calculi develop because of the excretion of certain metabolic products that precipitate in the urine and include oxalate, cysteine, and urate stones. Secondary calculi are caused by bladder infections and are usually composed of phosphate.

As in FLUTD, the first step that must be taken is the relief of the obstruction. Once the patency of the urinary tract is ensured, the uremia should be treated with fluid therapy and the patient prepared for surgery. Unlike cats, most dogs with urinary obstruction should be operated on to remove the calculi. If the urethral stone can be flushed into the bladder, a simple cystotomy will allow retrieval of the stone. If the uretheral stone cannot be dislodged, it may be necessary to perform a prescrotal urethrostomy to directly remove the calculi. Medical therapy is decided pending the results of chemical analysis of the stones. The primary calculi tend to recur because the causative metabolic disorder cannot be corrected. A permanent urethrostomy may be indicated to enlarge the urethral opening if primary urolithiasis recurs. This permanent opening may be large enough for the continuously formed small calculi to pass to the outside. Postoperatively these patients' urinations must be carefully monitored. Urethrostomy patients may bleed persistently from the incised cavernous tissue of the urethra. They should be closely watched for the development of anemia. Although it is uncommon, these patients may require transfusions.

■ REPRODUCTIVE EMERGENCIES
Male Genital Emergencies

Bite wounds, lacerations, and exposure to caustic chemicals constitute the most common forms of trauma to the external genitalia. Intact male dogs seem to be affected to a greater degree because of their territorial aggressions and tendency to roam. Af-

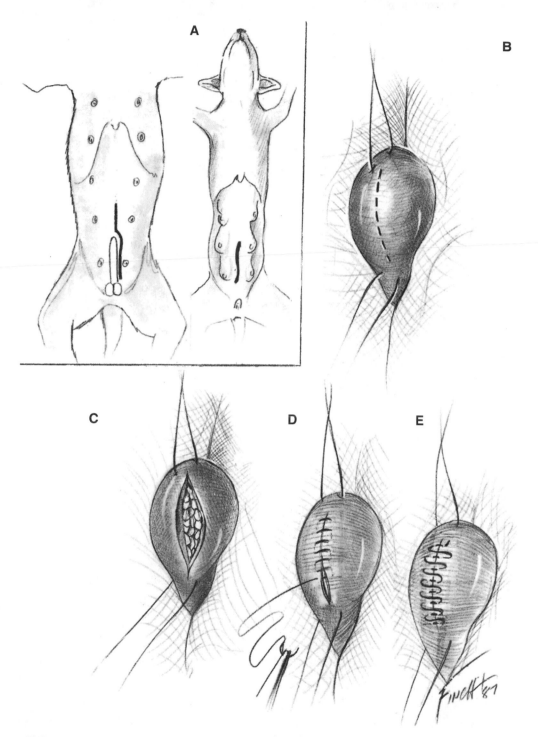

FIG. 5-14   Urinary cystotomy. **A,** Caudal ventral abdominal midline incision is made. **B,** Incision is made into the bladder. **C,** Incision may be extended with scissors. **D,** First layer of the bladder is closed. **E,** Second layer closure is placed over the first. (From Caywood DD, Lipowitz AJ: *Atlas of small animal surgery,* St Louis, 1989, Mosby.)

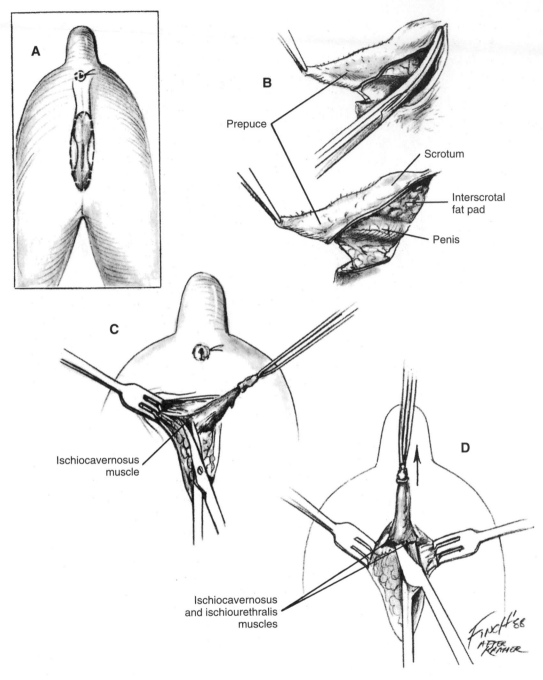

FIG. 5-15   Perineal urethrostomy (PU)—feline. **A,** Elliptical skin incision is made dorsoventrally around the scrotum and prepuce, which are excised. **B,** Cat is castrated, if intact. **C,** Penis is retracted laterally, and the ischiocavernosus muscle and penile crus are severed near the insertion on the ischium. **D,** Penile ligament is transected.

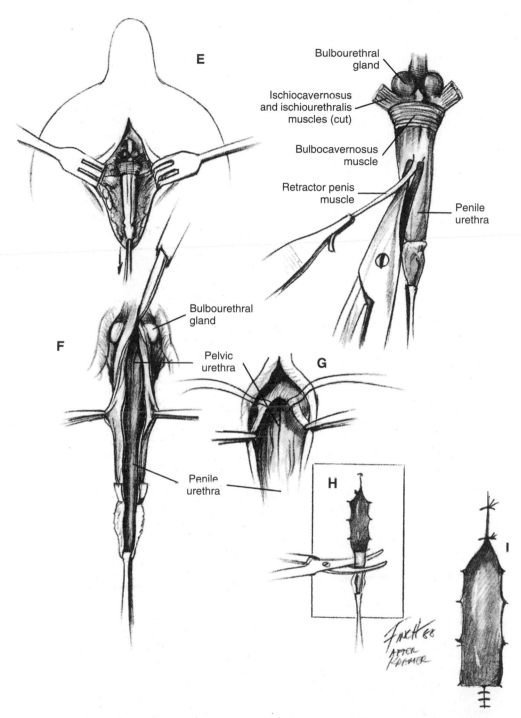

FIG. 5-15, cont'd   **E,** Penis is reflected ventrally, and the loose tissue on the dorsal surface is dissected. **F,** Incision is made through the corpus spongiosum penis muscle into the urethral lumen. **G,** Suturing is begun. **H,** Suture is placed through the penis, which is then amputated distally to the suture. **I,** Skin is to be sutured to cover the cut end of the penis. (From Caywood DD, Lipowitz AJ: *Atlas of small animal surgery,* St Louis, 1989, Mosby.)

ter patient evaluation, the first step is to control hemorrhage. Pressure or cold compresses can be applied to lacerations of the penis. Ligation and suturing may be necessary to arrest arterial bleeding. Large lacerations should be sutured, and puncture wounds should be surgically explored. Severe trauma to the penis can necessitate penile amputation, and injury to the scrotum or testicles may require castration. The patency of the lower urinary tract must always be ensured by catheterization or urethrostomy. The postoperative patient will often need hot compresses, antibiotics, and E-collars or sedatives to prevent self-trauma.

Paraphimosis is the inability to retract the penis within the prepuce. This may occur after sexual excitement and erection of the penis, and it may occur in lumbar disk patients because of the effect of anesthesia and the prolapse of the penis. The engorged distal portion of the penis becomes too large to retract, and constriction by the prepuce causes further swelling of the exposed part. With time, urethral obstruction, necrosis, and gangrene of the penis may develop. The immediate need is to replace the penis into the prepuce. The technician should keep the penis moist until veterinary help is available. The animal is anesthetized to allow adequate relaxation. The exposed penis is gently cleaned. Swelling can sometimes be reduced by bathing with cold hyperosmolar solutions. Gentle traction on the prepuce with pressure on the penis may be the only effort needed to replace the penis. At times, however, the prepucial os must be incised, the penis replaced, and the prepuce sutured. If there is any doubt about the viability of the penis, a urinary catheter should be inserted and the tissue watched for several days to determine if penile amputation is necessary. Postoperatively it is imperative to prevent erection of the penis. Tranquilizers and castration are advisable. Self-trauma is a common postoperative complication. E-collars and tranquilization may help. The technician should be aware that paraphimosis may recur and should notify the veterinarian of any postoperative problem.

Although it is infrequent, torsion of the testicles does occur in dogs and almost always involves a retained abdominal testicle. In the fetus, both testicles lie in the abdomen behind the kidneys. As birth approaches, the testicles begin to descend through the inguinal ring to eventually rest in the scrotum. Those testicles that fail to make this descent usually lie free in the abdomen and may be innocuous for a number of years. A twisting of the testicle around the spermatic cord will compromise the blood supply to and from the testicle and result in a surgical emergency. Clinical signs are indistinguishable from the other causes of the acute abdomen syndrome. Testicular torsion should be suspected if the animal is cryptorchid and if an abdominal mass can be palpated. A definitive diagnosis may depend on exploratory laparotomy. The treatment is the surgical removal of the affected testicle. Total castration is recommended because the tendency toward retained testicles is inherited. Owners of young cryptorchid dogs should be advised to castrate their dogs to prevent testicular torsion and because later in life retained abdominal testicles can become neoplastic, creating another threat to the animal.

Female Genital Emergencies

Although rupture of the pregnant uterus has been reported in dogs after automobile accidents, trauma to the female reproductive tract is rare. Lacerations of the vulva and vagina occur uncommonly from trauma and parturition. Any large lacerations should be sutured and patency of the urethra ensured.

A more common surgical emergency in the female dog is pyometra. Pyometra is the accumulation of pus within the uterus. In cats it is often associated with immunosuppressive viruses (feline leukemia virus and feline immunosuppresive virus). In dogs it most often occurs in middle-aged pets shortly after their heat cycles. Pyometra may present in two different forms. If the cervix is open, purulent vaginal discharge is obvious. If the cervix is closed, there may be no obvious external sign of uterine infection and the patient may have clinical signs referrable to secondary metabolic changes. These clinical signs are polydipsia, polyuria, lethargy, anorexia, and vomiting. Gram-negative bacterial pyelonephritis decreases the concentrating capacity of the kidney, producing polyuria. The dog will attempt to compensate for excessive fluid loss by becoming increasingly thirsty. Severe toxemia causing shock, coma, and death may develop because of untreated pyometra. Diagnosis of the closed form of pyometra may require laboratory tests and radiography.

Medical therapy for this form of endometritis has been successful in some cases; however, the therapy of choice is ovariohysterectomy. Any dehydration or shock should be treated with intravenous fluids, and the patient should be prepared for surgery. The urgency for surgery is greater in the closed form of pyometra because of the increased risk of toxemia. Anesthetizing these patients is also a high-risk endeavor. The technician should be prepared to deliver lower than normal doses of the anesthetic agents and to closely monitor heart rate and respirations during the surgical procedures. Postoperatively the pyometra patient should receive fluid therapy, antibiotics, and careful monitoring of body temperatures. Peritonitis from any contamination of the abdomen during surgery will usually develop within 3 days following surgery. If the uterus was found to be ruptured at the time of surgery, the likelihood of secondary peritonitis is increased and should be anticipated. Any elevation of temperature, onset of abdominal pain, or vomiting should be reported to the veterinarian.

Dystocia is defined as difficult or abnormal labor. It is uncommon in cats, but several of the toy breeds of dogs with large, dome-shaped heads are often affected. Maternal causes of dystocia include pelvic abnormalities, such as old fractures, torsion of the uterus, and uterine inertia, and emotional disorders. Deformed or dead fetuses, malpositioned fetuses, or abnormally large fetuses can also precipitate dystocia. Because the technician may actually be the person who receives inquiries from distraught owners, it is necessary to understand the sequence of events in a normal delivery. If this information is understood, the technician is in a better position to decide if an actual dystocia exists and to advise the owner of the need for veterinary attention.

The approach of parturition is heralded by restlessness and nesting activity by the mother. This occurs 24 to 48 hours before the onset of labor. Her body temperature drops to 98° F. True labor begins with obvious straining. A puppy or kitten should be produced within 4 to 6 hours after the onset of labor. The time between each delivery can vary from 10 minutes to 1 hour. The time actually spent by each offspring in the pelvic canal should be less than 5 minutes. The total delivery time may last from 4 to 6 hours for small litters and 12 to 14 hours for large litters.

Signs of impending dystocia
- Excessive walking, panting, or urinating on the part of the bitch
- Active labor for 3 hours without the production of a pup

- More than 4 hours between each delivery
- Signs of depression and toxicity in the bitch
- Passage of the due date by 3 days without signs of labor

After the diagnosis of dystocia is made, corrective measures should be taken. If a pup is caught in the pelvic canal, manual removal should be attempted. If the cervix is open and a fetus is presented to the brim of the pelvis, oxytocin (Pitocin) can be administered to induce labor. Ovariohysterectomy may be elected if the pelvic canal is narrowed, if the uterus is twisted or necrotic, or if it is requested by the owner. Cesarean section is performed if the retrieval of live fetuses is intended or if future breeding of the bitch is planned. All injectable or gas anesthetic agents will cross the placenta and secondarily depress the fetus. Therefore a minimal amount of time should occur between the induction of anesthesia and the delivery to allow the maximum survival of the offspring. Epidural anesthesia is perhaps the safest technique to use because fetal depression does not result, but this type of anesthesia is not in widespread use. If any of the general anesthetics are used, the animal should be clipped and scrubbed and the surgical site prepared before anesthetic induction. The surgery suite and surgeon should be ready to start surgery as soon as the patient is prepared. Once the patient is anesthetized, the cesarean section is performed through a ventral midline incision and an incision through one or both horns of the uterus. The technician should stand by to receive each pup from the veterinarian. The umbilical cord will already be closed by the surgeon. The fetal membrane should be stripped from the face and the pup stimulated to breathe by vigorous body massage. Fetal fluids can be removed from the airway passages by swinging the pup with its head down or by direct suction. If respirations do not begin, chemical stimulation by doxapram injected into the umbilical vein is used. Oxygen should be administered to any cyanotic pup. The pup should be placed with the mother when she is fully recovered. The technician should aid all pups in finding the mammary glands and nursing colostrum.

Uterine prolapse, although rare, can occur during or after parturition. Abdominal straining may produce an incomplete or complete eversion of the uterus. If found by the technician, the uterus should be cleaned and kept warm and moist. The uterus will need to be replaced when the animal is under general anesthesia. Hypertonic solutions may be helpful in shrinking the distended tissue before manual replacement. If portions of the uterus are severely damaged or necrotic, ovariohysterectomy may be indicated. Once the uterus is replaced, the vulva is often partially sutured to prevent reprolapse. Oxytocin (Pitocin) can be given to promote uterine involution, and tranquilizers will also help to decrease recurrence. Supportive nursing care should include fluid therapy and antibiotics.

Vaginal hyperplasia with prolapse is the protrusion of swollen vaginal tissue through the vulva. It is the result of edema of the floor of the vagina and vestibule that occurs in response to endogenous estrogen. It seems to occur in proestrus and estrus and often disappears with metestrus. It is a problem of large breeds of dogs, especially boxers. The discovery of a mass protruding from the vulva in a female in heat is suggestive of vaginal prolapse. It must be differentiated from the various vaginal tumors. Vaginal prolapse becomes an emergency when a large portion of the vagina is exposed and the tissue becomes dry, traumatized, or necrotic. An emergency also exists if urination is compromised. The treatment for this condition is threefold: decrease the influence of estrogen, replace or amputate the prolapse, and prevent self-trauma. Ideally the dog should be spayed at the time of replacement so that the hyperplasia will not recur. If the bitch is to be kept for breeding, exogenous progesterones or testosterone can be given in an attempt to override the estrogen influence. As in uterine prolapse, the patency of the urethra must be preserved, and the postoperative patient must be monitored for recurrence. The owner should be warned that the condition may return with subsequent heats.

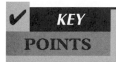

KEY POINTS

1. Shock refers to any condition in which there is inadequate tissue perfusion leading to cellular hypoxia, metabolic acidosis, and ultimately cell death.
2. Shock has been divided into four basic classes: hypovolemic, distributive, cardiogenic, and obstructive shock.
3. *Hypovolemic shock* is caused by loss of blood, plasma, or fluids leading to decreased circulating blood volume; *distributive shock* is caused by an increase in the intravascular space; *cardiogenic shock* is caused by the heart's inability to pump blood; *obstructive shock* is caused by a restriction in blood flow.
4. Clinical signs of shock may include tachycardia, hypotension, rapid respiration, hypothermia, weakness, restlessness, depression, reduced urine output, and coma and dilation of pupils.
5. Rather than speaking of target organs, it is more helpful to recognize that shock is a multisystem disorder and no part of the body remains unharmed.
6. The key role of the technician in a surgical emergency is assessment of the patient and anticipation of the therapy.
7. In most surgical emergencies tranquilizers are unnecessary and contraindicated.
8. Cardiac arrest is the absence or cessation of any effective contraction of the heart. The classic signs of cardiac arrest are the absence of pulse, heartbeat, and respiration.
9. The primary objectives in the treatment of cardiac arrest are to maintain the circulation that delivers oxygen to the tissues and to reestablish the normal electrical activity of the heart.
10. In respiratory tract trauma, the severity of the clinical signs is directly proportional to the amount of airway obstruction that develops after the injury.
11. The presence of loud breathing, dyspnea, and cyanosis should alert the technician to an impending crisis in which a tracheotomy may be necessary.
12. Fractures of the ribs become surgical emergencies when they directly lacerate the underlying lung parenchyma or seriously diminish excursions of the chest.
13. Pleural effusion in the trauma patient becomes an emergency when the lungs can no longer expand to provide adequate oxygenation of the blood.
14. *Pneumothorax* is the presence of air in the pleural cavity and usually results from rupture of the lung or a penetrating wound of the thorax. *Hemothorax* is the presence of blood in the chest.

Continued

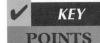

15. The primary aim in treating pleural effusion is to remove as much fluid as possible so that the functioning lung capacity can return to normal.

16. The ultimate priority in treatment of airway obstruction is to relieve the obstruction and return oxygenation to normal.

17. Evaluation of the patient with spinal cord trauma is based on the alterations of four spinal functions: (1) conscious proprioception, (2) voluntary leg movements, (3) superficial (skin) pain, and (4) deep pain.

18. A dorsal laminectomy refers to the removal of the dorsal bony roof of the spinal canal; a ventral slot procedure refers to the creation of an opening in the ventral aspect of the intervertebral space.

19. Two cardinal rules regarding eye injuries are (1) the eye must be kept moist and (2) immediate veterinary help should be sought.

20. Proptosis is a prolapse of the entire globe beyond the socket and eyelids.

21. All corneal injuries are emergencies.

22. Four common corneal injuries include an abrasion, an ulcer, a descemetocele, and an iris prolapse.

23. Lens luxation is movement of the lens from its normal position. It may cause secondary glaucoma or prolapse of the vitreous.

24. The primary therapeutic objective in treating oral foreign bodies is to remove the foreign material. An esophageal foreign body may be retrieved with an endoscope or by pushing the foreign body into the stomach.

25. The technician's sequential measurements of the animal's vital signs help determine the seriousness of blunt trauma.

26. *Acute abdomen* refers to any syndrome that causes severe abdominal pain. An *intussusception* is the prolapse or telescoping of a segment of intestine into the lumen of the adjacent intestine; *volvulus* refers to a twisting of the intestine; and *incarceration* refers to trapping of the intestines by hernias.

27. During intestinal obstruction surgery, the technician must isolate the gut section and must handle the intestinal tissue carefully so blood supply will not be compromised.

28. Three major objectives in the treatment of gastric dilation/volvulus (GDV) are (1) the reversal of shock, (2) the relief of gastric distention, and (3) the stabilization of the patient until surgery can be performed.

29. The ultimate objectives of therapy for blunt trauma to the kidney are to maintain adequate kidney function, control hemorrhage and shock, and repair the damage if possible.

30. Clinical signs of bladder rupture include shock, abdominal pain, hypothermia or hyperthermia, and hematuria or anuria.

31. Feline lower urinary tract disease (FLUTD) occurs as a result of cystitis and/or urethritis. Causative factors include infectious organisms, neoplasms, trauma, toxins, and irritation of the mucosa from urinary crystals or calculi; it is predominantly seen in the male cat. Urethral obstruction in dogs is also usually a disease of the males.

32. *Paraphimosis* is the inability to retract the penis within the prepuce. *Pyometra* is the accumulation of pus within the uterus. *Dystocia* is difficult or abnormal labor. *Vaginal hyperplasia with prolapse* is the protrusion of swollen vaginal tissue through the vulva.

1. What is shock?

2. What are the four basic classes of shock?

3. Define the following terms: hypovolemic shock, distributive shock, cardiogenic shock, and obstructive shock.

4. Identify the clinical signs of shock.

5. Describe the protocol to be followed in treatment of shock.

6. What is the key role of the technician in surgical emergency?

7. How should an animal that cannot walk or possibly has a spinal injury be transported?

8. What is the definition of cardiac arrest? What are the classic signs of cardiac arrest?

9. What sort of crisis signs may precede cardiac arrest?

10. What are the primary objectives in the treatment of cardiac arrest?

11. What is the protocol for treating cardiac arrest?

Continued

▼ REVIEW QUESTIONS—cont'd

12. What are the signs of an impending crisis requiring tracheotomy?

13. Define pneumothorax and hemothorax.

14. What is the primary aim in treating pleural effusion?

15. What is the ultimate priority in treatment of airway obstruction?

16. Evaluation of the neurologic patient is based on alterations of what four spinal functions?

17. What is the technician's role in treating the neurologic patient?

18. What is the technician's role in the postoperative care of the neurologic patient?

19. Name the two cardinal rules regarding eye injuries.

20. Describe appropriate assessment of the eye.

21. Which corneal injuries are emergencies?

22. Name and define four common corneal injuries.

▼ REVIEW QUESTIONS—cont'd

23. What is lens luxation?

24. Describe the protocol for the technician in treating ophthalmic emergencies.

25. What is the primary therapeutic objective in treating oral and esophageal foreign bodies?

26. What is meant by *acute abdomen?*

27. What special precaution must the technician take during intestinal obstruction surgery?

28. Define the following terms: *intussusception, volvulus,* and *incarceration.*

29. Describe three major objectives in the treatment of gastric dilation/volvulus (GDV).

30. What should the technician monitor for in suspected blunt trauma to the kidney?

31. What are the clinical signs of bladder rupture?

32. What is feline lower urinary tract disease (FLUTD), what is its cause, and how is it similar to urethral obstruction in dogs?

Continued

▼ REVIEW QUESTIONS—cont'd

33. What is paraphimosis and what is the proper response of the technician?

34. Describe pyometra and the technician's role in treating it.

35. What is dystocia and what are its clinical signs?

36. What is the technician's response to the animal with dystocia?

ANSWERS FOR CHAPTER 5

1. Shock refers to any condition in which there is inadequate tissue perfusion leading to cellular hypoxia, metabolic acidosis, and ultimately cell death.
2. Shock has been divided into four basic classes: hypovolemic, distributive, cardiogenic, and obstructive shock.
3. *Hypovolemic shock* is caused by loss of blood, plasma, or fluids leading to decreased circulating blood volume (see Key Point 3).
4. Clinical signs of shock include tachycardia, hypotension, rapid respiration, hypothermia, weakness, restlessness, depression, reduced urine output, and coma and dilation of pupils.
5. Protocol to be followed in shock therapy includes the following: (1) establish an airway; (2) insert an intravenous catheter; (3) control hemorrhage; (4) begin rapid fluid infusion; (5) prepare steroids and antibiotics; (6) maintain body temperature; (7) check mucous membrane color, capillary refill time, pulse, and respirations; and (8) monitor urine output.
6. The key role of the technician in surgical emergency is in assessment of the patient and anticipation of the therapy.
7. Any animal that cannot walk or has a possible spinal injury should be transported with a stretcher or any stiff object or blanket.
8. Cardiac arrest is the absence or cessation of any effective contraction of the heart. The classic signs of cardiac arrest are the absence of pulse, heartbeat, and respiration.
9. Crisis signs that may precede cardiac arrest include cyanosis, dysrhythmias with pulse irregularities, a decrease in blood pressure, and a prolonged capillary refill time. Respirations may become shallow and rapid, bleeding may stop, bladder and anus may relax, skin may cool, and pupils may dilate.
10. The primary objectives in the treatment of cardiac arrest are to maintain the circulation that delivers oxygen to the tissues and to reestablish the normal electrical activity of the heart.
11. Protocol for treating cardiac arrest is as follows: (1) call for help; (2) establish a patent airway; (3) begin external massage; (4) insert IV catheter and begin infusion of 5% dextrose in water or Ringer's lactate solution; (5) record the animal's ECG; (6) ready emergency drugs; (7) prepare monopulse machine for defibrillation; (8) when animal has stabilized, monitor ECG, respirations, pupils, pulse, urine output, and temperature.
12. The presence of loud breathing, dyspnea, and cyanosis should alert the technician to an impending crisis in which a tracheotomy may be necessary.
13. Pneumothorax is the presence of air in the pleural cavity and usually results from rupture of the lung. Hemothorax is the presence of blood in the chest.
14. The primary aim in treating pleural effusion is to remove as much fluid as possible so that the functioning lung capacity can return to normal. This can best be accomplished by thoracentesis and the insertion of a chest tube at the animal's seventh or eighth intercostal space with a local anesthetic.
15. The ultimate priority in treatment is to relieve the obstruction and return oxygenation to normal. The technician should aid the veterinarian in examining the mouth and pharynx quickly. If the obstruction cannot be relieved, it should be bypassed with a tracheotomy.
16. Evaluation of the neurologic patient is based on alterations of four spinal functions. These are, in order of their loss, conscious proprioception, voluntary leg movements, superficial (skin) pain, and deep pain.
17. The technician's role in treating the neurologic patient includes the following: (1) assisting in assessing extent of injury and deterioration of the patient's condition; (2) assisting in spinal surgery; and (3) providing postoperative nursing care.
18. In postoperative care of the neurologic patient, the technician must (1) monitor urination; (2) lift and turn the patient with a conscious effort to keep the spine straight; (3) check daily for improvement of each of the four spinal functions; and (4) prevent decubital sores in paralyzed patients.
19. Two cardinal rules regarding eye injuries are (1) the eye must be kept moist, and (2) immediate veterinary help should be sought.
20. Assessment of the eye includes a history of the trauma, assessment of the exterior eye (lids, conjunctiva, cornea), and assessment of the anterior chamber. Eye first aid measures may include hemorrhage control with pressure and cold packs and irrigation of the dry or exposed eye with eye wash, irrigating saline, or homemade solution.

21. All corneal injuries are emergencies.

22. Four common corneal injuries include an abrasion, an ulcer, a descemetocele, and an iris prolapse. A *corneal abrasion* is a superficial linear scratch in the corneal epithelium; a *corneal ulcer* is a denuded, craterlike lesion that is superficial and may only affect the epithelium or can also involve the stroma. A *descemetocele* is an ulcer that destroys stroma to Descemet's membrane. An *iris prolapse* occurs when the membrane is ruptured, the anterior chamber is penetrated, aqueous humor leaks from the eye, and the iris falls forward to plug the leak.

23. Lens luxation is movement of the lens from its normal position. It may cause secondary glaucoma or prolapse of the vitreous.

24. Protocol for the technician in treating ophthalmic emergencies is as follows: (1) obtain a quick, complete history from the owner; (2) perform a systematic examination of the structure of the eye; (3) lavage the eye vigorously, but gently; (4) correct any obvious problems (e.g., controlling hemorrhage and swelling, calming the animal and owner, assessing any other injuries); (5) seek immediate veterinary attention; and (6) keep the eye moist.

25. The primary therapeutic objective in treating oral foreign bodies is to remove the foreign material. An esophageal foreign body is retrieved with an endoscope or by pushing it into the stomach.

26. *Acute abdomen* refers to any syndrome that causes severe abdominal pain.

27. During intestinal obstruction surgery, the technician must pay strict attention to asepsis by isolating the gut section and must handle the intestinal tissue carefully so blood supply will not be compromised.

28. An *intussusception* is the prolapse or telescoping of a segment of intestine into the lumen of the adjacent intestine; *volvulus* refers to a twisting of the intestine, and *incarceration* refers to trapping of the intestines by hernias.

29. Three major objectives in the treatment of GDV are (1) the reversal of shock, (2) the immediate relief of gastric distention, and (3) the stabilization of the patient until surgery can be performed. The technician should first obtain a stomach tube and then assist the veterinarian in trying to pass the tube. At the same time that gastric distention is being relieved, shock should be treated, and the technician should also prepare IV fluids, sodium bicarbonate, and glucocorticoids for administration; the technician should prepare for the probability of surgery.

30. For suspected blunt trauma to the kidney, the technician should monitor for shock, pain near the kidneys, and an enlarging abdominal mass and hematuria as possible signs of a ruptured kidney. The ultimate objectives of therapy are to maintain adequate kidney function, control hemorrhage and shock, and repair the damage if possible.

31. Clinical signs of bladder rupture include shock, abdominal pain, hypothermia or hyperthermia, and hematuria or anuria.

32. Feline lower urinary tract disease (FLUTD) is the clinical condition resulting from cystitis and/or urethritis. Symptoms include frequent voiding of often bloody urine, urinating in inappropriate areas, and partial or complete obstruction of the urinary tract. Causative factors include infectious organisms, neoplasms, trauma, toxins, and irritation of the mucosa from crystals or calculi; it is predominantly seen in the male cat. Urethral obstruction in dogs is also usually a disease of males.

33. Paraphimosis is the inability to retract the penis within the prepuce. The immediate need is to replace it. The technician should keep the penis moist until veterinary help is available. The animal is anesthetized to allow adequate relaxation, and the penis is gently cleaned. Swelling can be reduced with cold hyperosmolar solutions. Gentle traction on the prepuce with pressure on the penis may be the only effort needed to replace the penis. However, at times surgery is necessary.

34. Pyometra, the accumulation of pus within the uterus, occurs in female dogs in two forms: open cervix and closed cervix. The urgency for surgery is greater in the closed form because of the increased risk of toxemia. Anesthetizing these patients is also a high-risk endeavor. The technician should be prepared to deliver lower than normal doses of anesthetics and to closely monitor heart rate and respirations in surgery. Postoperatively, the pyometra patient should receive fluid therapy, antibiotics, and careful monitoring of body temperature.

35. Dystocia is difficult or abnormal labor. Signs of impending dystocia include excessive walking, panting, or urination; active labor for 3 hours with no pups; more than 4 hours between each delivery; signs of depression or toxicity in the mother; and passage of the due date by 3 days without signs of labor.

36. If the animal with dystocia is anesthetized, it should be clipped and scrubbed. The technician should stand by during the cesarean section to receive each pup. The fetal membrane should be stripped from the face and the pup stimulated to breathe by vigorous body massage. Fetal fluids can be removed from airway passages by swinging the pup with its head down or by suction. The technician should aid all pups in finding the mammary glands.

SELECTED READINGS

Bojrab MJ, editor: *Current techniques in small animal surgery,* Philadelphia, 1990, Lea & Febiger.

Bongura: *Kirk's current veterinary therapy. XII. Small animal practice,* Philadelphia, 1995, WB Saunders.

Cunningham J: *Textbook of veterinary physiology,* 2nd ed, Philadelphia, 1997, WB Saunders.

Di Bartola SP, Chew DJ: *Fluid therapy in small animal practice,* Philadelphia, 1992, WB Saunders.

Dyce KM, Sack WO, Wensing CJG: *Textbook of veterinary anatomy,* 2nd ed, Philadelphia, 1996, WB Saunders.

Ettinger SJ: *Textbook of veterinary internal medicine,* Philadelphia, 1995, WB Saunders.

Fossum TW: *Small animal surgery,* St Louis, 1997, Mosby.

Leib M, Monroe W: *Practical small animal internal medicine.* Philadelphia, 1997, WB Saunders.

Nelson R, Couto C: *Small animal internal medicine,* 2nd ed, St Louis, 1998, Mosby.

Zazlow IM, editor: *Veterinary trauma and critical care,* Philadelphia, 1984, Lea & Febiger.

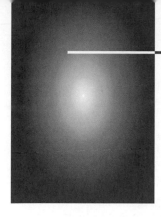

Index